BXB.A/Ahu

0180

Kostoris

R014

D1758458

THIS BOOK BELONGS TO:
Medical Library
Christie Hospital NHS Trust
Manchester
M20 4BX
Phone: 0161 446 3452

IMAGING OF HEAD AND NECK CANCER

IMAGING OF HEAD AND NECK CANCER

AT Ahuja
MBBS(Bom), MD(Bom), FRCR, FHKCR, FHKAM(Radiology)
Professor, Department of Diagnostic Radiology & Organ Imaging
Chinese University of Hong Kong, Prince of Wales Hospital, Shatin
Hong Kong, China

RM Evans
MBBCh, FRCR
Consultant Radiologist, Morriston Hospital
Swansea NHS Trust, Morriston
Swansea, Wales

AD King
MBChB, MRCP, FRCR, FHKAM(Radiology)
Associate Professor, Department of Diagnostic Radiology & Organ Imaging
Chinese University of Hong Kong, Prince of Wales Hospital, Shatin
Hong Kong, China

CA van Hasselt
MBChB, FRCS, FRCS(Edin), FCS(SA), Mmed(Otol), FHKAM(Otorhinolaryngology)
Professor of Surgery(Otor), Department of Surgery
Chinese University of Hong Kong, Prince of Wales Hospital, Shatin
Hong Kong, China

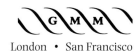
London • San Francisco

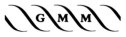

© 2003

Greenwich Medical Media Limited
4th Floor, 137 Euston Road,
London
NW1 2AA

870 Market Street, Ste 720
San Francisco
CA 94109, USA

ISBN 1 84110 090 0

First Published 2003

While the advice and information in this book is believed to be true and accurate, neither the authors nor the publisher can accept any legal responsibility or liability for any loss or damage arising from actions or decisions based in this book. The ultimate responsibility for the treatment of patients and the interpretation lies with the medical practitioner. The opinions expressed are those of the authors and the inclusion in this book of information relating to a particular product, method or technique does not amount to an endorsement of its value or quality, or of the claims made by its manufacturer. Every effort has been made to check drug dosages; however, it is still possible that errors have occurred. Furthermore, dosage schedules are constantly being revised and new side-effects recognised. For these reasons, the medical practitioner is strongly urged to consult the drug companies' printed instructions before administering any of the drugs mentioned in this book.

Apart from any fair dealing for the purposes of research or private study, or criticism or review, as permitted under the UK Copyright Designs and Patents Act 1988, this publication may not be reproduced, stored, or transmitted, in any form or by any means, without the prior permission in writing of the publishers, or in the case of reprographic reproduction only in accordance with the terms of the licences issued by the appropriate Reproduction Rights Organisations outside the UK. Enquiries concerning reproduction outside the terms stated here should be sent to the publishers at the London address printed above.

The rights of AT Ahuja, RM Evans, AD King and CA van Hasselt to be identified as editors of this work have been asserted by them in accordance with the Copyright Designs and Patents Act 1988.

The publisher makes no representation, express or implied, with regard to the accuracy of the information contained in this book and cannot accept any legal responsibility or liability for any errors or omissions that may be made.

A catalogue record for this book is available from the British Library.

www.greenwich-medical.co.uk

Distributed by Plymbridge Distribution Ltd and in the USA by JAMCO Distribution

Typeset by Charon Tec Pvt. Ltd, Chennai, India

Printed in China

CONTENTS

CONTRIBUTORS

AT Ahuja
MBBS(Bom), MD(Bom), FRCR, FHKCR,
FHKAM (Radiology)
Professor
Department of Diagnostic Radiology &
Organ Imaging
Chinese University of Hong Kong
Prince of Wales Hospital
Shatin
Hong Kong
China

I Birchall
MA (Hons, Cantab), MD(Cantab), FRCS(Gen),
FRCS(Oto), FRCS(Orl)
Professor of Laryngology
Honorary Consultant in Otolaryngology,
Head & Neck Surgery
University of Bristol & North Bristol NHS Trust
Southmead Hospital
Bristol
UK

M Castillo
MD
Professor & Chief of Neuroradiology
University of North Carolina
Chapel Hill
USA

ACW Chan
MBChB(Hons)(CUHK), MD(CUHK), FRCS(Edin),
FHKAM(Surgery), FACS
Associate Professor
Department of Surgery
Chinese University of Hong Kong
Prince of Wales Hospital
Shatin
Hong Kong
China

RM Evans
MBBCh, FRCR
Consultant Radiologist
Morriston Hospital
Swansea NHS Trust
Morriston
Swansea
Wales
UK

N Fischbein
MD
Associate Professor of Radiology
University of California San Francisco
San Francisco
USA

JF Griffith
MB, BCh, BAO, MRCP(UK), FRCR, FHKCR,
FHKAM(Radiology)
Associate Professor
Department of Diagnostic Radiology &
Organ Imaging
Chinese University of Hong Kong
Prince of Wales Hospital
Shatin
Hong Kong
China

SC Hodder
BDS, FDS, RCPS, MBChB, FRCS, DipFM
Consultant Oral Maxillo Facial Surgeon
Swansea NHS Trust
Honorary Senior Clinical Tutor
University of Wales
Medical School Swansea, Lead Clinician
Head & Neck
Cancer Services, South West Wales
UK

J Kew
BSc(SA), MBBCh(SA), FFRAD(SA), FRCR,
FHKCR, FRANZCR
Department of Radiology
The Queen Elizabeth Hospital
Woodville South
Adelaide
Australia

AD King
MBChB, MRCP, FRCR, FHKAM(Radiology)
Associate Professor
Department of Diagnostic Radiology &
Organ Imaging
Chinese University of Hong Kong
Prince of Wales Hospital
Shatin
Hong Kong
China

SF Leung
FRCR(UK)
Associate Professor
Department of Clinical Oncology
Chinese University of Hong Kong
Prince of Wales Hospital
Shatin
Hong Kong
China

EJ Loveday
MB, MRCP, FRCR, ILTM
Consultant Radiologist
Southmead Hospital
North Bristol NHS Trust
Bristol
UK

SK Mukherji
MD
Chief of Neuroradiology & Head & Neck Radiology
Neuroradiology Fellowship Program Director
University of Michigan Health System
Ann Arbor
Michigan
USA

CA van Hasselt
MBChB, FRCS, FRCS(Edin), FCS(SA), Mmed(Otol),
FHKAM(Otorhinolaryngology)
Professor of Surgery (Otor)
Department of Surgery
Chinese University of Hong Kong
Prince of Wales Hospital
Shatin
Hong Kong
China

AC Vlantis
MBBCh, DA(SA), FCS(SA)ORL, FCS(HK)
Assistant Professor
Department of Surgery
Chinese University of Hong Kong
Prince of Wales Hospital
Shatin
Hong Kong
China

M Ying
PhD, MPhil, PDip(DR)
Assistant Professor
Department of Optometry & Radiography
The Hong Kong Polytechnic University
Hunghom, Kowloon
Hong Kong
China

HY Yuen
MBChB(CUHK), FRCR(UK), FHKCR,
FHKAM(Radiology)
Senior Medical Officer
Department of Diagnostic Radiology &
Organ Imaging
Chinese University of Hong Kong
Shatin
Hong Kong
China

INTRODUCTION

At the very outset we would like to clarify that this is not an exhaustive reference book for specialists in Head and Neck Radiology. The aim of this book is to provide a practical guide to Head and Neck Radiology for clinicians and for general and trainee radiologists. The authors who have contributed all have extensive practical experience in the imaging and management of head and neck cancers.

The book is divided into two parts. The first part covers an introduction to the most common modalities that can be used for imaging the head and neck. The purpose is to familiarize the reader with basic concepts of the techniques and the essential anatomy of this complicated anatomical region. The second part of the book deals with the commonly encountered cancers in the head and neck, with an emphasis on the aspects of imaging that are relevant to clinical management.

While radiology practice may vary in different centres, depending on available expertise and equipment, this book should provide the necessary knowledge to facilitate imaging of common head and neck cancers, irrespective of local practice.

We owe a large debt of gratitude to our colleagues and staff of our respective hospitals. On a more personal level we would like to acknowledge the close support and help provided by our families (which in the case of three of the editors have expanded during the production of this book). For Anil this is, in particular, his wife Chu Wai Po, daughter Sanjali, mother, and late father. For Rhodri his wife Lynne, and his daughters Catrin and Bethan. For Ann her husband Guy, sons Tommy and Maxwell, parents and sister. For Andrew his wife Leonie, and daughters Katrina, Anna Greta and Carla Louise.

Anil Ahuja
Ann King
Rhodri Evans
Andrew van Hasselt

THE MAIN IMAGING MODALITIES

Ultrasound

RM Evans, M Ying and AT Ahuja

Introduction

Ultrasound (US) technology has made massive strides over the past decade and is now the second most common investigation carried out in hospitals worldwide after plain film examination. Modern high-resolution US has 3D-technology, extended field of view or panoramic facilities, excellent colour flow and power Doppler applications and a remarkably high near-field resolution. It is superior to both CT and MRI in near-field resolution, i.e. the ability to discriminate between two points in a superficial structure.

In head and neck imaging, US is playing an increasing role. The superficial nature of the structures of the neck readily lend themselves to US assessment, and the ability to carry out US-guided biopsy (either Fine Needle Aspiration Cytology (FNAC) or core biopsy) is an advantage over both CT and MRI.

US equipment is found in every major imaging department, worldwide. Despite its wide availability some clinicians have an innate distrust of US due to their difficulty in interpretation of US images as compared to the anatomical depictions of CT and MRI. However, with the newer extended field of view (panoramic image) applications, displaying the anatomy in a format that is intelligible to clinicians should become less of a problem. It is a dynamic tool,

the patient can tell the radiologist where he or she senses an abnormality allowing it to be assessed in multiple planes. Freehand US-guided biopsy techniques can also be easily performed by the radiologist. Clinicians have realised the capabilities of US in the neck and there is now increasing pressure to incorporate US into the setting of "one-stop clinics".

Key points

Advantages of US

- Non-invasive, non-ionising, good patient tolerance
- Universal, cost effective
- Real-time US-guided biopsy
- Colour flow applications
- Near-field resolution > MRI and CT

Disadvantages of US

- Image format may be difficult to comprehend
- Inability to depict deep structures
- May not define anatomic extent of large, complex masses

This chapter will highlight the three key areas in which US can make an impact in the head and neck, namely, salivary glands, thyroid and lymph nodes. We will look at anatomy, technique and the criteria that can be used in the interrogation of cervical lymph nodes.

Equipment and technique

An advanced US machine with a high-frequency transducer (7.5–12 MHz) is the basic level of equipment required. High-frequency transducers allow superior near-field resolution, though there is a trade-off in lack of penetration. Occasionally, lower-frequency transducers are required, e.g. 5 MHz for assessing the deep portion of the parotid gland. Colour flow applications are now standard, a high-sensitivity colour flow system and power Doppler colour system are ideal. When using colour flow and power Doppler the machine should be calibrated to allow depiction of the slow flowing vessels seen in the head and neck. A useful vascular landmark for calibration is the lingual artery, power Doppler settings should be geared towards accurate interrogation of intranodal vessels.

> ### Key points
>
> *Colour flow settings [1,2]*
>
> - High sensitivity
> - Low wall filter
> - Pulse repetition frequency (PRF) 700 Hz
> - Medium persistence
> - Colour gain – high but ↓ if background noise

A selection of standard gauge needles (19, 21, 23, 25 gauge) is needed for FNA procedures, together with syringes and short tubing. In our experience, the use of a short tube allows another operator to aspirate during the FNA, allowing the radiologist to have complete control for accurate needle placement. If core biopsies are carried out in the head and neck then advancing needles are contraindicated, non-advancing automated needles are available that ensure that the stylet does not advance during the cutting action – allowing core biopsies to be performed safely under direct US guidance.

> ### Key points
>
> *Technique and equipment*
>
> - High-frequency 7.5–12 MHz small footprint probes
> - Adjustable mobile table
> - Optimal patient positioning – biopsies
> - Fine needles, tubing and non-advancing core biopsy needle

Anatomy

We will now consider the following:

(a) salivary glands,
(b) thyroid,
(c) lymph nodes.

The key points that need to be covered during an US examination will be covered, highlighting the potential pitfalls where appropriate.

Salivary glands

Sublingual

The paired sublingual glands are identified by scanning floor of mouth in a transverse plane (Figure 1.1).

Identify the two "trouser legs" of the genioglossus muscles and the echogenic sublingual glands lie just

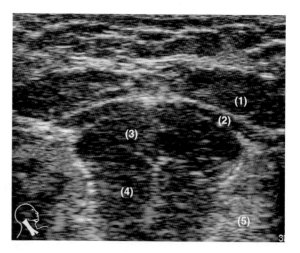

Fig. 1.1   Coronal images of the submental region: 1. anterior belly of digastric muscle, 2. mylohyoid, 3. geniohyoid, 4. genioglossus, 5. sublingual gland.

lateral, with the mylohyoid muscle forming its lateral boundary. If searching for a tumour or a retention cyst (ranula) of the sublingual gland use this plane and assess the symmetry of the two sublingual spaces, any mass effect will displace the central genioglossus muscles, helping to identify a sublingual mass.

Submandibular (Figures 1.2 and 1.3)

The submandibular gland is shaped like a saddle when viewed in a transverse plane. The posterior free border of the mylohyoid indenting its anterior surface. The plane of the mylohyoid acts as a division of the superficial and deep portions of the gland, though there is no true anatomical distinction. Do not rely only on the transverse scan plane for assessing the submandibular gland, also scan in the coronal plane. The deep portion of the submandibular gland will be seen sandwiched between the mylohyoid and hyoglossus muscles. This is the compartment where the submandibular duct, lingual vein and hypoglossal and lingual nerves are situated. Only the duct and vein can be identified routinely with US [3]. The other landmarks in this area are the facial vessels which can be identified superiorly, emerging from deep and posterior to the submandibular gland. The facial artery passes up and over the body of the mandible whereas the facial vein heads posteriorly to join the anterior division of the retromandibular vein (RMV). Identify the vessels prior to biopsy in this area, an anterior approach is safer than a posterior approach.

Parotid

The parotid is divided into superficial and deep portions or lobes, this is not a true anatomical division as there is no embryonic development of superficial and deep lobes. The division is an artificial one, created by the course of the facial nerve. It is the plane of dissection that is sought by surgeons in surgery of the parotid. The facial nerve is dissected out in order to preserve it when carrying out a superficial parotidectomy. If imaging places a tumour in the deep lobe of the parotid or identifies a superficial tumour encroaching into the deep lobe then this implies a potentially difficult dissection for the surgeons.

Several landmarks for the predicted course of the facial nerve have been proposed. Within the parotid gland courses the RMV, just lateral to the external carotid artery (ECA). It passes from the inferior tail in a cranial direction. The RMV is identified with US

and can be taken as a marker for the division of the parotid into superficial and deep lobes [4] (Figures 1.4 and 1.5).

As the facial nerve runs in close proximity to the RMV/ECA, its location and course within the parotid can be inferred by the location of RMV/ECA.

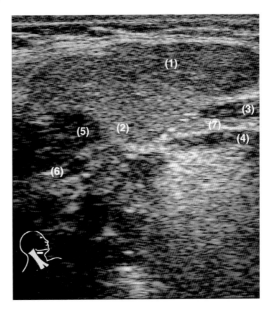

Fig. 1.2 Transverse view of the submandibular region: 1. superficial submandibular gland, 2. deep submandibular gland, 3. mylohyoid, 4. hyoglossus, 5. posterior belly of digastric muscle, 6. facial artery, 7. lingual vein.

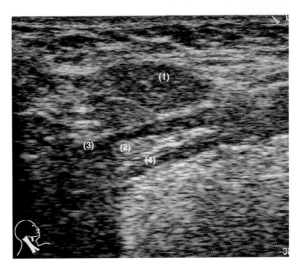

Fig. 1.3 Coronal view of the submandibular region: 1. superficial submandibular gland, 2. deep submandibular gland, 3. mylohyoid, 4. hyoglossus.

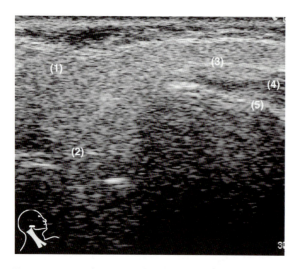

Fig. 1.4 Axial image of body of parotid: 1. superficial lobe parotid, 2. deep lobe parotid, 3. parotid duct, 4. masseter muscle, 5. mandible.

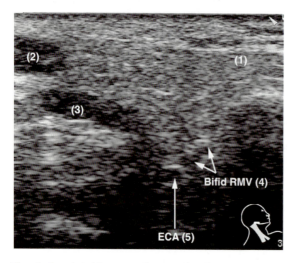

Fig. 1.5 Axial image of parotid tail: 1. superficial lobe parotid, 2. sternocleidomastoid muscle, 3. posterior belly of digastric muscle, 4. retromandibular vein (RMV), 5. external carotid artery (ECA).

In our experience another practical way to divide the parotid is to draw an imaginary line through the ramus of the mandible posteriorly (Figure 1.6); any mass which has its centre lateral to this line is deemed superficial, if it lies medial to the line it is encroaching into the deep lobe (Figure 1.7). This classification works for most surgeons, if an additional measurement is given, i.e. the distance between tumour and RMV then this is usually all the information required to plan the patient's surgery.

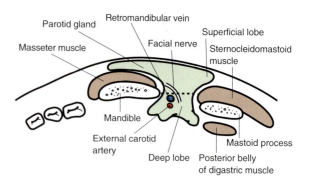

Fig. 1.6 Line drawing of a transverse section through the parotid gland. The dotted line indicates a practical method of dividing the parotid into superficial and deep lobes.

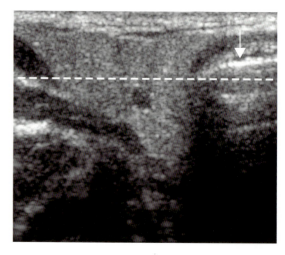

Fig. 1.7 Transverse sonogram showing a quick practical method of dividing the parotid into superficial and deep lobes. Arrow identifies the mandible.

Evaluate the parotid in both transverse and coronal planes, sweeping from cranial and caudal in the transverse plane. Drop the frequency or change to a lower-frequency probe to assess the deep lobe; however, one must note that US cannot assess all the deep lobe. If normal salivary tissue is seen all around a mass, it implies the mass is completely intra-glandular and no further imaging may be necessary. However, if normal salivary gland tissue is not seen around the mass, then further CT/MRI is mandatory to define the entire extent of the mass [5]. The superficial parotid gland extends anteriorly, rolling over the underlying masseter muscle. An assessory parotid gland may be found in 30% of patients in this anterior buccal location.

Key points

Salivary glands

1. Sublingual
   - Submental, transverse approach
2. Submandibular
   - Identify mylohyoid
     - Hyoglossus
     - Facial vessels
   - Transverse and coronal scans
3. Parotid
   - Superficial and deep
   - RMV, plane: ramus mandible
   - Accessory lobe in 30%
   - Cannot define deep extension of tumour → CT/MRI
   - Facial nerve (location inferred by position of RMV/ECA)

Thyroid (Figure 1.8)

The thyroid is unique among endocrine glands in its superficial location, the normal homogeneous echo-texture of the gland and the thin layer of overlying strap muscles and adipose tissue allow excellent evaluation with US.

The thyroid gland consists of a right and left lobe connected in the midline by a narrow isthmus. The gland is attached to trachea and larynx by a pre-tracheal layer of deep fascia. In 10–30% of the patients a third lobe (the pyramidal lobe) arises from the isthmus, projecting upwards in the midline or commonly just to the left of the midline, anterior to the thyroid cartilage.

The overlying strap muscles abut the anterior thyroid, it is important to assess these when staging thyroid tumours to identify extra-capsular spread (Figure 1.9).

Posterior to the thyroid the oesophagus is commonly identified, anterior to the longus colli muscle. The recurrent laryngeal nerve which may be invaded in thyroid carcinoma may be identified as a thin hypoechoic structure running north to south in the groove between thyroid and oesophagus. The lymphatic vessels from the thyroid form a subcapsular network and give rise to a medial and lateral collecting trunk. These drain primarily into the pre-tracheal and para-tracheal lymph node chains and secondarily into the nodes anterior and lateral to the internal jugular vein (IJV), i.e. the deep cervical chain. In thyroid cancer a diligent search in these areas for potential lymph node metastases is required [6–9].

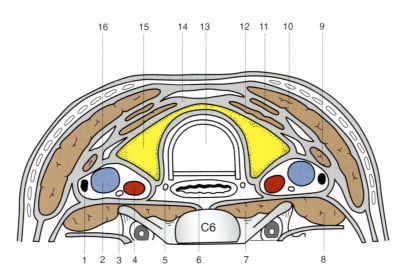

Fig. 1.8   Transverse section at the level of C6 showing relevant anatomy of the thyroid: 1. cervical lymph node, 2. internal jugular vein, 3. vagus nerve, 4. common carotid artery, 5. recurrent laryngeal nerve, 6. oesophagus, 7. longus colli, 8. scalenus anterior, 9. omohyoid, 10. sternocleidomastiod, 11. sternohyoid, 12. sternothyroid, 13. trachea, 14. pre-tracheal fascia, 15. thyroid gland and 16. carotid sheath.

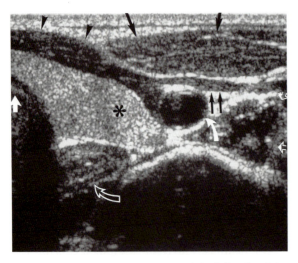

Fig. 1.9 Transverse sonogram of the left side of the neck demonstrating relevant anatomy: • bold white arrow – trachea, • curved white arrow – common carotid artery (CCA), • open curved white arrow – oesophagus, • open white arrows – scalenus anterior, • black arrowheads – strap muscles, • small black arrows – omohyoid muscle, • large black arrows – sternocleidomastoid muscle, • asterisk – left lobe of thyroid gland.

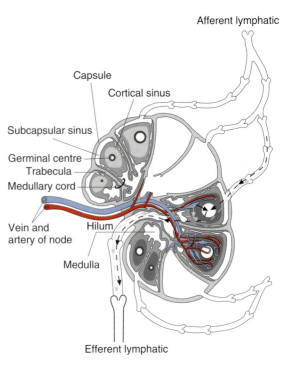

Fig. 1.10 Lymph node anatomy.

In evaluating the thyroid transverse scans are the key, scanning the thyroid from superior to inferior, adjusting the depth and gain settings to ensure that the whole of both lobes and the superficial isthmus are assessed. To evaluate large goiters a lower-frequency (5 MHz) probe may be required to assess extension into retroclavicular region. Adequate extension of the neck is required to ensure complete assessment of the inferior aspect of the thyroid, this may be difficult in the elderly.

Key points

Thyroid

1. Neck extension for adequate assessment
2. Tumour invasion
    - Strap muscles
    - Oesophagus/trachea
    - Recurrent laryngeal nerve
3. Lymph nodes
    - Pre- and para-tracheal
    - Deep cervical nodes

Lymph nodes

In the normal adult neck there may be up to 300 lymph nodes, ranging in size from 3 to 4 mm. The lymphatic anatomy of the neck is complex, the many classification systems that exist for the cervical lymphatics also add to the confusion. A full description of the complete anatomical examination technique is beyond the scope of this text, however, a brief description of the key areas to examine is given. Once familiar with the anatomy, the operator must then develop a set of criteria to determine whether the nodes identified are benign or malignant, a spectrum of criteria are discussed.

The anatomy of the individual node is important if one is to understand the changes in vascularity that occur during malignant transformation. A normal node has central hilar vessels, other points of note are that the afferent lymphatics enter the periphery of the node, leaving the node via a larger efferent lymphatic (Figure 1.10).

The major lymphatic groups and chains are displayed in Figure 1.11. These chains or groups form a

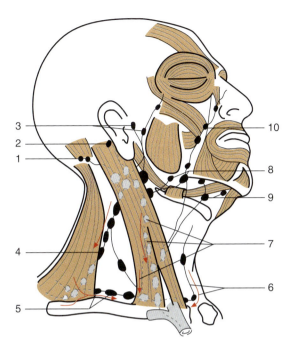

Fig. 1.11 Rouviere's original schematic representation of the lymphatic chains of the neck: 1. occipital nodes, 2. mastoid nodes, 3. parotid nodes, 4. spinal accessory lymphatic chain, 5. transverse cervical lymphatic chain, 6. anterior jugular lymphatic chain, 7. internal jugular lymphatic chain, 8. submaxillary nodes, 9. submental nodes and 10. facial node.

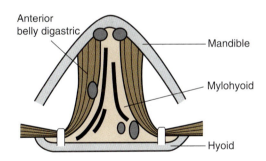

Fig. 1.12 Submental region.

continuous network whereby lymph drains from the neck into the central thoracic ducts. We will consider each key area, allowing a comprehensive evaluation of the neck.

Submental group

Nodes are commonly seen anteriorly between the two digastric muscle insertions, superficial to mylohyoid, and less commonly; off midline and

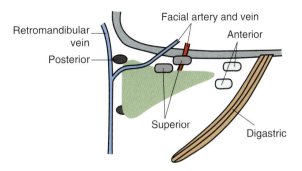

Fig. 1.13 Submandibular region.

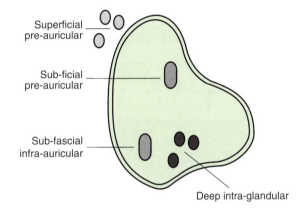

Fig. 1.14 Parotid region.

adjacent to the hyoid. Cancers of the lips, buccal region, anterior mandible, floor of mouth and anterior tongue drain to these nodes (Figure 1.12).

Submandibular group

The submandibular gland is the key structure, nodes are commonly seen superior and anterior to the gland, less commonly: posterior and inferior. These nodes are extra-glandular. Submandibular nodes drain the anterior facial structures, floor of mouth and anterior oral cavity (Figure 1.13).

Parotid region

Due to late embryonic encapsulation of the gland, lymph nodes may be found outside the parotid, just deep to the capsule or within the gland. Intraparotid nodes can cause diagnostic problems, identification of an echogenic hilus or the typical central, hilar blood flow pattern on colour flow aids in their identification. The forehead, temporal region, external auditory meatus and buccal region drain into the parotid nodes (Figure 1.14).

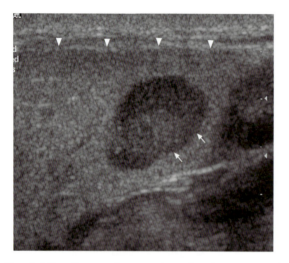

Fig. 1.15 Grey scale sonogram showing a parotid lymph node (arrows). Arrowheads indicate the superficial lobe of the parotid gland.

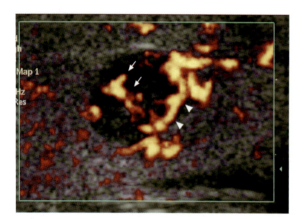

Fig. 1.16 Power Doppler sonogram of a parotid node showing hilar (arrows) and peripheral (arrowheads) vascularity.

Figure 1.15 and Figure 1.16 shows intraparotid node & hilar vascularity.

Facial nodes

A small cluster of nodes are found anterior to the masseter and superficial to the buccinator muscle in the buccal space. These nodes receive lymph from the maxillary region and lips (Figure 1.17).

Deep cervical chain

This is the main lymphatic chain of the neck. The most superior node is the jugulo-digastric node which lies inferior to the posterior belly of the digastric

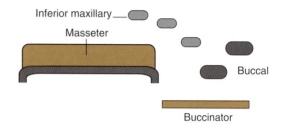

Fig. 1.17 Facial region.

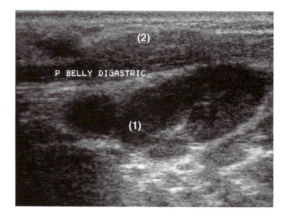

Fig. 1.18 Benign jugulo-digastric node: 1. underlying posterior belly of digastric muscle, 2.

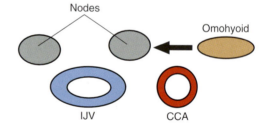

Fig. 1.19 Deep cervical chain.

muscle. It is the largest lymph node in the neck (Figure 1.18).

Deep cervical nodes lie anterior and lateral to the IJV, more inferiorly they may lie posterior. The deep cervical chain is divided into upper, middle and inferior portions by the level of the hyoid and cricoid cartilage (or cricothyroid membrane [10]). The deep cervical nodes receive lymph from the parotid, retropharyngeal and submandibular nodes (Figure 1.19).

Spinal accessory chain

The spinal accessory chain or posterior triangle chain is a superficial lymph node chain, running

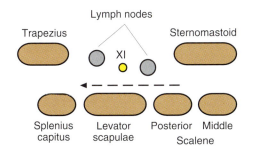

Fig. 1.20   Posterior triangle.

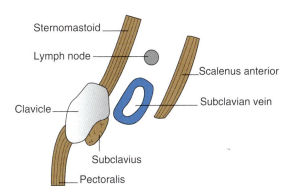

Fig. 1.22   Transverse cervical chain.

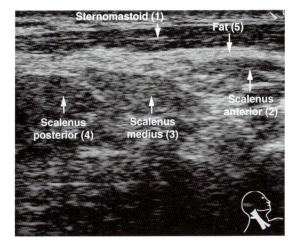

Fig. 1.21   Axial view of the posterior triangle region: 1. sternocleidomastoid, 2. scalenus anterior, 3. scalenus medius, 4. scalenus posterior, 5. fat.

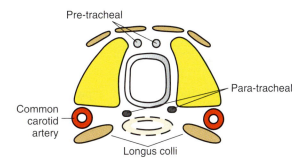

Fig. 1.23   Anterior cervical nodes.

from mastoid to acromion in direction. The nodes lie superficial to the underlying scalene muscles, identifying the superficial fat plane between sternomastoid and the muscles of the floor of the posterior triangle is the key to this area (Figures 1.20 and 1.21). The spinal accessory chain merges with the deep cervical chain superiorly and the supraclavicular nodes inferiorly. They drain the mastoid, occipital, parietal scalp and lateral neck.

Supraclavicular region

The supraclavicular or transverse cervical chain links the spinal accessory chain laterally with the deep cervical chain medially (Figure 1.22). They also receive lymph from below the clavicle, and primary tumours from chest and abdomen may metastasize to these nodes.

Anterior cervical nodes

There are two lymphatic chains in the anterior cervical group: the pre-tracheal nodes, which are situated directly anterior to the trachea and the para-tracheal nodes, which are situated medial to the common carotid artery. Inferiorly, these nodes may lie directly behind the thyroid, between thyroid and longus colli (Figure 1.23).

These nodes receive lymph from the larynx, trachea, pyriform fossae, thyroid and cervical oesophagus.

These are the major lymphatic groups and chains of the neck, and a standard US examination can cover these lymph node territories.

While radiologists tend to describe nodes according to their correct anatomical classification [11], surgeons and oncologists use the "level" concept to stage their patients. The levels concept is driven by the fact that the extent and level of cervical node involvement is probably the most important prognostic factor for patients with a SCC primary. Radiologists need to be aware of the levels system in order to

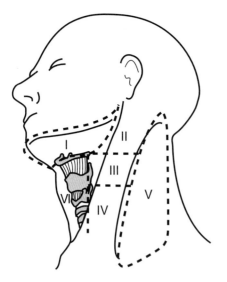

Fig. 1.24 AJCC level classification.

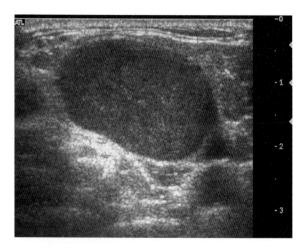

Fig. 1.25 Grey scale sonogram showing a round, hypoechoic malignant lymph node.

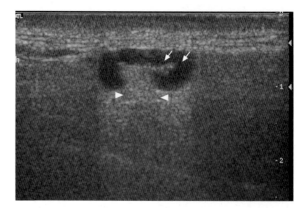

Fig. 1.26 Grey scale sonogram showing an elliptical, hypoechoic normal node with echogenic hilus (arrows) continuous with the adjacent fat (arrowheads).

provide the information, which allows surgeons and oncologists to accurately stage their patients – allowing the correct treatment options to be chosen (Figure 1.24).

Criteria of malignancy

US is a sensitive examination for lymphadenopathy, however, in order to develop specificity, a set of criteria are needed to help differentiate benign from malignant lymphadenopathy. We will briefly consider the main criteria.

Size

Size alone is a poor criterion. Minimum axial diameters are the most specific dimension for predicting malignancy. van den Brekel et al. [12] recommend a minimal axial diameter of 7 mm for submental and submandibular nodes and 8 mm for other cervical nodes, giving an overall accuracy of 70% for this sole criterion.

Increasing size of a lymph node on serial follow-up of patients with head and neck cancer should be viewed with suspicion.

Shape (Figure 1.25)

A round shape is more characteristic of a malignant node than the normal elliptical shape of benign nodes [13–16]. While ratios (either short/long or long/short axis) [17,18] can be measured, an eyeball assessment of shape is a reliable and robust sign of malignancy.

Hilus

The echogenic hilus is a good sign of a benign node, its presence is a manifestation of the normal sinusoidal architecture of the node [18,19]. It is not seen in every benign node, but when seen in an ellipsoid node – it is a good sign of benignity (Figure 1.26). The hilus is often visible in lymphomatous nodes, however, reflecting the lack of disruption of the lymphatic architecture [20] that occurs as distinct from that which occurs in metastatic SCC nodes. The presence of a round node with absent hilus is suspicious for malignancy (Figure 1.27).

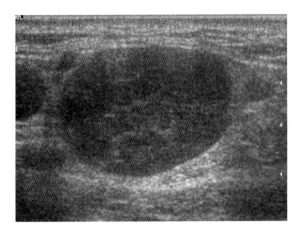

Fig. 1.27   Grey scale sonogram of a round, hypoechoic malignant node without echogenic hilus.

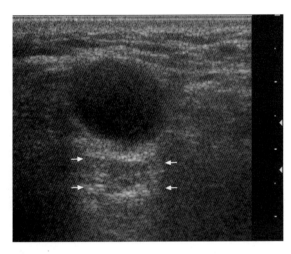

Fig. 1.28   Grey scale sonogram showing a hypoechoic node with posterior enhancement (arrows), i.e. a pseudocystic appearance. The internal architecture of the node is not clear.

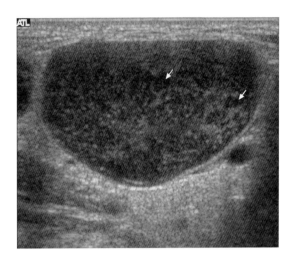

Fig. 1.29   Grey scale sonogram with high resolution transducer showing a lymphomatous node with reticulation, i.e. micronodular pattern. Note the hypertrophied follicles are demonstrated (arrows).

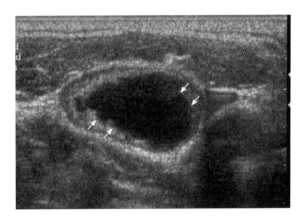

Fig. 1.30   Grey scale sonogram of malignant node with intranodal cystic necrosis (arrows).

Echogenicity

A diffusely hypoechoic node, or "pseudocystic" appearance of a lymph node is characteristic of lymphoma [21] (Figure 1.28). The typical distal enhancement is seen in 90% of nodes involved in non-Hodgkin's lymphoma [22]. This "pseudocystic" appearance is less noticeable on the newer generation machines, however, it is a valid sign of lymphoma. A reticulated intranodal pattern is seen with newer generation of tranducers [23] (Figure 1.29). If such an appearance is seen (and depending on local practice) a decision to proceed to US-guided core biopsy will be of benefit to the patient. Such an approach will hasten diagnosis and may obviate an excision biopsy [24,25].

Necrosis

In patients with SCC primary, the presence of necrosis within a node is a very strong indicator of malignancy [26]. Necrosis may manifest itself as a truly cystic area (Figure 1.30) or as a central, ill-defined area of relative hyperechogenicity (Figure 1.31). Cystic necrosis may be florid, causing a potential pitfall, i.e. mimicking a branchial cleft cyst. Tuberculous nodes also tend to undergo cystic degeneration [27,28], creating another potential pitfall.

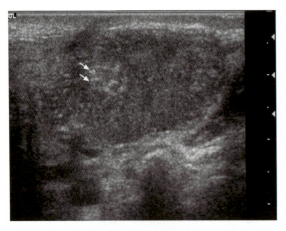

Fig. 1.31 Sonogram of a round, hypoechoic malignant node with intranodal coagulation necrosis (arrows).

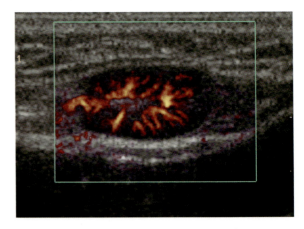

Fig. 1.33 Power Doppler sonogram of a reactive node with hilar vascularity.

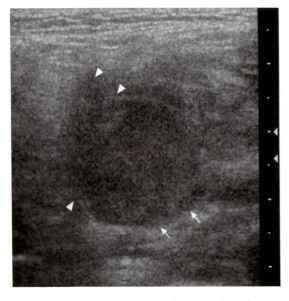

Fig. 1.32 Transverse scan of a round malignant node (arrows). Note the adjacent soft tissue involvement due to extra-capsular spread (arrowheads).

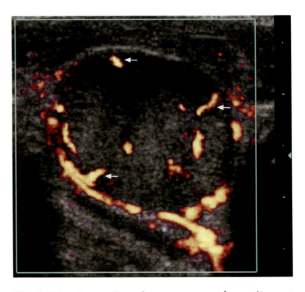

Fig. 1.34 Power Doppler sonogram of a malignant node with peripheral vascularity (arrows).

Extra-capsular spread

An ill-defined border or frank invasion of neighbouring structures can be detected with US (Figure 1.32). The impact on the patient's prognosis is grave (a 50% reduction in 2-year survival [29]).

Colour flow

The pattern of colour flow distribution within a node is more reliable than the various vascular and resistive indices that can be measured in intranodal vessels [30]. Benign nodes have a central hilar flow pattern (Figure 1.33) whereas malignant nodes have a disorganised, peripheral pattern with areas of relative avascularity (reflecting necrosis) and peripheral subcapsular vessels (an excellent sign of malignancy) [30–33] (Figure 1.34).

Spectacular colour flow is often seen in lymphomatous nodes, this is usually an exaggerated benign (i.e. hilar) type pattern (Figure 1.35). This again reflects the lack of disruption of the architecture of the node

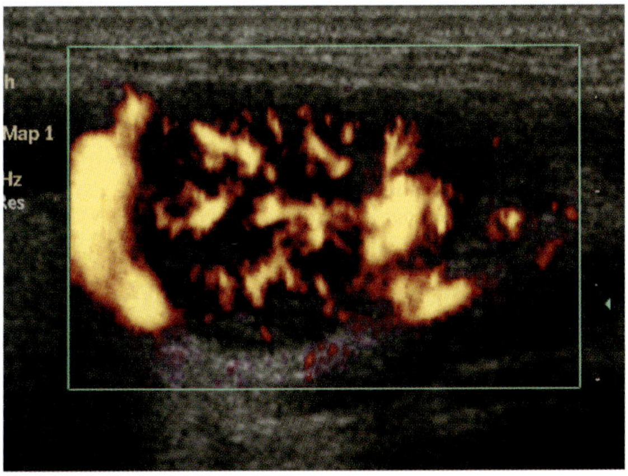

Fig. 1.35 Power Doppler sonogram of a lympho-matous node with exaggerated vascularity.

that occurs in lymphoma. Despite the profound vascularity seen, core biopsy can be carried out safely.

Key points

Colour flow distribution

1. Benign
   - Central, hilar
   - No peripheral flow
2. Malignant
   - Aberrant, multiple central vessels
   - Focal absence of perfusion
   - Subcapsular vessels

Number

The presence of multiple nodes in a draining region from a primary tumour would be regarded by some authors as a sign of malignancy [12,34]. However, the high sensitivity of US means that this is a common finding in the neck and number of nodes present is a poor indicator of malignancy.

Calcification

The typical punctate pattern of calcification (micro-calcification) seen in a papillary thyroid carcinoma is also seen in lymph node metastases from papillary carcinoma [6] (Figure 1.36). When seen, the sign is specific and a diligent search for the thyroid primary should ensue.

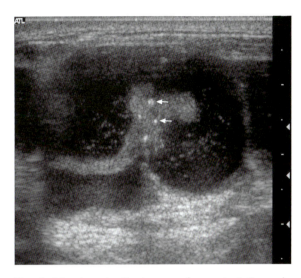

Fig. 1.36 Longitudinal scan of a metastatic node from papillary carcinoma of the thyroid with punctate calcification (arrows).

No one criterion is absolute, these criteria should be used in summation. These signs may point to a specific diagnosis (e.g. lymphoma) or help in determining which lymph node to aspirate if staging the neck using US-guided FNAC.

US criteria

	Benign	Malignant
Size		+
Shape		
Ellipsoid	++	
Round		++
Hilus	++	
Hypo-echogenicity (lymphoma)		+++
Necrosis	(+TB)	+++
Extra-capsular spread		+++
Colour flow		
Hilar	++	
Peripheral		+++
Number		+
Micro-calcification (papillary carcinoma thyroid)		+++

Summary

Anatomy is the key to solving the problems that present in the head and neck. Ultrasound (±FNAC) can provide most of the answers that the radiologist and surgeon require, and is a very cost-effective method of triage for the various pathologies that occur in the neck. It will not provide the answer in every case but it allows a more appropriate limited/focused use of MRI and CT.

References

1. Ahuja A, Ying M, Yuen YH and Metreweli C. Power Doppler sonography to differentiate tuberculous cervical lymphadenopathy from nasopharyngeal carcinoma. *Am. J. Neuroradiol.* 2001; **22**: 735–740.
2. Ying M, Ahuja A, Brook F and Metreweli C. Power Doppler sonography of normal cervical lymph nodes. *J. Ultrasound Med.* 2000; **19**: 511–517.
3. Evans RM. Salivary glands. *BMUS Bull.* 2001; **9**: 20–25.
4. Laing MR and McKerrow WS. Intraparotid anatomy of the facial nerve and retromandibular vein. *Br. J. Surg.* 1988; **75**: 310–312.
5. Zhao Y and Zhang R. Differential diagnosis of parotid gland masses by gray scale real-time ultrasound. *Hua Xi Yi Ke Da Xue Xue Bao* 1990; **21**: 92–95.
6. Ahuja AT, Chow L, Chick W, King W and Metreweli C. Metastatic cervical nodes in papillary carcinoma of the thyroid: ultrasound and histological correlation. *Clin. Radiol.* 1995; **50**: 229–231.
7. Bruneton JN and Normand F. Thyroid gland. In: JN Bruneton (Ed.) *Ultrasonography of the Neck.* Springer-Verlag, Berlin, 1987, 22–50.
8. Compagno J. Diseases of the thyroid. In: L Barnes (Ed.) *Surgical Pathology of the Head and Neck.* Marcel Dekker, New York. 1985; 1435–1486.
9. Yousem DM and Scheff AM. Thyroid and parathyroid. In: PM Som and HD Curtin (Eds) *Head and Neck Imaging.* Mosby, St Louis. 1996, 952–975.
10. American Joint Committee on Cancer, *AJCC Cancer Staging Manual*, 5th edition. Lippincott-Raven, New York. 1997.
11. Hajek PC, Salomonowitz E, Turk R, Tscholakoff D, Kumpan W and Czembirek H. Lymph nodes of the neck: evaluation with US. *Radiology* 1986; **158**: 739–742.
12. van den Brekel MW, Castelijns JA, Stel HV, Luth WJ, Valk J, van der Waal I and Snow GB. Occult metastatic neck disease: detection with US and US-guided fine-needle aspiration cytology. *Radiology* 1991; **180**: 457–461.
13. Vassallo P, Wernecke K, Roos N and Peters PE. Differentiation of benign from malignant superficial lymphadenopathy: the role of high-resolution US. *Radiology* 1992; **183**: 215–220.
14. Sakai F, Kiyono K, Sone S, Kondo Y, Oguchi M, Watanabe T, Sakai Y, Imai Y, Takeda S, Yamamoto K and Ohta H. Ultrasonic evaluation of cervical metastatic lymphadenopathy. *J. Ultrasound Med.* 1988; **7**: 305–310.
15. Ying M, Ahuja A, Brook F, Brown B and Metreweli C. Sonographic appearance and distribution of normal cervical lymph nodes in a Chinese population. *J. Ultrasound Med.* 1996; **15**: 431–436.
16. Ahuja A, Ying M, King W and Metreweli C. A practical approach to ultrasound of cervical lymph nodes. *J. Laryngol. Otol.* 1997; **111**: 245–256.
17. Tohnosu N, Onoda S and Isono K. Ultrasonographic evaluation of cervical lymph node metastases in esophageal cancer with special reference to the relationship between the short to long axis ratio (S/L) and the cancer content. *J. Clin. Ultrasound* 1989; **17**: 101–106.
18. Solbiati L, Rizzatto G, Bellotti E, Montali G, Cioffi V and Croce F. High-resolution sonography of cervical lymph nodes in head and neck cancer: criteria for differentiation of reactive versus malignant nodes. *Radiology* 1988; **169**(P): 113.
19. Rubaltelli L, Proto E, Salmaso R, Bortoletto P, Candiani F and Cagol P. Sonography of abnormal lymph nodes in vitro: correlation of sonographic and histologic findings. *Am. J. Roentgenol.* 1990; **155**: 1241–1244.
20. Evans RM, Ahuja A and Metreweli C. The linear echogenic hilus in cervical lymphadenopathy – a sign of benignity or malignancy? *Clin. Radiol.* 1993; **47**: 262–264.
21. Bruneton JN, Normand F, Balu-Maestro C, Kerboul P, Santini N, Thyss A and Schneider M. Lymphomatous superficial lymph nodes: US detection. *Radiology* 1987; **165**: 233–235.
22. Ahuja A, Ying M, Yang WT, Evans R, King W and Metreweli C. The use of sonography in differentiating cervical lymphomatous lymph nodes from cervical metastatic lymph nodes. *Clin. Radiol.* 1996; **51**: 186–190.
23. Ahuja AT, Ying M, Yuen HY and Metreweli C. "Pseudocystic" appearance of non-Hodgkin's lymphomatous nodes: an infrequent finding with high-resolution transducers. *Clin. Radiol.* 2001; **56**: 111–115.
24. Bearcroft PW, Berman LH and Grant J. The use of ultrasound-guided cutting-needle biopsy in the neck. *Clin. Radiol.* 1995; **50**: 690–695.
25. Cozens NJA and Berman L. Fine-needle aspiration or core biopsy? In: AT Ahuja and RM Evans (Eds) *Practical Head and Neck Ultrasound.* Greenwich Medical Media Limited, London. 2000, 129–144.
26. Som PM. Lymph nodes of the neck. *Radiology* 1987; **165**: 593–600.
27. Ying M, Ahuja AT, Evans R, King W and Metreweli C. Cervical lymphadenopathy: sonographic differentiation between tuberculous nodes and nodal metastases from non-head and neck carcinomas. *J. Clin. Ultrasound* 1998; **26**: 383–389.
28. Ahuja A, Ying M, Evans R, King W and Metreweli C. The application of ultrasound criteria for malignancy in differentiating tuberculous cervical adenitis from metastatic nasopharyngeal carcinoma. *Clin. Radiol.* 1995; **50**: 391–395.
29. Johnson JT. A surgeon looks at cervical lymph nodes. *Radiology* 1990; **175**: 607–610.
30. Ahuja AT, Ying M, Ho SS and Metreweli C. Distribution of intranodal vessels in differentiating benign from metastatic neck nodes. *Clin. Radiol.* 2001; **56**: 197–201.
31. Ariji Y, Kimura Y, Hayashi N, Onitsuka T, Yonetsu K, Hayashi K, Ariji E, Kobayashi T and Nakamura T. Power Doppler sonography of cervical lymph nodes in patients with head and neck cancer. *Am. J. Neuroradiol.* 1998; **19**: 303–307.
32. Wu CH, Chang YL, Hsu WC, Ko JY, Sheen TS and Hsieh FJ. Usefulness of Doppler spectral analysis and power Doppler sonography in the differentiation of cervical lymphadenopathies. *Am. J. Roentgenol.* 1998; **171**: 503–509.
33. Na DG, Lim HK, Byun HS, Kim HD, Ko YH and Baek JH. Differential diagnosis of cervical lymphadenopathy: usefulness of color Doppler sonography. *Am. J. Roentgenol.* 1997; **168**: 1311–1316.
34. van den Brekel MW, Stel HV, Castelijns JA, Croll GJ and Snow GB. Lymph node staging in patients with clinically negative neck examinations by ultrasound and ultrasound-guided aspiration cytology. *Am. J. Surg.* 1991; **162**: 362–366.

Computed Tomography

AD King and AT Ahuja

Introduction

Computed tomography (CT) provides a rapid, readily available technique for imaging all regions of the head and neck at relatively low cost. The images can be displayed to show both the soft tissue and bone detail, and reconstructed into three-dimensional images. The disadvantages of CT are that it involves radiation, thereby limiting its role in regular follow-up studies, requires the injection of an iodine-based contrast agent, which is not without the risk of side effects, and the images may be degraded by dental amalgam.

CT technique

CT images are acquired using either a conventional, spiral or multislice technique. Spiral CT, also known as helical CT, is the most commonly employed technique at present, although it is being superseded by multislice CT. Spiral CT scans the head and neck rapidly, enabling a full set of data to be acquired from a large volume of the patient at one time. The data that is acquired can be reconstructed retrospectively at any interval and in any plane or into three-dimensional reconstructions. Rapid scanning means

(a) there is less artefact from respiration and swallowing, which can significantly degrade images of the pharynx and larynx; particularly, in patients who are ill, breathless, or have a compromised aerodigestive tract;

(b) improved ability to scan the head and neck during optimum vascular contrast enhancement.

Acquisition of a large volume at one time also means that there is less likelihood of missing a lesion because of misregistration or partial volume artefact. Multislice CT provides even better resolution and better multiplanar and three-dimensional

Table 2.1 CT technique.

	Standard technique	Additional techniques and information
Patient preparation	Patient lies supine with the neck extended and shoulders pulled down; the scan is performed in quiet or suspended respiration	
Scan coverage	Skull base to lung apices	Scan may be limited to the region of direct interest only (i.e. sinuses, larynx and salivary glands); but for all malignant lesions, the scan must cover the primary tumour and relevant sites of the lymph node metastases
Scan plane	Axial plane: gantry tilted parallel to the inferior orbitomeatal line (IOML) Coronal plane: as an additional plane for assessment of the skull base, orbital floor, palate and paranasal sinuses. Gantry tilted perpendicular to the IOML	Gantry may need to be tilted parallel to the body of the mandible to reduce artefact from dental amalgam and parallel to the vocal cords for imaging of the larynx Coronal images may be obtained (a) by direct scanning in the coronal plane with the patient's neck hyperextended or (b) by reconstructing the images from the axial scan
Slice thickness/ collimation	3–5 mm with a pitch of 1–1.5 and reconstruction increment of 3–5 mm (spiral CT)	
IV Intravenous (contrast)	Scans may be performed pre- and post-contrast injection or post-contrast injection only; 100–150 ml of IV non-ionic contrast is injected via a pump at 2–2.5 ml/s	Dynamic contrast-enhanced scans are required for glomus tumours
Image display	Hard copy images: all images are displayed with a soft tissue window Multislice CT provides multiple images that are usually reviewed at a workstation	Specific sites of bony interest such as the skull base, sinuses, mandible and larynx are displayed on bone windows, which are obtained by reconstructing the original data into a bone algorithm and displaying on a bone window setting
Multiplanar and three-dimensional reconstruction	These techniques are best performed with multislice CT, but can also be performed from spiral CT reconstructed from thin overlapping sections obtained without tilting of the gantry	Multiplanar images are useful, if the coronal plane cannot be obtained directly, a sagittal plane is required, or the images in one plane are degraded by dental amalgam; three-dimensional reconstruction can be performed for the mandible, skull base, larynx and facial bones
Functional CT	Imaging during phonation or Valsalva's manoeuver for assessment of the vocal cords	

reconstructions. The scanning is even faster, allowing a further reduction in aquisition time and an increase in the volume that can be scanned with thin slices at one time.

The basic techniques for CT scanning is shown in Table 2.1.

The role of CT in imaging the head and neck

CT is used to evaluate the extent of the primary tumour and metastatic lymph nodes at diagnosis and to detect tumour recurrence and post-treatment complications.

Evaluation of the primary tumour

The conspicuity of most head and neck tumours is enhanced by the use of IV contrast. However, even after enhancement, the contrast between the tumour and adjacent tissues is not always optimal and a clear appreciation of the full extent of the lesion may be sometimes difficult, especially in regions such as the oral cavity, nasopharynx and oropharynx. Further problems arise in areas of normal lymphoid tissue found in Waldeyer's ring (nasopharynx, palate, tonsils and tongue base), which normally enhance following contrast, thereby reducing visualisation of the tumour in those sites. CT demonstrates fine bony detail and is, especially, valuable in the paranasal sinuses and petrous temporal bone. Small cortical breaches can be identified when thin CT sections are obtained, but once the tumour has gained access to the marrow cavity, delineation of the full extent of marrow involvement may be more difficult. CT demonstrates the presence and pattern of calcification within a tumour, which aids in characterisation. When imaging the primary tumour, careful assessment of other regions of the head and neck must be made because of the increased risk of a second tumour. Tumours of the oropharynx, oral cavity, hypopharynx and larynx are most commonly associated with second tumours. Tumours at these primary sites have an overall prevelance of a second tumour in 13% (20% are synchronous and 80% metachronous) of which nearly half occur also in the head and neck region [1].

Evaluation of metastatic lymphadenopathy

The identification of metastatic nodes by CT is based on finding one or more of the following features.

Enlarged node

The use of nodal size as a criterion for identification of a metastatic node has many problems. Non-enlarged nodes may harbour tumour, while enlarged nodes may be reactive and not metastatic in nature. The cut-off value for the upper limit of normal size, therefore, is controversial, and is a trade-off between specificity and sensitivity. When a high cut-off value is applied, nodes that are identified as being abnormal on imaging are likely to be metastatic, but this is at the expense of missing some smaller metastatic nodes. On the other hand, when a low cut-off value is used, there is less chance of missing metastatic nodes, but this is at the expense of mistaking normal nodes for metastatic nodes. Currently, some radiologists use a maximum diameter of 15 mm in the jugulodiagastric region and 10 mm in the other regions as the upper limit of normal size [2], however, diagnosis may be inaccurate in 20–28% using this criterion [2]. Using the measurement from the maximum diameter, it has been shown that choosing a cut-off value of nodes of 10 mm produces a sensitivity of 88% and a specificity of 39%, while reducing the cut-off value to 5 mm increases the sensitivity to 98%, but at the expense of a very low specificity of only 13% [3]. There is further controversy regarding which dimension of the node should be measured. Most normal nodes in the neck are oval in shape, while metastatic nodes tend to be more rounded. The diameter of a normal node in its maximum plane, usually the vertical plane, may frequently be greater than 1 cm, whereas the diameter of the same node in its minimum plane, usually the transverse plane, is considerably smaller. For this reason, the dimension in the minimum plane is often used for assessment, using 11 mm in the jugulodiagastric region and 10 mm in the other regions [4] apart from the retropharyngeal nodes, which should not exceed 5 mm [5]. However, measurement is further complicated by the finding that normal nodes in the upper neck are larger than normal nodes in the lower neck, with the result that some centres advocate using different values in the upper and lower neck [6]. Finally, there are two further considerations when using measurement as a criterion for a metastatic node. Firstly, the histology of the primary tumour can influence the size of metastatic nodes; for example, the papillary carcinoma is well known to produce very small metastatic nodes, out of which 50% are less than 3 mm in diameter [7]. Secondly, the compromise between sensitivity and specificity will depend on which of these two factors will have a greater influence and impact on the treatment in a particular patient.

Clearly, there is no one correct size when assessing metastatic nodes. We measure the dimension in the minimum plane, using 5 mm in the retropharyngeal region, 11 mm in the jugulodiagastric region and 10 mm in the other regions. However, it must be stressed that it is important for the clinician and radiologist to agree between themselves about which size criteria should be used in which patient.

Nodal necrosis

Nodal necrosis is the most accurate sign of a metastatic node in a patient with a known primary malignancy [2]. This feature is, particularly, valuable in the head and neck, where necrosis is a common finding in metastatic nodes from cancers of this region. The signs of nodal necrosis on CT are the presence of a low attenuation centre with or without peripheral enhancement [4] (Figure 2.1). Normal fat within the hilum of a node may produce an area of low attenuation; but, in practice, this rarely causes confusion with necrosis.

Extracapsular tumour spread

Identification of extracapsular tumour spread (ECS) is an accurate sign of a metastatic node provided there is no previous radiotherapy and no infection. The signs of ECS on CT are nodal capsular enhancement, with irregularity and infiltration of adjacent tissues [8] (Figure 2.1).

Sites of metastatic nodes

When describing the position of nodes, it may be preferable to name the anatomical site (Figure 2.2)

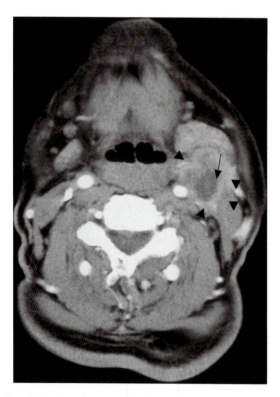

Fig. 2.1   Axial contrast-enhanced CT scan showing a malignant cervical node with nercosis (arrow) and ECS (arrowheads).

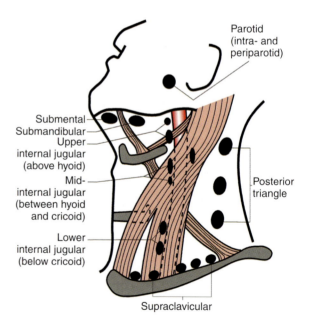

Fig. 2.2   This figure plus the following groups: 1. Facial. 2. Mastoid. 3. Central – nodes in the anterior infrahyoid neck between the right and left common carotid arteries. These nodes lie adjacent to the anterior jugular vein and around the larynx, thyroid and trachea. 4. Retropharyngeal – lateral retropharyngeal nodes which lie medial to the internal carotid artery between C1 and C3 (the median group is not identified as a discrete nodal chain).

rather than refer to numerical levels. The reason for this is that there are several different systems in practice for the numerical designation of nodal levels. Different classifications may be found not only in radiology but also in clinical practice leading to confusion when communicating the results of imaging investigations. However, for the most widely used surgical classification please refer to the chapter on the oral cavity and oropharynx.

Evaluation of tumour recurrence

Most patients with head and neck tumours require follow-up imaging to identify local and nodal recurrence. Recurrent tumour is often difficult to detect clinically, this being especially so when patients have undergone reconstructive surgery and the site of the tumour recurrence is deep seated.

The distinction between tumour recurrence and post-surgical scarring is difficult; particularly, early on when immature scarring may demonstrate contrast enhancement similar to that seen in tumour. To assist with the interpretation of follow-up studies, a baseline scan should be performed. The timing of this baseline study is controversial, but is usually at 6 weeks to 3 months after treatment. Indeterminate lesions may be accessible to a CT-guided biopsy.

Summary of advantages of CT for evaluating head and neck tumours

In general, MR imaging is used for assessing most head and neck tumours, however, CT does have advantages in specific cases. These are listed in Table 2.2.

Summary of disadvantages of CT for evaluating head and neck tumours

The disadvantages of CT for evaluating head and neck tumours are given in Table 2.3.

Table 2.2 Advantages of CT for evaluating head and neck tumours.

Faster scan	1. This is important for imaging patients who are unable to remain still for any length of time because they are sick or have difficulty with breathing, coughing or swallowing saliva 2. This is important for imaging the larynx, especially, for functional information
Bony detail and calcification	CT should be used as an additional complimentary examination to MR for demonstrating cortical bony erosion in the paranasal sinuses and petrous temporal bones, and should be used for further evaluation of suspicious cortical or cartilage invasion on MR CT is superior to MR for identifying calcification within a tumour
Metallic implants	CT can be used when MR is contraindicated
Biopsy	CT can be used for image-guided biopsy
Availability	CT is often used because it is more readily available

Table 2.3 Disadvantages of CT for evaluating head and neck tumours.

Radiation dose	The absorbed radiation doses to patients undergoing CT is relatively high compared to other diagnostic radiology techniques, and is an important consideration that must be taken into account when deciding on the benefits of the examination; the dose may be increased still further with the new multislice techniques that can increase the absorbed dose by up to 40%
Metallic artefact	Artefact from dental work may severely degrade the images in the oral cavity (Figure 2.3)
IV contrast	Adverse reactions to contrast occur in 3.13% (non-ionic) and 12.66% (ionic) of patients of which 0.04% and 0.22%, respectively, are serious reactions (dyspnoea, hypotension, cardiac arrest and loss of consciousness)

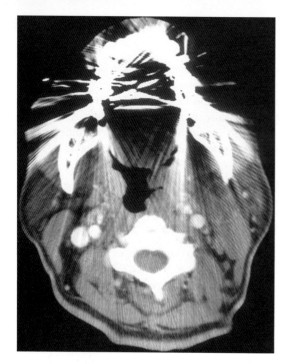

Fig. 2.3 Artefact from dental work.

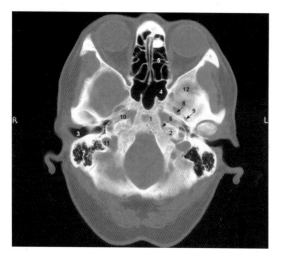

Fig. 2.4 Axial CT scan (bone window) at the level of the skull base: 1. clivus, 2. apex of petrous temporal bone, 3. external auditory canal, 4. sphenoid sinus, 5. ethmoid sinus, 6. petroclival fissure, 7. mastoid air cells, 8. foramen ovale, 9. foramen spinosum, 10. horizontal portion of carotid artery above foramen lacerum, 11. jugular fossa and 12. greater wing of sphenoid.

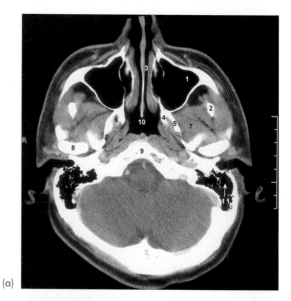

(a)

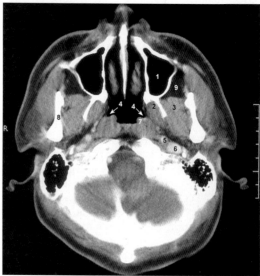

(b)

Fig. 2.5 Axial CT scan at the level of the nasopharynx: (a) – 1. maxillary sinus, 2. mandible (coronoid process), 3. nasal septum, 4. medial pterygoid plate, 5. lateral pterygoid plate, 6. pterygoid fossa, 7. lateral pterygoid, 8. mandible (condyle), 9. clivus, 10. nasopharynx and 11. mastoid air cells; (b) – 1. maxillary sinus, 2. medial pterygoid, 3. lateral pterygoid, 4. opening of the Eustachian tube, 5. internal carotid artery, 6. internal jugular vein, 7. torus tubarius, 8. mandible (ramus) and 9. retroantral fat.

Normal CT anatomy of the head and neck

The anatomy of the head and neck is demonstrated in the contrast-enhanced axial plane from the skull base to the lung apices (Figures 2.4–2.11). More detailed anatomy of specific regions, including anatomy in the coronal plane, is provided in the relevant chapters in Section 2 of this book.

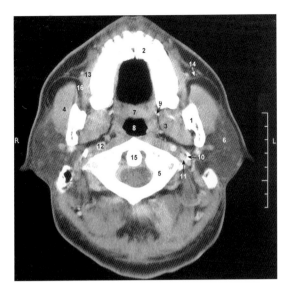

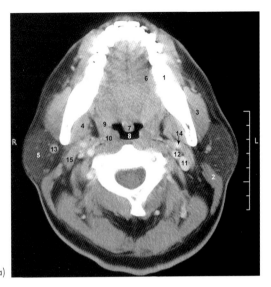

(a)

Fig. 2.6   Axial CT scan at the level of the maxilla and oropharynx: 1. mandible (ramus), 2. alveolar process of maxilla, 3. medial pterygoid, 4. masseter, 5. C1, 6. parotid gland, 7. soft palate, 8. oropharynx, 9. hook of the hamulus, 10. styloid process, 11. internal jugular vein, 12. internal carotid artery, 13. buccinator, 14. parotid duct, 15. dens of C2 and 16. buccal fat pad.

Fig. 2.7(a)   Axial CT scan at the level of the oral cavity and oropharynx: 1. mandible (body), 2. sternocleidomastoid, 3. masseter, 4. medial pterygoid, 5. parotid, 6. oral tongue, 7. uvula, 8. oropharynx, 9. anterior tonsillar pillar, 10. posterior tonsillar pillar, 11. internal jugular vein, 12. internal carotid artery, 13. retromandibular vein, 14. external carotid artery and 15. posterior belly of digastric.

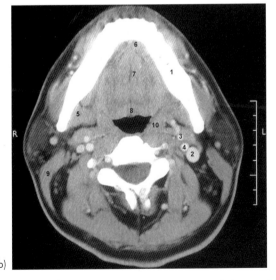

(b)

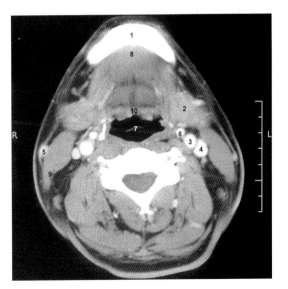

Fig. 2.7(b)   Axial CT scan at the level of the oral cavity and oropharynx: 1. mandible (body), 2. internal jugular vein, 3. external carotid artery, 4. internal carotid artery, 5. submandibular gland, 6. sublingual gland, 7. lingual septum, 8. tongue base, 9. sternocleidomastoid and 10. palatine tonsil.

Fig. 2.8   Axial CT scan at the level of the tongue base: 1. mandible (symphsis), 2. submandibular gland, 3. internal carotid artery, 4. internal jugular vein, 5. external jugular vein, 6. external carotid artery, 7. epiglottis, 8. geniohyoid/anterior belly of digastric, 9. sternocleidomastoid and 10. tongue base.

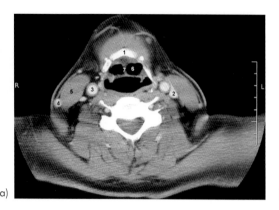 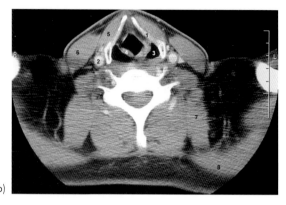

(a) (b)

Fig. 2.9 Axial CT scan at the level of the hypopharynx: (a) – 1. hyoid bone, 2. internal jugular vein, 3. common carotid artery, 4. external jugular vein, 5. sternocleidomastoid, 6. valleculae, 7. median glossoepiglottic fold; (b) – 1. thyroid cartilage, 2. common carotid artery, 3. pyriform sinus, 4. aryepiglottic folds, 5. strap muscles, 6. sternocleidomastoid, 7. levator scapulae and 8. trapezius.

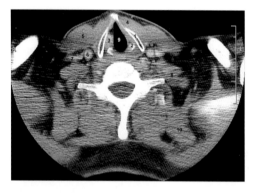 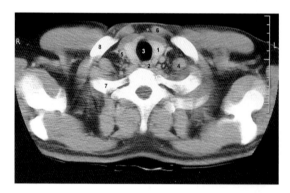

Fig. 2.10 Axial CT scan at the level of the larynx: 1. thyroid cartilage, 2. cricoid/arytenoid cartilage, 3. true vocal cord, 4. strap muscles, 5. sternocleidomastoid, 6. common carotid artery, 7. internal jugular vein, 8. scalene muscles, 9. glottic airway and 10. levator scapulae.

Fig. 2.11 Axial CT scan at the level of the thyroid: 1. thyroid gland, 2. cervical oesphagus, 3. trachea, 4. internal jugular vein, 5. common carotid artery, 6. sternocleidomastoid, 7. first rib and 8. clavicle.

References

1. Haughey BH, Gates GA, Arfken CL and Harvey J. Meta-analysis of second malignant tumors in head and neck cancer: the case for an endoscopic screening protocol. *Ann. Otol. Rhinol. Laryngol.* 1992; **101**: 105–112.
2. Saki O, Curtin HD, Romo LV and Som PM. Lymph node pathology. Benign and proliferative lymphoma and metastatic disease. *Radiol. Clin. N. Am.* 2000; **38**: 980–981.
3. Curtin HD, Ishwaren H, Mancuso AA, Dalley RW, Caudry DJ and McNeil BJ. Comparison of CT and MR imaging in staging of neck metastases. *Radiology* 1998; **207**: 123–130.
4. van den Brekel MWM, Stel HV, Castelijns JA, Nauta JP, van der Waal I, Valk J, Meyer CJ and Snow GB. Cervical lymph node metastasis: assessment of radiologic criteria. *Radiology* 1990; **177**: 379–384.
5. Lam WWM, Chan YL, Leung SF and Metreweli C. Retropharyngeal lymphadenopathy in nasopharyngeal carcinoma. *Head Neck* 1997; **19**: 176–181.
6. van den Brekel MWM, Castelijns JA and Snow GB. The size of lymph nodes in the neck on sonograms as a radiologic criteria for metastasis: how reliable is it? AJNR 1998; **19**: 695–700.
7. Noguchi S, Noguchi A and Murakami N. Papillary carcinoma of the thyroid. Developing pattern of metastasis. *Cancer* 1970; **26**: 1053–1060.
8. Yousem DM, Som PM, Hackney DB, Schwaibold F and Hendrix RA. Central nodal necrosis and extracapsular neoplastic spread in cervical lymph nodes: MR imaging versus CT. *Radiology* 1992; **182**: 733–759.

Magnetic Resonance Imaging

AD King

Introduction

Magnetic resonance (MR) imaging produces excellent quality images with superb contrast, good spatial resolution, and direct multiplanar formats without using ionising radiation. It is the best imaging technique for characterising and mapping the extent of tumour. The disadvantages are that it is relatively expensive, time consuming, and susceptible to motion artefact. In addition, there are contraindications to MR imaging, which are listed in Table 3.1.

The list of metallic implants and foreign bodies is extensive and cannot be covered in this text. Most are non-ferromagnetic and are compatible with MR, but some are not and are contraindicated. Therefore, each patient needs to be assessed on an individual basis before arranging a scan.

Table 3.1 Contraindications to MR imaging.

Absolute contraindications	Relative contraindications
Cardiac pacemaker	Pregnancy (especially first trimester). Scan is performed when investigation cannot wait until after pregnancy and other forms of diagnostic imaging are inadequate or require exposure to ionising radiation
Intracranial aneurysm and haemostatic clips (ferromagnetic)	Claustrophobia (usually, this can be overcome by several techniques including patient positioning, the use of mirrors and headphones, or sedation)
Metallic foreign body in the eye	
Cochlear implant	

MR technique

Standard sequences for MR imaging of the head and neck

There are many sequences utilised in MR imaging, but only a few standard sequences are frequently employed in head and neck imaging. These are the T1-weighted sequence before and after intravenous (IV) gadolinium, and the T2-weighted sequence. These sequences can be combined with a technique to saturate the signal from fat.

T1-weighted sequence

The T1-weighted sequence produces images with excellent anatomical detail because of the good spatial resolution and contrast between the many soft tissue interfaces in the head and neck. T1-weighted images are dependent on the TR (repetition time) and TE (echo time). Increasing the TR decreases the T1 effect in the scan; therefore, a relatively short TR of about 500 ms is used. The TE is kept as short as possible, about 20 ms, to reduce the T2 effects, but at the same time it cannot be too short or the quality of the image will suffer from a decrease in the signal-to-noise ratio. A spin-echo technique may be used to produce T1-weighted images. This is one of the original techniques used in MR imaging, and is relatively slow, but is still preferred in some centres, in preference to the faster or turbo spin-echo techniques, because of the higher quality of the anatomic detail. Most of head and neck cancers are of low or intermediate signal intensity on T1-weighted images. Tumours containing fat, blood products, or secretions with a high protein content have areas of high signal intensity.

T1-weighted sequence post-IV gadolinium

The T1-weighted sequence is repeated after the IV injection of gadolinium to demonstrate an increase in the signal intensity in normal and abnormal enhancing tissues. Normal structures that enhance include mucosal linings, soft palate, tonsils, and tongue base. Most of head and neck cancers show enhancement after contrast. Enhancement also improves the detection of necrosis by revealing areas of non-enhancing tissue within a tumour. Tumours, such as paragangliomas and angiofibromas, show intense enhancement on dynamic images, aiding to the characterisation of the tumour. One area of caution is the interpretation of tumour infiltration in bone marrow. Following the IV contrast, enhancing tumour may have the same high signal intensity as the fatty bone marrow, rendering the tumour inconspicuous. The post-contrast T1-weighted images, therefore, should be accompanied either by fat suppression or interpreted side by side with the pre-contrast study.

T2-weighted sequence

The anatomical detail on a T2-weighted sequence is not as good as that on the T1-weighted sequence, but the T2-weighted sequence accentuates the difference between the contrast of normal and abnormal tissues. The T2-weighted images are produced using a long TE to maximise the T2 differences and a long TR to minimise the T1 differences. Fast spin-echo, also known as turbo spin-echo, and gradient-echo sequences have largely replaced the conventional T2-weighted spin-echo sequence in the head and neck. These sequences produce comparable quality for a T2-weighted image, but are faster decreasing the risk of movement artefacts. The majority of the tumours in the head and neck are highly cellular and produce images with an intermediate or mildly increased signal rather than very high signal intensity. This is useful in the paranasal sinuses where inflammatory changes have a very high signal intensity, thereby differentiating them from tumour. Cancers may contain very high signal regions, if they are cystic or necrotic and the T2-weighted images help to accentuate this difference between the solid and necrotic portion of a tumour.

Fat-saturation sequence

This is an additional technique that can be combined with a T1- or a T2-weighted image to suppress the signal from fat. Fat suppression is used to characterise fatty tissue or to increase the conspicuity of tumours surrounded by fat. Fat suppression may increase the conspicuity of tumour on both the contrast-enhanced T1-weighted sequence and on the fast spin-echo T2-weighted sequence. In the first case, a high signal intensity enhancing tumour on a T1-weighted sequence becomes less conspicuous as it blends with the high signal intensity of the surrounding fat. By suppressing the signal of fat, the areas of tumour enhancement stand out more readily. This is, particularly, valuable in the identification of perineural tumour spread and tumour invasion of the fatty bone marrow. In the second case, fat suppression is required with the fast T2-spin-echo techniques because, unlike conventional spin-echo images, the fat has a high-signal intensity, thereby obscuring adjacent pathological processes with a high-T2-signal intensity. Once again suppressing the signal from fat may improve conspicuity of the lesion.

Other MR techniques

The sequences described above are the standard technique for producing cross-sectional images. However, MR can also be employed to produce angiographic images with or without IV contrast, spectroscopic information, and imaging guidance for interventional procedures. The IV contrast agent, dextran-covered ultrasmall iron oxide, can be combined with the standard MR imaging to detect the malignant nodes. While this technique is frequently cited in the literature, it is rarely used in clinical practice.

Image quality and artefacts

The overall quality of a scan depends on many inter-related parameters that influence contrast, spatial resolution, signal-to-noise ratio, and scanning time. Discussion of these parameters is beyond the scope of this chapter, but in general it is not possible to optimise all these factors and there is always a trade-off, especially with scanning time. To increase the coverage or the quality (signal-to-noise ratio) of the images, scanning time is prolonged. A longer scanning time increases the chance of motion during acquisition; thereby the images may contain motion artefacts. Movement is a particular problem for patients with head and neck tumours, because of the difficulty with breathing, coughing, and swallowing saliva. Physiological factors may also cause movement such as pulsation from major vessels in the neck. If the movement is marked, the images will be severely affected by a ghosting artefact that occurs in the phase encoding direction (AP in the axial plane) (Figure 3.1). Lesser degrees of movement lead to blurring of the images (Figure 3.2). Comfortable positioning of the patient with immobilisation of the head, instructions to breathe quietly using abdominal respiration, and avoidance of movements such as

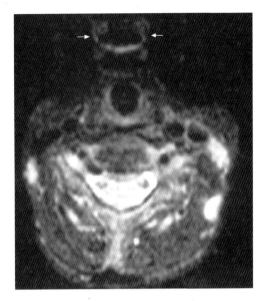

Fig. 3.1 Ghosting artefact (arrows) caused by swallowing.

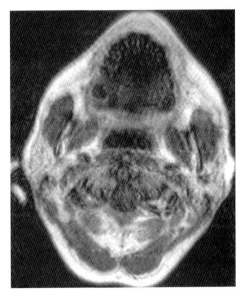

Fig. 3.2 Blurred image caused by patient movement.

swallowing are helpful to reduce the chance of image degradation. However, even the most co-operative patient will find it difficult to lie completely still for more than 5–8 min per scan. Sick patients, who are breathless or have a compromised aerodigestive tract, may not be able to tolerate even the shortest of the MR scans. In these cases, computed tomography (CT) is a better alternative.

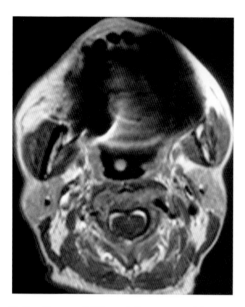

Fig. 3.3 Susceptibility artefact caused by metallic dental work.

MR images are degraded also by susceptibility arte-fact caused by metallic foreign bodies (Figure 3.3) and by air–tissue interfaces. The artefact from metallic foreign bodies may cause less degradation of the image on MR than on CT, and, while metallic dental bridges distort the MR image, dental amalgam is less of a problem. In general, ferromagnetic mater-ial such as iron and nickel cause major distortion of the magnetic field and the resulting image. Paramag-netic materials such as titanium, from which many implants in the maxillofacial region are now made, cause very little distortion, while diamagnetic mater-ials such as gold, zinc, copper, and mercury have the least effect. Susceptibility artefact from air–tissue interfaces is found especially around the paranasal sinuses and at the junction of the chin and upper neck. Avoiding T2-weighted fat-saturation and gradient-echo sequences can reduce susceptibility artefact. Fat-saturation images can be degraded by any inhomogeneity in the magnetic field leading to asymmetrical fat suppression (Figure 3.4).

MR imaging protocols for the head and neck

The choice of protocol depends upon position and size of the tumour, general status of the patient, equipment, and the radiologist's own preferences.

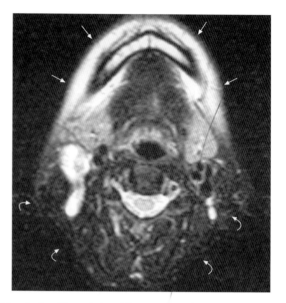

Fig. 3.4 T2-weighted fat supressed image showing suppression of the high signal intensity of fat in the posterior neck (curved arrows), but failure of fat sup-pression in the anterior neck (straight arrows).

Therefore, in this complex region, there is no stand-ard sequence or plane that will be suitable for all patients. When scanning the head and neck region, it is always tempting to perform just one more sequence or plane, but this comes at the expense, not only of cost, but also of increasing the likelihood of patient movement. In addition, the more images that are available, the more difficult it becomes for the radiologist to meticulously scrutinise all the areas. The suggested protocols that are shown in Table 3.2 provide a broad guide only.

The role of MR in imaging the head and neck

MR is used to evaluate the extent of the primary tumour and metastatic lymph nodes at diagnosis and to detect tumour recurrence and post-treatment complications.

Evaluation of the primary tumour

Accurate mapping of tumour extent is required for treatment, especially planning radiotherapy fields and surgery. MR imaging is the best modality for

Table 3.2   MR protocols using a 1.5 T magnet.

	Technique
MR coil	The options are to use 1. dedicated combined head and neck coil (not widely available), 2. head coil to cover the primary tumour and nodes from the skull base to oral cavity, 3. neck coil to cover the primary tumour and nodes from the oral cavity to suprastenal notch, 4. surface coil: additional coil to examine superficial structures such as the larynx, salivary glands, and thyroid.
Scan plane	A sagittal localiser is used to plan the scan plane. In general, at least two planes are required. These are most frequently the axial and coronal planes. A sagittal plane can be used as an alternative or additional plane in regions such as the skull base, tongue base, floor of mouth, and posterior wall of the hypopharynx.
MR sequences	1. T1-weighted spin-echo sequence, 2. T2-weighted fast spin-echo sequence with or without fat saturation, 3. T1-weighted spin-echo sequence post-contrast. Post-contrast scans are obtained in at least two planes and we prefer to use a 512 high-resolution matrix. One of the planes may be substituted for a 256 matrix with fat saturation.
Image parameters	1. Slice thickness should be 4–5 mm (3 mm for some regions, such as the larynx). 2. Field of view is small as possible (14–16 cm for T1 and 18–20 cm for T2-weighted images). 3. Matrix size: preferably a 512 matrix for at least some of the sequences such as the T1-weighted images with a 256 matrix for the other images. 4. Number of signal averages is equal to 2.

demonstrating the extent of the majority of head and neck cancers because of the multiplanar capacity and superior soft tissue contrast, although multislice CT may challenge MR in the future.

MR identifies deep-seated tumours as well as some superficial tumours, in regions such as the pyriform fossa and subglottis, that are difficult to visualise by endoscopy. However, some small superficial mucosal tumours may produce a normal or only a subtle abnormality on MR imaging. Imaging should, therefore, always be correlated to the endoscopy findings. The radiologist also should be made aware of any recent biopsy that has the potential to produce abnormal signal that may be misinterpreted as tumour. Preferably, the MR scan should be performed at least 10–14 days after a biopsy, but the timing is controversial and is also influenced by the clinical management. Small tumours in the soft palate, tongue base, and palatine tonsils may be obscured because of their similar signal intensity to normal tissue at these sites [1]. MR has specific advantages over other imaging techniques in most regions of the head and neck (see advantages of MR for evaluating head and neck tumours).

When imaging the primary tumour, other regions of the head and neck must be carefully inspected, because of the increased risk of synchronous tumours (see Chapters 2 and 6).

Evaluation of metastatic lymphadenopathy

The identification of a metastatic node by MR is based on the finding of one or more of the following features.

Enlarged node

In general, the size criterion employed for assessing a metastatic node by MR is the same as that employed by CT [2–5]. The size criterion and difficulties in selecting an optimum "cut-off" size are discussed under enlarged nodes in Chapter 2.

Nodal necrosis

Nodal necrosis is the most accurate sign of a metastatic node in a patient with a known primary

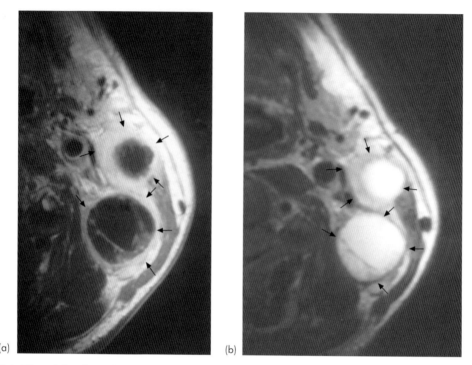

(a)   (b)

Fig. 3.5 (a) T1-weighted axial image post-contrast and (b) T2-weighted axial image showing necrotic metastatic cervical lymph nodes (arrows).

malignancy. This feature is particularly valuable in the head and neck, where necrosis is a common finding in metastatic nodes from cancers of this region. The generally accepted criteria for nodal necrosis on MR are the presence of inhomogeneous signal intensity, usually a high signal focus on T2-weighted images, a low signal focus on T1-weighted images, or a non-enhancing focus on T1-weighted images with peripheral enhancement following contrast [6,7] (Figure 3.5a and b).

Extracapsular tumour spread

Identification of extracapsular tumour spread (ECS) is an accurate sign of a metastatic node, provided there is no previous radiotherapy and infection. The sign of ECS on MR is nodal capsular enhancement, with irregularity and infiltration of adjacent tissues [7] (Figure 3.6).

Disruption of normal nodal architecture

Focal areas of tumour invasion within a node may appear similar to necrosis on MR imaging.

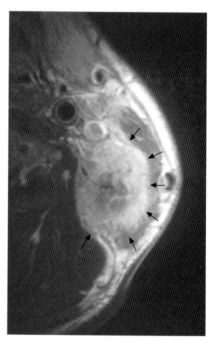

Fig. 3.6 Axial T1-weighted image post-contrast showing a large necrotic metastatic node with ECS (arrows).

Evaluation of tumour recurrence

Patients with head and neck tumours require follow-up imaging to detect the local and nodal recurrence. Recurrent tumour is often difficult to detect clinically, especially when patients have undergone reconstructive surgery and the site of the tumour recurrence is deep seated. Tumour recurrence has a similar signal to the original tumour. In the head and neck, it is often of low signal intensity on T1, intermediate signal intensity on T2 and demonstrates moderate enhancement after contrast on the T1-weighted images. However, interpretation of post-operative scans is difficult because tumour recurrence may have similar appearances to post-radiation necrotic tissue or to immature scar tissue. As the scar tissue matures, the enhancement disappears, usually after 6 months although in some cases it may persist for longer, and the signal intensity on T2-weighted images becomes low. To assist the interpretation of follow-up studies, a baseline scan is mandatory and is usually performed at 6 weeks to 3 months after treatment. The radiologist interpreting the scan needs to be acquainted with the imaging features of the surgical flaps and the expected changes following radiotherapy in the different regions of the head and neck (please refer to chapters in Section 2).

Table 3.3   Advantages of MR imaging.

Pharynx (naso-, oro-, and hypo-) and oral cavity	Superior delineation of soft tissue anatomical detail, allowing better depiction of tumour invasion
Sinonasal region	Distinction of tumour from inflammatory changes
Neural structures	Relationship of tumour to the cranium, especially to dura and cavernous sinus, and to the cranial nerves, including demonstration of perineural tumour spread
Vascular structures	Relationship of tumour to major arteries and venous structures
Bone marrow	Extent of tumour invasion within bone marrow (except on the T1-weighted image post-contrast where tumour may be masked)
Nodes	MR is better for depiction of retropharyngeal nodes
Tumour characterisation	Distinguishing necrotic/cystic from solid regions within a tumour Enhancement pattern, some tumours are highly vascular with marked enhancement and signal voids, most notably paragangliomas and angiofibromas

Table 3.4   Disadvantages of MR imaging.

Availability, time, and expense	For these reasons some centres continue to use CT
MR contraindicated	See Introduction for specific contraindications
Patient unable to remain motionless	Image quality may be severely degraded. CT is a better option for these patients
Superficial tumours (thyroid and salivary glands)	Ultrasound may be a better initial investigation
Larynx	CT may be preferred as initial investigation because it is less prone to movement artefact
Cortical bone	CT should be used as an additional complimentary examination to MR for demonstrating cortical bony erosion in the paranasal sinuses and petrous temporal bones, and may be used for further evaluation of suspicious cortical or cartilage invasion on MR
Calcification	CT is superior to MR for demonstrating tumour calcification
Nodes	MR has no advantage over ultrasound or CT for the examination of neck nodes (excluding retropharyngeal nodes)

Summary of the advantages of MR for evaluating head and neck tumours

For the majority of head and neck tumours MR should be the imaging modality of choice.

Table 3.3 lists some of the specific advantages of MR and Table 3.4 some of the disadvantages of MR.

Normal MR anatomy of the head and neck

The anatomy of the head and neck is demonstrated in the axial plane on T1-weighted high-resolution images after contrast from the skull base to the lung apices (Figures 3.7a–n). More detailed anatomy of specific regions, including anatomy in the coronal and sagittal planes, is provided in the relevant chapters in Section 2 of this book.

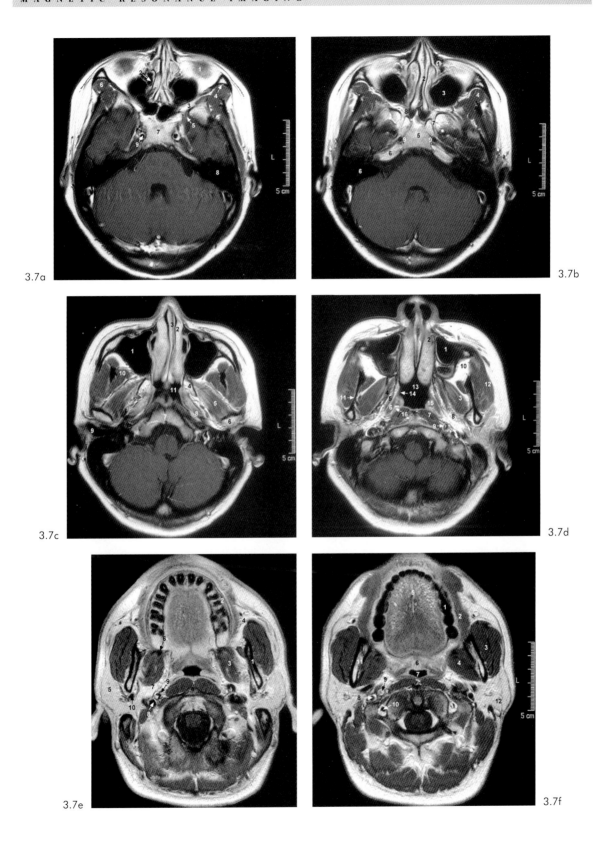

3.7a

3.7b

3.7c

3.7d

3.7e

3.7f

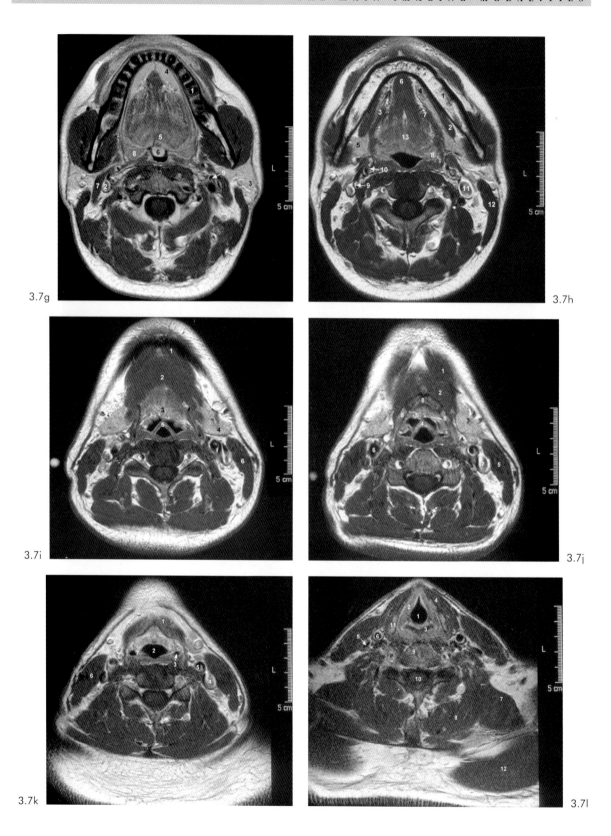

3.7g

3.7h

3.7i

3.7j

3.7k

3.7l

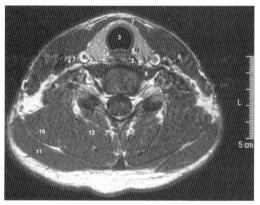 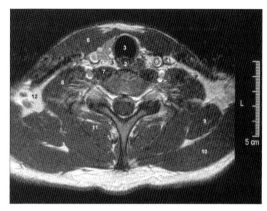

3.7m

3.7n

Fig. 3.7 *Axial T1-weighted image at the level of the skull base:* (a) – 1. globe, 2. ethmoid sinus, 3. ptery-gomaxillary fissure, 4. zygomatic bone, 5. foramen rotundum, 6. temporalis, 7. clivus, 8. petrous temporal bone, and 9. internal carotid artery; (b) – 1. nasolacrimal duct, 2. nasal septum, 3. maxillary sinus, 4. temporalis, 5. clivus, 6. petrous temporal bone, 7. vidian canal, 8. pterygopalatine fossa, and 9. petrocli-val fissure. *Axial T1-weighted image at the level of the nasopharynx:* (c) – 1. maxillary sinus, 2. middle nasal turbinate, 3. nasal septum, 4. pterygoid process, 5. lateral pterygoid, 6. condyle of the mandible, 7. clivus, 8. eustachian tube, 9. external auditory canal, 10. temporalis, and 11. nasopharynx; (d) – 1. maxillary sinus, 2. inferior nasal turbinate, 3. lateral pterygoid, 4. medial pteryoid, 5. tensor veli palatini, 6. levator veli palatini, 7. prevertebral muscles, 8. pharapharyngeal fat space, 9. internal carotid artery, 10. retroantral fat, 11. ramus of the mandible, 12. masseter, 13. nasopharynx, 14. opening of Eusthacian tube, 15. torus tubar-ius, and 16. fossa of Rosenmuller. *Axial T1-weighted image at the level of the maxilla:* (e) – 1. ramus of mandible, 2. maxillary alveolar ridge, 3. medial pterygoid, 4. parotid duct, 5. parotid gland, 6. hook of the hamulus, 7. parapharyngeal fat space, 8. internal jugular vein, 9. internal carotid artery, and 10. retromandibular vein. *Axial T1-weighted image at the level of the oropharynx and oral cavity:* (f) – 1. maxillary alveolar ridge, 2. buccinator, 3. masseter, 4. medial pterygoid, 5. oral tongue, 6. uvula, 7. oropharynx, 8. internal jugular vein, 9. internal carotid artery, 10. vertebral artery, 11. ramus of mandible, and 12. parotid gland; (g) – 1. body of the mandible, 2. internal jugular vein, 3. parotid gland, 4. sublingual gland, 5. tongue base, 6. uvula, 7. posterior belly of digastric, 8. palatine tonsil, and 9. internal carotid artery; (h) – 1. mandible, 2. mylohyoid, 3. hyoglossus, 4. sublingual gland, 5. submandibular gland, 6. genioglossus, 7. lingual artery, 8. palatine tonsil, 9. internal carotid artery, 10. external carotid artery, 11. internal jugular vein, 12. sterno-cleidomastoid, and 13. tongue base. *Axial T1-weighted image at the level of the tongue base:* (i) – 1. anterior belly of digastric, 2. geniohyoid, 3. tongue base, 4. submandibular gland, 5. epiglottis, and 6. sternocleido-mastoid. *Axial T1-weighted image at the level of the hypopharynx:* (j) – 1. anterior belly of digastric, 2. genio-hyoid, 3. submandibular gland, 4. epiglottis, 5. sternocleidomastoid, 6. common carotid artery, 7. internal jugular vein, and 8. hyoid; (k) – 1. strap muscles, 2. laryngeal vestibule, 3. piriform sinus, 4. internal jugular vein, 5. common carotid artery, 6. sternocleidomastoid, and 7. aryepiglottic fold. *Axial T1-weighted image at the level of the larynx:* (l) – 1. glottic airway, 2. true cord, 3. cricoid cartilage, 4. strap muscles, 5. internal jugu-lar vein, 6. common carotid artery, 7. levator scapulae, 8. paraspinal muscles, 9. vertebral body, 10. spinal cord, 11. thyroid cartilage, and 12. trapezius. *Axial T1-weighted image at the level of the thyroid:* (m) – 1. thyroid gland, 2. cervical oesphagus, 3. trachea, 4. internal jugular vein, 5. common carotid artery, 6. sternocleido-mastoid, 7. strap muscles, 8. prevertebral muscles, 9. scalene muscles, 10. levator scapulae, 11. trapezius, and 12. paraspinal muscles. *Axial T1-weighted image at the level of the supraclavicular fossa:* (n) – 1. thyroid gland, 2. cervical oesphagus, 3. trachea, 4. internal jugular vein, 5. common carotid artery, 6. sternocleido-mastoid, 7. prevertebral muscles, 8. scalene muscle, 9. levator scapulae muscles, 10. trapezius muscle, 11. paraspinal muscles, and 12. supraclavicular fossa.

References

1. King AD, Lei IK, and Ahuja AT. MR imaging of primary non-Hodgkin's lymphoma of the palatine tonsil. *Br. J. Radiol.* 2001; **74**: 226–229.
2. Curtin HD, Ishwaren H, Mancuso AA, Dalley RW, Caudry DJ, and McNeil BJ. Comparison of CT and MR imaging in staging of neck metastases. *Radiology* 1998; **207**: 123–130.
3. Van den Brekel MWM, Stel HV, Castelijns JA, Nauta JP, van der Waal I, Valk J, Meyer CJ, and Snow GB. Cervical lymph node metastasis: assessment of radiologic criteria. *Radiology* 1990; **177**: 379–384.
4. Lam WWM, Chan YL, Leung SF, and Metreweli C. Retropharyngeal lymphadenopathy in nasopharyngeal carcinoma. *Head Neck* 1997; **19**: 176–181.
5. Van den Brekel MWM, Castelijns JA, and Snow GB. The size of lymph nodes in the neck on sonograms as a radiologic criteria for metastasis: how reliable is it? *AJNR* 1998; **19**: 695–700.
6. Saki O, Curtin HD, Romo LV, and Som PM. Lymph node pathology. Benign and proliferative lymphoma and metastatic disease. *Radiol. Clin. N. Am.* 2000; **38**: 980–981.
7. Yousem DM, Som PM, Hackney DB, Schwaibold F, and Hendrix RA. Central nodal necrosis and extracapsular neoplastic spread in cervical lymph nodes: MR imaging versus CT. *Radiology* 1992; **182**: 733–759.

Positron Emission Tomography

SK Mukherji, N Fischbein and M Castillo

Introduction

The past decade has seen dramatic changes in imaging of head and neck cancer. Active areas of investigation include metabolic and functional imaging. The goal of these techniques is to provide information that clinicians cannot identify on physical examination. Results of metabolic imaging techniques suggest that they may improve our ability to identify metastases and recurrent tumour and to monitor treatment. In this chapter, we review the positron emission tomography (PET) and its potential applications in head and neck imaging.

Physics and technique

Unlike other anatomical imaging techniques, PET is a functional imaging technique that depicts tissue metabolic activity. Most tumours show increased glycolytic activity compared with non-neoplastic tissues and ^{18}F-labelled fluorodeoxyglucose (a glucose analogue), is a useful marker of tumour activity. We review the basic physics and technical aspects of PET and the radiopharmaceuticals which can be used in head and neck imaging.

PET imaging uses radioisotopes which are unstable as their nuclei contain an excess of protons that decay with emission of positively charged particles (positrons). These radioisotopes are short lived and cyclotron produced. Positrons travel a short distance (1–2 mm) in tissue before combining with negatively charged electrons resulting in mutual annihilation with conversion of mass to energy and the emission of two 511 keV photons at approximately 180° to each other. These photons are more penetrating than positrons and exit the body easily and can be detected. Annihilation and photon emission explain the resolution limitations of PET. Annihilation happens at a distance from the decaying radionuclide and is determined by both the density of the matter and by the energy of the positron. The two annihilation photons are not emitted in perfect collinearity. This divergence results from requirements of conservation of momentum [1]. These two factors lead to a lower limit of unsharpness (2–3 mm).

The metabolism of cancer cells is abnormal when compared to normal cells of the same tissue. Glucose metabolism and the rate of protein synthesis are high and there is an increased need for fatty acids and nucleic acids by rapidly proliferating cells. Short-lived positron emitters such as ^{18}F and ^{11}C can label biological substrates without altering their character. These substrates are used to study many physiological processes. The most widely used tracer for PET is 2-[^{18}F]fluoro-2-deoxy-D-glucose (FDG). FDG is a glucose analogue with a fluorine-for-hydroxyl substitution of D-glucose. ^{18}F is cyclotron-produced and has a half-life of 110 min. The typical dose of FDG in adult is approximately 370 MBq (10 mCi). FDG is taken up by glucose transporters and phosphorylated by hexokinase to FDG-6-phosphate. Further metabolism is blocked by the extra hydroxyl moiety. FDG-6-phosphate thus accumulates in the cells providing a marker for glucose uptake and utilisation. FDG and serum glucose compete for uptake, therefore, patients should fast for 4 h prior to FDG-PET study. Tumour cells have high glycolysis even in the presence of oxygen [2]. Uptake of glucose and FDG is facilitated by increased expression of glucose transporter molecules at the tumour cell surface [3], and activity of hexokinase has been shown to be higher in tumour cells [4]. Tumour concentration of FDG generally reaches a peak at 30 min, remains constant up to 60 min and then declines [4]. Non-tumours, but rapidly metabolising cells, such as macrophages may also accumulate FDG [5].

As stated previously, PET relies on the detection of photons travelling at 180° to each other (annihilation reaction). Detectors used in PET consist of a scintillator (typically bismuth-germanate, or BGO), photomultiplier tubes, and an amplifier. The mechanical gantry holds the detectors and shielding. There are septa between detectors for interplane shielding in multiring detector systems [6]. Most PET scanners use multiple rings of detectors that produce multiple slices. Scanners can be operated in either a high-resolution mode or a high-sensitivity mode [7].

At present, images are generally displayed and interpreted directly on a computer console which allows simultaneous viewing of axial, sagittal and coronal planes, as well as rotation.

PET does not provide the same anatomic detail provided by computed tomography (CT) or magnetic resonance (MR) imaging and does not allow for precise localisation of pathology. Computerised co-registration of PET and CT/MR images helps circumvent this limitation and provides additional information [8]. One method of registration makes use of an iterative surface-fit algorithm that performs scaling, translation and rotation of one of the surfaces and obtains the best fit of the two surfaces under comparison after manual alignment [9]. Anatomical landmarks such as the nasal profile or the convexities of the brain or external markers may be used to guide registration. The recent development of combined CT/PET scanners has eased the difficulty of anatomical correlation [10].

Positron emission events are imaged efficiently and with high resolution using a PET scanner with full-ring bismuth-germanate crystal block detectors. Since these scanners are of limited availability, interest has focused on the use of conventional or modified gamma cameras to image positron emission events. Conventional multiheaded single photon emission computed tomography (SPECT) cameras are in widespread use, but attempts to image FDG using them has proven to be of limited value due to low spatial resolution and low sensitivity [11,12]. Their poor performance is a consequence mostly of limited efficiency for detection of 511 keV photons using a camera optimised for detection of 140 keV photons. Results are improved by operating a modified gamma camera fitted with thicker (1.6 cm versus 0.95 cm) NaI crystals in coincidence mode. In this situation, there are limitations due to count rate and the contribution of accidental coincidence [11]. Several recent studies have demonstrated that a dual-head camera with PET capability is sensitive for the detection of primary head and neck cancers and accurate in the preoperative assessment of lymph node metastases and detection of local recurrences [13–15].

Clinical applications

Literature on the role of PET scanning in head and neck oncology is rapidly expanding. The majority of studies are based on the use of FDG and they will be the focus of our review.

On a whole body scan, the most intense activity is located in the brain, followed by myocardium, renal collecting systems and bladder. There is moderate activity in the liver, spleen, and bone marrow, and variable activity in the bowel, breast and muscle [16]. In the head and neck, there is marked accumulation of FDG in the floor of mouth, generally attributed to the sublingual glands and the lymphoid tissue of Waldeyer's ring. Moderate activity is present in the parotid and submandibular glands, the extraocular muscles, and the nasal turbinates. The thyroid gland may demonstrate striking FDG uptake. Muscle uptake is usually mild unless the patient is talking or has recently exerted his neck or shoulder muscles. Bones and fat show no uptake [17].

Normal FDG uptake in head and neck:

1. Sublingual glands ↑↑↑
2. Waldeyers ring especially, lingual tonsil ↑↑↑
3. Parotid and submandibular glands ↑↑
4. Extraocular muscles ↑↑
5. Nasal tubinates ↑↑
6. Cervical muscles ↑↑
7. Thyroid gland ↑

Radiation therapy causes little or no change in normal uptake patterns of FDG in the head and neck except for a mild generalised increase in soft tissue uptake. In a series of 11 patients with squamous cell carcinoma (SCC) of the head and neck studied before, during, and after 6 weeks of radiation, Rege *et al.* [18] found that the average metabolic ratio in the tonsils, nasal turbinates, soft palate and gingiva did not change significantly while FDG uptake decreased dramatically in tumours. Salivary glands maintained normal FDG uptake, though their function decreased following radiation therapy.

Initial evaluation of primary tumours

FDG-PET has valuable applications in the assessment of head and neck cancers. FDG-PET can find unknown primary lesions and second primaries and stage disease prior to therapy. It can detect residual and/or recurrent disease and assess response to therapy and detect metastases. FDG-PET detects over 95% of SCC with volumes greater or equal to 1 cc (Figure 4.1). The degree of uptake is unrelated to the histological grade of the lesions [19–21]. Small superficial lesions may go undetected by FDG-PET [22].

Unknown primary tumours

About 5% of patients with SCC present only with cervical nodal metastases and no identifiable primary tumour. Evaluation with CT/MR and endoscopy with random biopsy of likely primary sites identify primary sites in 10–20% of these patients [23]. If no primary tumour site is found on CT/MR or endoscopy with

biopsy the three therapeutic approaches available are as follows: a patient may undergo neck dissection followed by watchful waiting (controversial), neck dissection followed by radiation therapy to one or both sides of the neck and all possible primary tumour sites, including the nasopharynx, or radiation therapy to all likely primary sites and the neck possibly followed by neck dissection. Identification of a primary tumour allows for more appropriately directed treatment which significantly reduces morbidity and is of benefit to the patient.

> **Key points**
>
> *Unknown primary therapeutic approaches*
> - Neck dissection, then "wait and see"
> - Neck dissection and radiation therapy → possible primary sites and both sides of neck
> - Radiation therapy → possible primary sites and neck, then surgery

The recently reported success of FDG-PET in identifying unknown primary lesions in patients presenting with metastatic cervical adenopathy is promising. A number of series (number of patient 4–18) report successful localisation of unknown primary lesions in 20–50% of cases [20,24–28] (Figure 4.2). Most but not all of these lesions were not seen on other imaging studies. One of these reports [25] made use of FDG-SPECT rather than FDG-PET with good success. In one report [24], a 4 mm lesion was missed with PET and found endoscopically, and in another [27] a nasopharyngeal primary was identified at postradiation therapy follow-up PET. There was also a 20–30% rate of presumed false-positive diagnoses [25, 26], assuming biopsy to be the gold standard (an assumption not necessarily valid as biopsy is operator-dependent and may miss small or deep submucosal deposits). In each series there were a number of patients in whom no primary site was ever identified by PET, endoscopic biopsy, or clinical follow-up. It is assumed that some small primary tumours might have been eliminated by the body's own immune surveillance system, cured by radiation therapy, or that prior SCC of the skin may be the primary site. The fact that a number of primary lesions are never identified by any method makes it difficult to calculate accurate values for sensitivity and specificity.

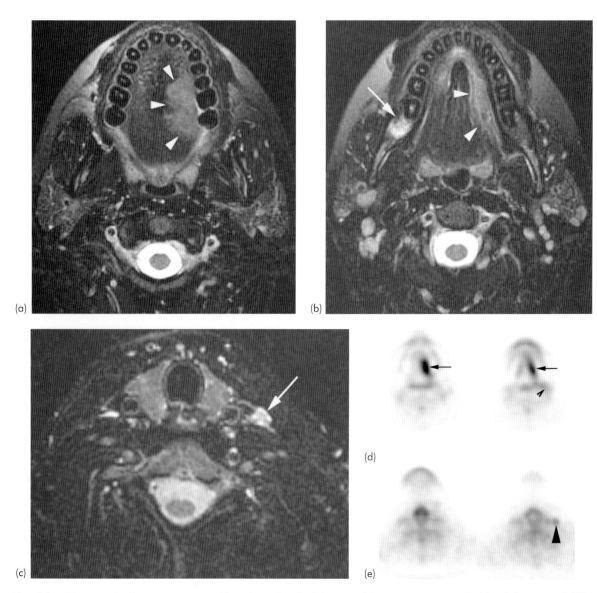

Fig. 4.1   Untreated primary tumour and lymph node of a 34-year-old woman presented with a left tongue SCC. (a) Axial fast spin-echo T2-weighted image with fat saturation shows an irregular and deeply invasive lesion of the left lateral tongue (white arrowheads). (b) More inferiorly, the tumours extends into the left floor of mouth (white arrowheads). A bright lesion in the right mandible (white arrow) was odontogenic in origin. Small lymph nodes are seen in the neck, none of which appear pathological. (c) Axial T2-weighted image through the level of the thyroid gland demonstrates a level IV lymph node (white arrow) which was nicely shown but not clearly pathologic by size criteria or the presence of necrosis. (d) An FDG-PET study was performed. Images through the oral cavity (PET) show asymmetrical activity in the left tongue, extending into the left floor of mouth (black arrows), consistent with the known primary tumour. Asymmetrical activity in the left submandibular gland (oblique arrowhead) is related to obstruction of the submandibular duct by tumour. No upper cervical lymph nodes are seen. (e) FDG-PET images though the lower neck show an asymmetrical focus of activity in the left lower neck, which seemed to correspond to the lymph node seen on MR. A left hemiglossectomy and modified radical neck dissection were performed. The primary site was completely excised, and the neck dissection yielded a single positive lymph node in the upper aspect of level IV. The patient was then treated with post-operative radiation therapy and has remained free of disease.

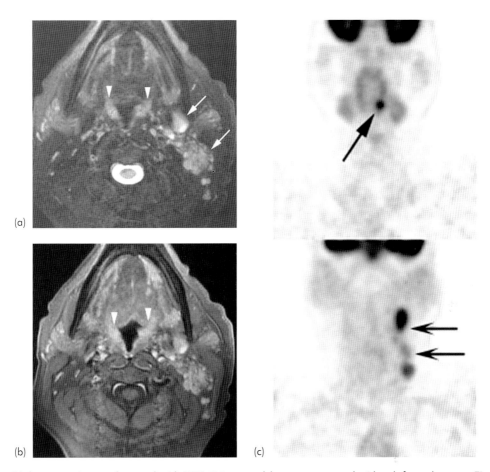

Fig. 4.2 Unknown primary detected with PET: 54-year-old man presented with a left-neck mass. Fine needle aspiration of the mass yielded SCC. (a) Axial fast spin-echo T2-weighted image with fat saturation shows multiple abnormally enlarged and heterogeneous lymph nodes in the left neck (white arrows). Tonsils (white arrowheads), nasopharynx, tongue base, and the remainder of the upper aerodigestive tract was unremarkable as visualised. (b) Axial T1-weighted image post-gadolinium with fat saturation shows similar findings, with the tonsils (white arrowheads) again appearing quite symmetrical. (c) An FDG-PET scan shows multiple foci of abnormal activity in left-sided lymph nodes (lower image, horizontal arrows), as well as an asymmetrical focus of activity in the left tonsil (upper image, oblique arrow). A biopsy directed at the lower pole of the left tonsil yielded SCC.

Key points

Unknown primary

- Accuracy PET for unknown primary 10–60%
- False-positive diagnoses 20–46%

One recent study [29] reported a much poorer performance for FDG-PET in the search for an unknown primary, with a primary site correctly identified in only 1/13 patients and apparent false-positive results in 6/13 patients. Suggested reasons for these findings include the relative poor resolution of the PET system used, the small size of two of the primary lesions identified by endoscopy and biopsy, and the possibility of biopsy sampling errors. When searching for an unknown primary it is preferable that imaging studies be obtained before endoscopy and biopsy, since sites of recent tissue sampling may be mistaken for tumour on post-biopsy images. Also, imaging will help to focus the endoscopic evaluation to the area most likely to yield positive tissue.

Synchronous tumours

The issue of a second primary tumour is also relevant for patients with head and neck cancer as many of these patients abuse tobacco and alcohol and are at risk for synchronous or metachronous cancers of the head and neck, lung, and oesophagus. The risk of second tumours in patients with head and neck cancer is 4% per year, with second tumours located predominantly in the oral cavity, pharynx, or larynx (40%), lungs (31%), and oesophagus (9%) [30]. The added value of including the chest and abdomen in imaging studies is debatable [31] given FDG-PET's sensitivity to inflammatory as well as neoplastic conditions (i.e. high false positives). In one study [13], 68 patients with head and neck cancer studied using dual-head FDG-PET of the head, neck and chest, showed a second simultaneous primary malignant tumour and only five were detected by clinical or routine imaging. We believe that inclusion of the chest and abdomen in the PET study is useful in the evaluation of patients with head and neck cancers.

Lymph nodes

Accurate staging of the neck is essential for the oncologist and surgeon. Most primary tumour subsites of the head and neck have a relatively high incidence of nodal metastases and must always be accounted for when therapy is planned. Staging is traditionally done by clinical palpation and anatomic imaging. Clinical examination is limited by patient body habitus, inaccessibility of certain nodal groups to palpation and tissue changes induced by prior therapy. CT and MR allow assessment of areas that cannot be palpated and may demonstrate metastatic nodes. Imaging techniques are limited by the fact that normal-sized, non-necrotic nodes may harbour tumour and that enlarged nodes may be reactive rather than neoplastic. Size criteria for determination of nodal metastases have been extensively reviewed in the literature [32]. The performance of CT and MR for detecting metastatic foci in non-necrotic nodes varies with the size criteria selected for labelling a node as abnormal. Considering a size of 5 mm to be abnormal yields a sensitivity of 92–98% for CT/MR but a specificity of only 13–20%, while considering a size of 10 mm to be abnormal reduces sensitivity to 81–88% but increases specificity to 39–48% [32].

PET affords an opportunity to detect metastatic nodes based on abnormal accumulation of FDG by tumour. The sensitivity of FDG-PET for detection of cervical nodal metastases ranges from 50% to 100% (Figures 4.1 and 4.3). FDG-PET can detect neoplastic nodes

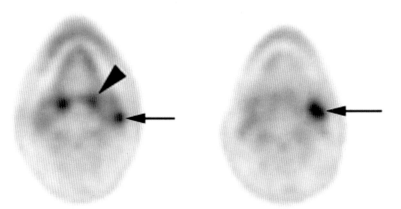

Fig. 4.3 Untreated metastatic lymph node of a 44-year-old man presented with a left-sided sore throat. A tonsillectomy was performed, which demonstrated SCC. No clearly pathological nodes were identified on palpation or CT, and an FDG-PET was performed for staging. The activity in the left tonsil (black arrowhead) is decreased compared with the right, presumably as a consequence of prior surgery (and demonstrating the potential pitfall of interpreting the right tonsil as pathologic, the equivalent of a "pseudomass"). Two foci of abnormal uptake were identified in the left neck (black arrows), corresponding to levels I and II lymph nodes. At the time of neck dissection, both nodes were found to contain metastatic deposits.

as small as 4 mm. Histopathological studies show that more than 40% of all metastases are found in nodes smaller than 1 cm [33]. The specificity of FDG-PET in detection of cervical nodal metastases ranges from 80% to 100%, with false-positive results due to reactive nodes.

FDG-PET has been used in the management of the "N0" neck. The N0 neck shows no evidence of pathologic lymphadenopathy by clinical palpation. These N0 patients may, however, harbour subclinical metastases in 20–30% of instances [34], and thus the neck is often treated surgically or with radiation therapy in order to eradicate subclinical disease. A negative PET study may be considered reassuring enough that a more conservative approach could be adopted in the N0 patient. One study [35] evaluated 11 N0 patients with SCC of the oral cavity who underwent 19 neck dissections and found that FDG-PET had 100% sensitivity and specificity in the detection of presence or absence of disease. Given that FDG-PET is relatively insensitive to metastatic foci smaller than 3–4 mm, these numbers will likely fall as more patients are studied. However, whether or not to treat micrometastases is contentious, they may not necessarily develop into nodal metastases. The nodal lymphatic system may well destroy (micrometastases, hence adding to the dilemma of overtreating the N0 neck).

In the evaluation of lymph nodes, the use of other PET radiopharmaceuticals, such as "C-methionine" or "C-tyrosine", might be more suitable than FDG given their better specificity in differentiating between malignant and inflammatory tissue [36] and could guide fine needle aspiration. "C-amino-acids" are avidly taken up by salivary glands, however, which would mask parotid and submandibular nodes.

Post-treatment evaluation

Following surgery and/or radiation therapy it may be difficult to detect residual or recurrent tumour clinically. Disease may also be difficult to detect on post-therapeutic CT and MR [37,38]. Early detection of persistent or recurrent tumour allows for salvage therapy. Biopsy of suspicious and previously irradiated areas may show only tissue necrosis [39]. FDG-PET is more accurate than CT/MR imaging in differentiating recurrent laryngeal cancer from post-irradiation soft tissue sequalae (85% versus

42%) [40]. Biopsy is also not a perfect gold standard, as failure to biopsy deep enough or in the correct location may miss tumour located in desmoplastic, poorly vascularised tissue. FDG-PET is effective in this setting as is not limited by anatomic distortion as are CT and MR.

Key points

Residual/recurrent disease [41]

	PET	CT/MR
Sensitivity (%)	80–100	70–92
Specificity (%)	43–100	50–57

The utility of FDG-PET in detection of residual/recurrent disease following primary therapy has been assessed in multiple studies. Sensitivity for detection of disease ranges from 80% to 100% and specificity ranges from 43% to 100% (Figures 4.4 and 4.5). The high sensitivity suggests that disease is unlikely to be missed if present, though false-positives are a significant issue necessitating close clinical and imaging correlation. A negative result is generally reassuring as the negative predictive value of FDG-PET is high [15,42]. At present, most FDG-PET scans obtained in patients at risk for recurrent disease are done because of a clinical suspicion of disease. The role of FDG-PET in routine surveillance of the post-therapy neck is not yet determined, though it has been suggested as a cost-effective means [43]. One report [15] suggests that in patients suspected of having recurrent laryngeal or hypopharyngeal cancer in whom FDG-PET is negative, endoscopy may be omitted for at least 6–12 months. At our institution we carry out the following protocol in the follow-up of head and neck cancer patients: regular clinical follow-up, baseline post-therapy (surgery and/or radiation) imaging, and serial FDG-PET, with additional anatomic imaging performed if findings on FDG-PET require correlation.

PET can assess the early effects of chemotherapy in advanced inoperable malignancy, different authors [44] studied 28 patients with stage III/IV head and neck cancers who were participating in organ preservation protocols. FDG-PET was performed before and 1–2 weeks after chemotherapy. Sensitivity and specificity of PET for residual cancer after therapy

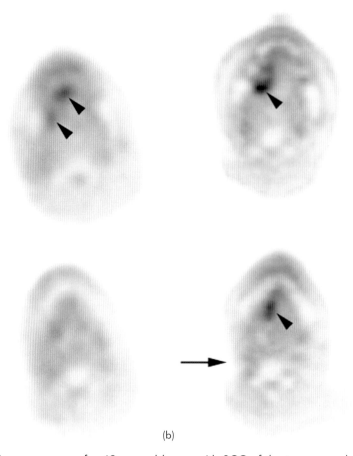

(a)   (b)

Fig. 4.4   True positive recurrence of a 49-year-old man with SCC of the tongue and neck was treated with radiation therapy and modified radical neck dissection. It was elected to follow him with serial FDG-PET scans. (a) PET study performed 6 months following the completion of radiation therapy shows two areas of mildly asymmetrical activity in the right lateral and anterior tongue (black arrowheads). There is also a mild generalised increase in soft tissues of the head and neck related to radiation therapy and soft tissue edema and inflammation. The clinical examination was negative, and it was elected to follow the patient, with the thought being that this was likely a false-positive examination. (b) Follow-up FDG-PET scan was performed 4 months later. The areas of focal uptake were increased in intensity, though the clinical examination remained negative. A biopsy directed to the site of PET abnormality yielded SCC, and a salvage surgery was performed. Note the right neck deformity (black arrow) due to the prior neck dissection, better appreciated than on the prior study as some of the cervical edema has resolved.

were 90% and 83%, respectively. They recommend that PET be done when biopsy access is difficult, when post-therapeutic biopsy results are questionable and when the tumour site has a normal re-epithelialised appearance post-therapy.

Distant metastases

Patients with recurrent or advanced-stage head and neck cancers are at particularly high risk for distant metastases. Exclusion of distant metastases is important in staging and prognosis. This is also important when a major surgical procedure is contemplated as presence of distant metastases contraindicate aggressive surgical and radiotherapeutic procedures aimed at cure rather than palliation. Keyes *et al.* [31] reported that using a modified scanning protocol to include the lungs, but in only one case did PET show a lesion not found by routine evaluation. Different authors [45] looked at detection of occult metastatic disease in 29 patients. Ten cases of metastases were confirmed and PET was positive in 9 out of 10 instances. One false-positive

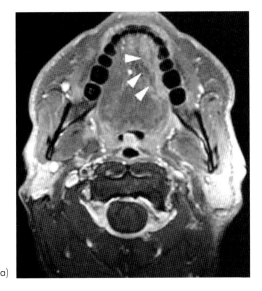

(a)

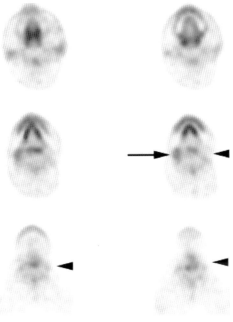

(b)

Fig. 4.5 True negative PET of a 25-year-old man status post left partial glossectomy. (a) Follow-up MR 6 months after surgery showed asymmetrical enhancement along the left lateral tongue extending down toward the floor of mouth (white arrowheads). It was uncertain whether this represented post-surgical change or recurrent tumour. Clinical examination was negative. (b) An FDG-PET scan showed symmetrical activity in the tongue and floor of mouth. The activity posterior to the right mandible (long arrow) represents the submandibular gland, with the contralateral gland surgically absent and hence showing no activity. The deformity related to the prior left neck dissection is evident on multiple slices (black arrowhead).

and one false-negative result occurred making the sensitivity of PET for detecting distant metastases 90%, specificity 94%, positive predictive value 90%, and negative predictive value 94%.

Salivary tumours and melanoma

Most of the above-referenced publications contain a mix of histologies under the rubric of "head and neck cancer". The general experience in the evaluation of the less common types of tumours reflects similar results when using FDG-PET, e.g. salivary gland tumours can be separated into benign and malignant disease [46]. Subjective PET findings correctly differentiated malignant from benign disease in 69% of cases, with 100% of malignant lesions correctly classified but only 42% of benign lesions correctly classified. False-positive PET findings for malignancy in 30% of cases and SUV analysis and ratios failed to distinguish benign from malignant. These authors concluded that FDG-PET was not useful in distinguishing malignant salivary gland tumours from benign ones. FDG-PET is useful in evaluating metastases from mucosal and non-mucosal melanoma [47].

Key points	
Distant metastases [45]	
PET	
Sensitivity	90%
Specificity	94%
PPV (Positive Predictive Value)	90%
NPV (Negative Predictive Value)	94%

Recurrent thyroid cancer

Determination of management and therapeutic options in patients with differentiated thyroid cancer post-thyroidectomy and radioactive iodine ablative therapy can be reliably made using whole body ^{131}I scintigraphy (WBS). Unfortunately, in many patients thyroid cancer does not concentrate ^{131}I and cannot be localised by this method. The loss of iodine concentrating ability results in false-negative WBS in approximately 20% of cases of metastatic thyroid cancer [48]. There is evidence [48–54] that FDG-PET is useful in the follow-up of thyroid cancer patients with negative WBS. In patients with either papillary/follicular or medullary thyroid cancer suspected of having recurrent or metastatic disease, FDG-PET demonstrates the ability to identify residual/ recurrent disease when conventional imaging with WBS fails. Grunwald *et al.* [49] found that FDG-PET had over 80% sensitivity for recurrence and/or metastases in the setting of negative WBS. Chung *et al.* [51] found that FDG-PET was 94% sensitive and 95% specific for localisation of metastatic sites in 33 patients with negative ^{131}I scans. FDG-PET may not; however, be sensitive to detect minimal disease in cervical lymph nodes [48] or to reliably demonstrate pulmonary metastases smaller than 1 cm [52]. If thyroglobulin level (or calcitonin level with medullary carcinoma of the thyroid) is elevated and a WBS is negative, FDG-PET may be used to detect disease. When dissection of iodine-negative lymph node metastases is contemplated, CT of the lungs is probably useful to assess for pulmonary metastases [52].

Lymphoma

Early results using FDG-PET to assess malignant lymphoma of the head and neck suggested that FDG uptake correlated with proliferative activity and that it was useful in prognosis [55,56]. A small study [57] evaluated four patients with non-Hodgkin's lymphoma of the head and neck and found that FDG-PET mapped the extent of disease. FDG-PET may play a role in staging of lymphoma and it has been suggested as a replacement for CT scan and bone scintigraphy [58,59]. A residual mass after treatment of lymphoma may represent tumour or fibrosis.

Key points

PET: Recurrent thyroid carcinoma

- Useful in differentiated papillary/follicular and medullary carcinoma
- Indicated if whole body ^{131}I scan negative
- 80–94% sensitivity for recurrence/metastases reported
- False-positives: reactive nodes, inflammatory disease
- Cannot detect small lymph node metastases or pulmonary metastases less than 1 cm

---

FDG-PET offers the advantage of functional tissue characterisation independent of morphology [60, 61]. A potential caveat of FDG-PET is in staging of extranodal B-cell lymphoma of the mucosa-associated lymphoid tissue (MALT) type. This tumour and other low-grade malignancies do not show up well on FDG-PET leading to false-negative results [62].

Limitations and pitfalls

FDG-PET is subject to limitations and pitfalls. To interpret FDG-PET images correctly one must be aware of normal distribution of the tracer, normal variations of uptake and benign causes of uptake that may be confused with malignancy [16]. Also, one must be aware of the circumstances under which disease may be occult or subtle on FDG-PET. Knowledge of prior therapy is important as surgery may result in significant tissue asymmetry that makes the normal side appear diseased in comparison with low activity on the side of prior surgery.

FDG is taken up non-specifically by glycolytically-active cells and because of its uptake by macrophages and other inflammatory cells it accumulates in areas of inflammation and tumours [5,63–65]. It is possible that dynamic imaging may be useful to distinguish granulation tissue from tumour tissue [66]. Reactive or inflamed lymph nodes are a common cause of false-positive results limiting the specificity of FDG-PET for detecting metastases. Inflammation at the site of a previously treated tumour also accounts for false-positive readings and makes it difficult to determine if a patient harbours residual/recurrent disease [67]. Muscle uptake is also confusing and patients generally should lie quietly and refrain from speaking in order to avoid uptake in the cricopharyngeal area. Muscle relaxants may be necessary to avoid muscular uptake [22]. Other false-positive findings in the head and neck include healing bone and paranasal sinus inflammatory disease. Foreign body granuloma has also been reported to cause a false-positive result [22].

A limitation of FDG-PET is its lack of sensitivity to small tumour deposits (3–4 mm or less). Micrometastases are not reliably detected with FDG-PET and some cervical nodal disease in patients with head and neck cancer may not be detected. Larger necrotic nodes with thin rims of viable neoplastic tissue may be overlooked by FDG-PET. False-negative scans may occur if FDG-PET imaging is done too soon after radiation therapy [68].

Summary

> ### Key points
>
> *Uses of PET*
>
> - Locating unknown primary
> - Detecting residual/recurrent disease
> - Locating synchronous tumours
> - Detection of distal metastases
> - ? role in monitoring treatment response

In conclusion, FDG-PET is a powerful tool in oncologic imaging. In head and neck cancer it is useful in locating unknown primary and second primary lesions, staging nodal disease, detecting residual/recurrent disease following surgical and/or radiation therapy, monitoring response to organ preservation therapy, and detection of distant metastases. FDG-PET may prove to be a cost-effective cancer surveillance tool in patients with a prior diagnosis of head and neck cancer. It also has a significant role in the evaluation and treatment planning of patients with thyroid cancer and negative ^{131}I whole-body scans. Both false-positive and false-negative scans occur and knowledge of these issues allows for an accurate interpretation of FDG-PET scans.

Acknowledgements

The authors appreciate the assistance of Gary Caputo, MD, in reviewing the PET section of this chapter, the assistance of Carole Schreck, R.T., C.N.M.T., in figure preparation, and the clinical comments of Michael J. Kaplan, MD.

References

1. Ter-Pogossian MM. Positron emission tomography instrumentation. In: M Reivich, A Alalavi (Eds) *Positron Emission Tomography*. Alan R. Liss, Inc., New York. 1985, 43–61.
2. Warburg O. On the origin of cancer cells. *Science* 1956; **123**: 309–314.
3. Reisser C, Eichhorn K, Herold-Mende C, Born AI and Bannasch P. Expression of facilitative glucose transport proteins during development of squamous cell carcinomas of the head and neck. *Int. J. Cancer* 1999; **80**: 194–198.
4. Som P, Atkins HL, Bandoypadhyay D *et al.* A fluorinated glucose analog, 2-fluoro-2-deoxy-D-glucose (F-18): nontoxic tracer for rapid tumor detection. *J. Nucl. Med.* 1980; **21**: 670–675.
5. Kubota R, Yamada S, Kubota K, Ishiwata K, Tamahashi N and Ido T. Intratumoral distribution of fluorine-18-fluorodeoxyglucose *in vivo*: high accumulation in macrophages and granulation tissues studied by microautoradiography. *J. Nucl. Med.* 1992; **33**: 1972–1980.
6. Ahluwalia BD. Positron emission tomography imaging systems and applications. In: BD Ahluwalia (Ed.) *Tomographic Methods in Nuclear Medicine: Physical Principles, Instruments, and Clinical Applications*. CRC Press, Boca Raton. 1989, 105–122.
7. DeGrado TR, Turkington TG, Williams JJ, Stearns CW, Hoffman JM and Coleman RE. Performance characteristics of a whole-body PET scanner. *J. Nucl. Med.* 1994; **35**: 1398–1406.
8. Wong WL, Hussain K, Chevretton E *et al.* Validation and clinical application of computer-combined computed tomography and positron emission tomography with 2-[18F] fluoro-2-deoxy-D-glucose head and neck images. *Am. J. Surg.* 1996; **172**: 628–632.
9. Sercarz JA, Bailet JW, Abemayor E, Anzai Y, Hoh CK and Lufkin RB. Computer coregistration of positron emission tomography and magnetic resonance images in head and neck cancer. *Am. J. Otolaryngol.* 1998; **19**: 130–135.
10. Kinahan PE, Townsend DW, Beyer T and Sashin D. Attenuation correction for a combined 3D PET/CT scanner. *Med. Phys.* 1998; **25**: 2046–2053.
11. Shreve PD, Steventon RS, Deters EC, Kison PV, Gross MD and Wahl RL. Oncologic diagnosis with 2-[fluorine-18]fluoro-2-deoxy-D-glucose imaging: dual-head coincidence gamma camera versus positron emission tomographic scanner. *Radiology* 1998; **207**: 431–437.
12. Macfarlane DJ, Cotton L, Ackermann RJ, Minn H, Ficaro EP, Shreve PD and Wahl RL. Triple-head SPECT with 2-[fluorine-18]fluoro-2-deoxy-D-glucose (FDG): initial evaluation in oncology and comparison with FDG PET. *Radiology* 1995; **194**: 425–429.
13. Stokkel MP, Moons KG, ten Broek FW, van Rijk PP and Hordijk GJ. 18F-fluorodeoxyglucose dual-head positron emission tomography as a procedure for detecting simultaneous primary tumors in cases of head and neck cancer. *Cancer* 1999; **86**: 2370–2377.
14. Stokkel MPM, ten Broek FW and van Rijk PP. Preoperative assessment of cervical lymph nodes in head and neck cancer with fluorine-18 fluorodeoxyglucose using a dual-head coincidence camera: a pilot study. *Eur. J. Nucl. Med.* 1999; **26**: 499–503.
15. Stokkel MPM, Terhaard CHJ, Hordijk GJ and van Rijk PP. The detection of local recurrent head and neck cancer with fluorine-18 fluorodeoxyglucose dual-head positron emission tomography. *Eur. J. Nucl. Med.* 1999; **26**: 767–773.
16. Shreve PD, Anzai Y and Wahl RL. Pitfalls in oncologic diagnosis with FDG PET imaging: physiologic and benign variants. *Radiographics* 1999; **19**: 61–77.
17. Jabour BA, Choi Y, Hoh CK *et al.* Extracranial head and neck: PET imaging with 2-[F-18] fluoro-2-deoxy-D-glucose and MR imaging correlation. *Radiology* 1993; **186**: 27–35.
18. Rege SD, Chaiken L, Hoh CK *et al.* Change induced by radiation therapy in FDG uptake in normal and malignant structures of the head and neck: quantitation with PET. *Radiology* 1993; **189**: 807–812.
19. Bailet JW, Abemayor E, Jabour BA *et al.* Positron emission tomography: a new, precise imaging modality for detection of primary head and neck tumors and assessment of cervical adenopathy. *Laryngoscope* 1992; **102**: 281–288.
20. Rege S, Maass A, Chaiken L *et al.* Use of positron emission tomography with fluorodeoxyglucose in patients with extracranial head and neck cancer. *Cancer* 1994; **73**: 3047–3058.
21. Wong WL, Chevretton EB, McGurk M *et al.* A prospective study of PET-FDG imaging for the assessment of head and

neck squamous cell carcinoma. *Clin. Otolaryngol.* 1997; **22**: 209–214.

22. Paulus P, Sambon A, Vivegnis D, Hustinx R, Moreau P, Collignon J, Deneufbourg JM and Rigo P. 18-FDG-PET for the assessment of primary head and neck tumors: clinical, computed tomography, and histopathological correlation in 38 patients. *Laryngoscope* 1998; **108**: 1578–1583.

23. Muraki AS, Mancuso AA and Harnsberger HR. Metastatic cervical adenopathy from tumors of unknown origin: the role of CT. *Radiology* 1984; **152**: 749–753.

24. Braams JW, Pruim J, Kole AC *et al.* Detection of unknown primary head and neck tumors by positron emission tomography. *Int. J. Oral. Maxillofac. Surg.* 1997; **26**: 112–115.

25. Mukherji SK, Drane WE, Mancuso AA, Parsons JT, Mendenhall WM and Stringer S. Occult primary tumors of the head and neck: detection with 2-[F-18] fluoro-2-deoxy-D-glucose SPECT. *Radiology* 1996; **199**: 761–766.

26. AAssar OS, Fischbein NJ, Caputo GR *et al.* Metastatic head and neck cancer: role and usefulness of FDG-PET in localizing occult primary tumors. *Radiology* (in press).

27. Safa AA, Tran LM, Rege S *et al.* The role of positron emission tomography in occult primary head and neck cancers. *Cancer J. Sci. Am.* 1999; **5**: 214–218.

28. Hanasono MM, Kunda LD, Segall GM, Ku GH and Terris DJ. Uses and limitations of FDG positron emission tomography in patients with head and neck cancer. *Laryngoscope* 1999; **109**: 880–885.

29. Greven KM, Keyes JW Jr, Williams DW III, McGuirt WF and Joyce WT III. Occult primary tumors of the head and neck: lack of benefit from positron emission tomography imaging with 2-[F-18]Fluoro-2-deoxy-D-glucose. *Cancer* 1999; **86**: 114–118.

30. Leon X, Quer M, Diez S, Orus C, Lopez-Pousa A and Burgues J. Second neoplasm in patients with head and neck cancer. *Head Neck* 1999; **21**: 204–210.

31. Keyes JW Jr, Watson NE Jr, Williams DW III, Greven KM and McGuirt WF. FDG-PET in head and neck cancer. *AJR* 1997; **169**: 1663–1669.

32. Curtin HD, Ishwaran H, Mancuso AA, Dalley RW, Caudry DJ and McNeil BJ. Comparison of CT and MR imaging in staging of neck metastases. *Radiology* 1998; **207**: 123–130.

33. Eichhorn T, Schroeder HG, Glanz H and Schwerk WB. Histologically controlled comparison of palpation and sonography in the diagnosis of cervical lymph node metastases. *Laryngol. Rhinol. Otol.* 1987; **66**: 266–274.

34. McGuirt WF Jr, Johnson JT, Myers EN, Rothfield R and Wagner R. Floor of mouth carcinoma. The management of the clinically negative neck. *Arch. Otolaryngol. Head Neck Surg.* 1995; **121**: 278–282.

35. Myers LL and Wax MK. Positron emission tomography in the evaluation of the negative neck in patients with oral cavity cancer. *J. Otolaryngol.* 1998; **27**: 342–347.

36. Braams JW, Pruim J, Freling NJM *et al.* Detection of lymph node metastases of squamous cell cancer of the head and neck with FDG-PET and MRI. *J. Nucl. Med.* 1995; **36**: 211–216.

37. Mukherji SK, Mancuso AA, Kotzur IM *et al.* Radiologic appearance of the irradiated larynx. Part I: expected changes. *Radiology* 1994; **193**: 141–148.

38. Hudgins PA, Burson JG, Gussack GS and Grist WJ. CT and MR appearance of recurrent malignant head and neck neoplasms after resection and flap reconstruction. *AJNR. Am. J. Neuroradiol.* 1994; **15**: 1689–1694.

39. Fu KK, Woodhouse RJ, Quivey JM, Phillips TL and Dedo HH. The significance of laryngeal edema following radiotherapy of carcinoma of the vocal cord. *Cancer* 1982; **49**: 655–658.

40. McQuit WR, Greven WM, Keyer JW *et al.* PET in the evaluation of laryngeal carcinoma. *Ann. Otol. Rhinol. Laryngol.* 1995; **104**: 274–278.

41. Chisin R and Macapiulac HA. The indications of FDG-PET in neck oncology. *Radiol. Clin. N. Am.* 2000; **38**: 999–1012.

42. Fischbein NJ, AAssar OS, Caputo GR *et al.* Clinical utility of positron emission tomography with 18F-fluorodeoxyglucose in detecting residual/recurrent squamous cell carcinoma of the head and neck. *AJNR Am. J. Neuroradiol.* 1998; **19**: 1189–1196.

43. Anzai Y, Carroll WR, Quint DJ *et al.* Recurrence of head and neck cancer after surgery or irradiation: prospective comparison of 2-deoxy-2-[F-18] fluoro-D-glucose PET and MR imaging diagnoses. *Radiology* 1996; **200**: 135–141.

44. Lowe VJ, Dunphy FR, Varvares M *et al.* Evaluation of chemotherapy response in patients with advanced head and neck cancer using [F-18] fluorodeoxyglucose positron emission tomography. *Head Neck* 1997; **19**: 666–674.

45. Manolidis S, Donald PJ, Valk P and Pounds TR. The use of positron emission tomography scanning in occult and recurrent head and neck cancer. *Acta Otolaryngol. (Stockh.)* 1998; Suppl. 534: 1–11.

46. Keyes JW Jr, Harkness BA, Greven KM, Williams DW III, Watson NE Jr and McGuirt WF. Salivary gland tumors: pretherapy evaluation with PET. *Radiology* 1994; **192**: 99–102.

47. Holder WD Jr, White RL Jr, Zuger JH, Easton EJ Jr and Greene FL. Effectiveness of positron emission tomography for the detection of melanoma metastases. *Ann. Surg.* 1998; **227**: 764–769.

48. Wang W, Macapinlac H, Larson SM, Yeh SD, Akhurst T, Finn RD, Rosai J and Robbins RJ. [18F]-2-fluoro-2-deoxy-D-glucose positron emission tomography localizes residual thyroid cancer in patients with negative diagnostic (131)I whole body scans and elevated serum thyroglobulin levels. *J. Clin. Endocrinol. Metab.* 1999; **84**: 2291–2302.

49. Grunwald F, Briele B and Biersack HJ. Non-131I-scintigraphy in the treatment and follow-up of thyroid cancer. Single-photon-emitters or FDG-PET? *Quart. J. Nucl. Med.* 1999; **43**: 195–206.

50. Conti PS, Durski JM, Bacqai F, Grafton ST and Singer PA. Imaging of locally recurrent and metastatic thyroid cancer with positron emission tomography. *Thyroid* 1999; **9**: 797–804.

51. Chung JK, So Y, Lee JS, Choi CW, Lim SM, Lee DS, Hong SW, Youn YK, Lee MC and Cho BY. Value of FDG PET in papillary thyroid carcinoma with negative ^{131}I whole-body scan. *J. Nucl. Med.* 1999; **40**: 986–992.

52. Dietlein M, Scheidhauer K, Voth E, Theissen P and Schicha H. Fluorine-18 fluorodeoxyglucose positron emission tomography and iodine-131 whole-body scintigraphy in the follow-up of differentiated thyroid cancer. *Eur. J. Nucl. Med.* 1997; **24**: 1342–1348.

53. Feine U, Lietzenmayer R, Hanke JP, Held J, Wohrle H and Muller-Schauenburg W. Fluorine-18-FDG and iodine-131-iodide uptake in thyroid cancer. *J. Nucl. Med.* 1996; **37**: 1468–1472.

54. Grunwald F, Schomburg A, Bender H, Klemm E, Menzel C, Bultmann T, Palmedo H, Ruhlmann J, Kozak B and Biersack HJ. Fluorine-18 fluorodeoxyglucose positron emission tomography in the follow-up of differentiated thyroid cancer. *Eur. J. Nucl. Med.* 1996; **23**: 312–319.

55. Okada J, Oonishi H, Yoshikawa K, Itami J, Uno K, Imaseki K and Arimizu N. FDG-PET for predicting the prognosis of malignant lymphoma. *Ann. Nucl. Med.* 1994; **8**: 187–191.

56. Okada J, Yoshikawa K, Itami M, Imaseki K, Uno K, Itami J, Kuyama J, Mikata A and Arimizu N. Positron emission tomography using fluorine-18-fluorodeoxyglucose in malignant lymphoma: a comparison with proliferative activity. *J. Nucl. Med.* 1992; **33**: 325–329.

57. Walsh RM, Wong WL, Chevretton EB and Beaney RP. The use of PET-18FDG imaging in the clinical evaluation of head and neck lymphoma. *Clin. Oncol.* 1996; **8**: 51–54.

58. Moog F, Kotzerke J and Reske SN. FDG-PET can replace bone scintigraphy in primary staging of malignant lymphoma. *J. Nucl. Med.* 1999; **40**: 1407–1413.

59. Wiedmann E, Baican B, Hertel A, Baum RP, Chow KU, Knupp B, Adams S, Hor G, Hoelzer D and Mitrou PS. Positron emission tomography (PET) for staging and evaluation of response to

treatment in patients with Hodgkin's disease. *Leuk. Lymphom.* 1999; **34**: 545–551.

60. Jerusalem G, Beguin Y, Fassotte MF, Najjar F, Paulus P, Rigo P and Fillet G. Whole-body positron emission tomography using 18F-fluorodeoxyglucose for posttreatment evaluation in Hodgkin's disease and non-Hodgkin's lymphoma has higher diagnostic and prognostic value than classical computed tomography scan imaging. *Blood* 1999; **94**: 429–433.

61. Zinzani PL, Magagnoli M, Chierichetti F, Zompatori M, Garraffa G, Bendandi M, Gherlinzoni F, Cellini C, Stefoni V, Ferlin G *et al.* The role of positron emission tomography (PET) in the management of lymphoma patients. *Ann. Oncol.* 1999; **10**: 1181–1184.

62. Hoffmann M, Kletter K, Diemling M, Becherer A, Pfeffel F, Petkov V, Chott A and Raderer M. Positron emission tomography with fluorine-18-2-fluoro-2-deoxy-D-glucose (F18-FDG) does not visualize extranodal B-cell lymphoma of the mucosa-associated lymphoid tissue (MALT)-type. *Ann. Oncol.* 1999; **10**: 1185–1189.

63. Hautzel H and Muller-Gartner HW. Early changes in fluorine-18-FDG uptake during radiotherapy. *J. Nucl. Med.* 1997; **38**: 1384–1386.

64. Yamada S, Kubota K, Kubota R, Ido T and Tamahashi N. High accumulation of fluorine-18-fluorodeoxyglucose in turpentine-induced inflammatory tissue. *J. Nucl. Med.* 1995; **36**: 1301–1306.

65. Palmer WE, Rosenthal DI, Schoenberg OI, Fischman AJ, Simon LS, Rubin RH and Polisson RP. Quantification of inflammation in the wrist with gadolinium-enhanced MR imaging and PET with 2-[F-18]-fluoro-2-deoxy-D-glucose. *Radiology* 1995; **196**: 647–655.

66. Kubota R, Kubota K, Yamada S, Tada M, Ido T and Tamahashi N. Microautoradiographic study for the differentiation of intratumoral macrophages, granulation tissues and cancer cells by the dynamics of fluorine-18-fluorodeoxyglucose uptake. *J. Nucl. Med.* 1994; **35**: 104–112.

67. Strauss LG. Fluroine-18 deoxyglucose and false-positive results: a major problem in the diagnostics of oncological patients. *Eur. J. Nucl. Med.* 1996; **23**: 1409–1415.

68. Greven KM, Williams DW III, Keyes JW Jr *et al.* Distinguishing tumour recurrence from irradiation sequelae with positron emission tomography in patients treated for larynx cancer. *Int. J. Radiat. Oncol. Biol. Phys.* 1994; **29**: 841–845.

COMMON HEAD AND NECK TUMOURS

Cancer of the Nasopharynx

AD King and SF Leung

The most frequent cancer to involve the nasopharynx is an undifferentiated or squamous cell carcinoma. Other cancers that arise in the nasopharynx include lymphoma, plasmacytoma, adenocarcinoma, adenoid cystic carcinoma, metastases, melanoma, chordoma and sarcomas, such as rhabdomyosarcoma. This chapter focuses on nasopharyngeal carcinoma (NPC). This cancer is endemic in the southern Chinese population, being the third most common cancer in Hong Kong. The incidence remains high in the Chinese population, even after emigration; therefore, NPC may be encountered worldwide. NPC has a propensity to invade the complex structures bordering the nasopharynx including the skull base. Discussion of this tumour will illustrate the complex radiological anatomy of this region and the imaging techniques that are employed. This is the key to understanding all cancers in this region.

Nasopharyngeal carcinoma

Introduction

NPC is most commonly an undifferentiated carcinoma or a poorly differentiated squamous cell carcinoma that has a close relationship to the Epstein–Barr virus

(EBV). NPC has a high incidence in regions of Africa, Greenland and, southern China.

Clinical presentation [1]

- Peak age incidence 40–70 years.
- Males > females.
- A family history of NPC may occasionally be present.

Symptoms

- Neck mass (especially, in the upper neck).
- Blood-stained nasal discharge, nasal obstruction, post-nasal drip and epistaxis.
- Hearing loss and tinnitus.

Signs

- Cervical lymphadenopathy (especially, in the upper neck).
- Conductive hearing loss (secondary to a middle ear effusion resulting from obstruction of the Eustachian tube).
- Cranial nerve palsies in advanced disease, most commonly, involving the V and VI cranial

nerves. The III, IV and IX to XII may also be involved.

Investigation, staging and treatment

The first examination to be performed in a patient with suspected NPC is nasopharyngoscopy, under topical anaesthesia. This will identify the tumour, assess the mucosal limits of the tumour and allow for an endoscopically controlled biopsy of the lesion to be taken. Once the diagnosis is established, patients undergo blood tests including serum alkaline phosphatase and serum tumour marker EBV–DNA. Imaging of the primary tumour, nodal metastases and distant metastases is then performed to stage the disease and plan therapy (see Table 5.1). Patients also undergo a dental review in order to minimise the need for dental surgery after treatment.

The primary treatment for NPC is radiotherapy. Radiotherapy is given to the primary tumour and both sides of the neck. The radiation field covers the "imaging visible" primary tumour (gross tumour volume) with a safety margin that covers possible microscopic tumour extension (clinical target volume). Nodal metastases are covered to at least one level inferior to the lowest groups of nodes that are involved. Surgery is rarely employed and used only in selected cases of local tumour recurrence or persistent/recurrent neck node metastases. Chemotherapy is being used, concurrently, with radiotherapy for advanced stage disease. Brachytherapy may be used as a supplement to external radiotherapy for early stage disease. Intensity-modulated radiotherapy is expected to be

Table 5.1   T-stage.

Staging UICC/AJCC Cancer Staging Manual,
5th edition, 1997:

- T1 tumour confined to the nasopharynx.
- T2 tumour extends to soft tissues of the oropharynx and/or nasal cavity
  - T2a without parapharyngeal extension,
  - T2b with parapharyngeal extension.
- T3 tumour invades bony structures and/or paranasal sinuses.
- T4 tumour with intracranial extension and/or involvement of cranial nerves, infratemporal fossa, hypopharynx or orbit.

increasingly used in all stages of disease, to spare the parotids in early stage disease and to give more conformed coverage for T3 and T4 disease.

Imaging

Which imaging modality should be used?

Magnetic resonance (MR) is the imaging modality of choice for the nasopharynx and the complex anatomical regions that border the nasopharynx.

MR imaging has the following advantages over computed tomography (CT):

1. Differentiation of the small nasopharyngeal wall tumours from retained secretions and normal lymphoid tissue.
2. Diagnosis of early tumour extension outside the nasopharynx into the prevertebral region and parapharyngeal regions.
3. Diagnosis of tumour invasion into the posterior nasal cavity.
4. Diagnosis of tumour invasion into the cranium (dural and cavernous sinus).
5. Differentiation of the tumour from inflammatory mucosal changes in the paranasal sinuses.
6. Diagnosis of perineural tumour invasion/ extension.
7. Diagnosis of the extent of skull base involvement. MR is superior for the demonstration of marrow infiltration of the skull base and is now considered equal to CT for cortical invasion. MR is, particularly, useful in delineating the exact extent of postero-lateral tumour extension to the foramen lacerum, petro-occipital fissure and petrous temporal bone.
8. Diagnosis of the retropharyngeal nodes and differentiation of nodes from the primary tumour.

CT imaging has the following advantages over MR:

1. Availability and cost.
2. Some radiologists prefer CT for detail of cortical bone invasion:

– Ultrasound cannot be used to image the primary tumour and retropharyngeal nodes, but in some centres, it has a role in imaging nodes in the neck. It is, particularly, useful for indeterminate nodes that can be biopsied under ultrasound guidance.

Imaging the primary tumour

Tumour within the nasopharynx

Cross-sectional imaging is usually employed to stage NPC after the diagnosis has been established by direct nasopharyngoscopy and biopsy. Occasionally, it may be used to screen the nasopharynx for cancer in those patients who present with metastatic lymphadenopathy from an unknown primary tumour. The fossa of Rosenmuller is the most common site for NPC (Figure 5.1). The shape and size of the fossa may be variable; although, in general, it becomes more prominent with age. Asymmetry should be regarded with suspicion and may require careful evaluation with nasopharyngoscopy; however, it should be noted that it is not unusual for normal patients to show asymmetry of the fossae, particularly, on CT imaging. This is one of the areas that is more accurately assessed by MR, which is able to differentiate between the mucosa and small muscles in this region (Figure 5.1). Any increase in the mucosal thickness, especially with reduced enhancement compared to normal mucosa,

may indicate a small tumour (Figure 5.2). However, in the majority of cases NPC is usually extensive at the time of diagnosis with involvement of several or all walls of the nasopharynx (roof, posterior and lateral walls). The number of nasopharyngeal walls (subsites) involved by the tumour is no longer used for staging purposes. This is not only because of the technical difficulties in defining the boundaries of each subsite, but also because it lacks prognostic significance. In rare cases, tumour may be submucosal and not identified on endoscopy. NPC within the nasopharynx can invade the intra-nasopharyngeal portion of the levator palatini muscle, while the cartilaginous tip of the Eustachian tube is relatively resistant to invasion. The normal lymphoid tissue of the adenoids (pharyngeal tonsil) in the roof and upper posterior wall of the nasopharynx may be mistaken for a tumour. However, on MR imaging the normal lymphoid tissue can be differentiated from a carcinoma by the presence of "stripes" on the T2-weighted and T1-weighted image post-contrast (Figure 5.3).

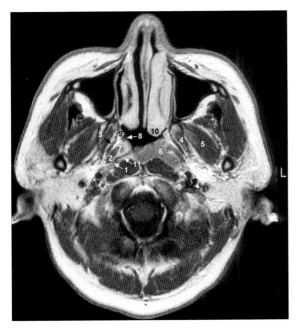

Fig. 5.1 Axial MR of tumour confined to nasopharynx: 1. fossa of Rosenmuller, 2. levator palatini, 3. tensor palatini, 4. medial pterygoid, 5. lateral pterygoid, 6. tumour in nasopharynx, 7. torus tubarius, 8. opening of Eustachian tube, 9. choanal ridge, 10. posterior aspect of nasal turbinate and 11. mucosa.

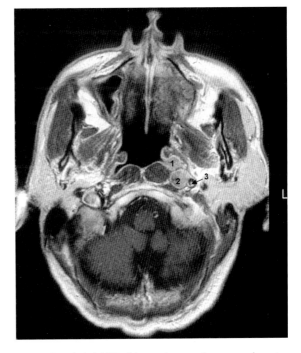

Fig. 5.2 Axial MR of lateral retropharyngeal metastatic node and early primary tumour in the fossa of Rosenmuller: 1. tumour in the fossa of Rosenmuller, 2. retropharyngeal node and 3. carotid artery.

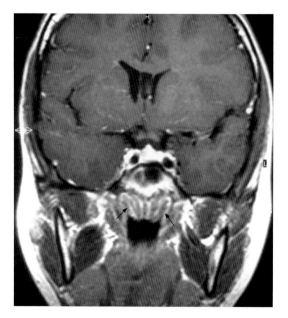

Fig. 5.3 Coronal post-gadolinium T1-weighted MR. Normal lymphoid tissue in the nasopharynx (arrows).

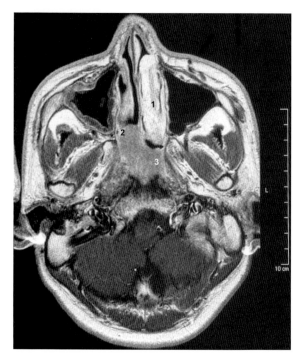

Fig. 5.4 Axial MR of tumour extending into nasal cavity: 1. nasal turbinate, 2. tumour in nasal cavity and 3. tumour in nasopharynx.

Important imaging points for oncological management

The confirmation of early stage disease (T1 and T2a) is important as it may influence the decision to use brachytherapy as part of the treatment; these cases are also ideal for parotid sparing radiotherapy techniques.

Tumour extending outside the nasopharynx

NPC is often extensive at diagnosis, not only involving a large part of the nasopharynx, but also spreading into the adjacent areas that make-up the complex anatomy of this region. The sites of local tumour extension are described according to the system of staging (T2–T4).

Nasal cavity (stage T2a)

The anatomical boundary between the nasopharynx and nasal cavity is controversial on imaging. Tumour invasion of the nasal cavity (Figure 5.4) may be defined as tumour extending beyond the choanal ridge or tumour extending beyond the posterior aspect of the inferior or middle nasal turbinates (Figure 5.1). In the majority of cases, tumour invades the posterior aspect of the nasal cavity to just beyond the boundary,

while extensive involvement, especially into the anterior nasal cavity is far less common [2]. When nasal cavity tumour is present, a careful inspection of the pterygopalatine fossa and pterygomaxillary fissure should be made, because these structures will be involved in over a third of cases. In some patients, invasion of the nasal cavity actually occurs indirectly via the pterygopalatine fossa and sphenopalatine foramen rather than directly from the nasopharynx [2]. Involvement of the superior recess of the nasal cavity is a difficult area to assess on endoscopy, but can be appreciated on coronal MR imaging.

Important imaging points for oncological management

The exact anterior extent of tumour into the nasal cavity influences the anterior field border of radiotherapy.

Oropharynx (stage T2a)

The clinical definition of oropharyngeal involvement is the presence of tumour identified by examination of the oral cavity/oropharynx and may be due to mucosal disease or nodal disease causing

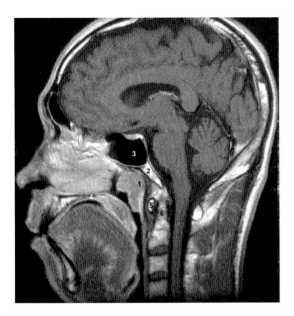

Fig. 5.5 Sagittal MR of tumour in the nasopharynx and normal skull base: 1. NPC, 2. clivus, 3. sphenoid sinus, 4. hard palate, 5. C1 and 6. C2.

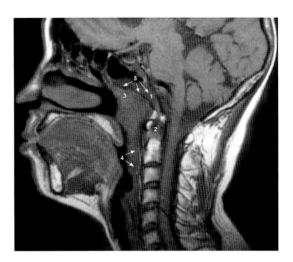

Fig. 5.6 Sagittal MR of tumour extending into oropharynx and skull base: 1. clivus, 2. C1/C2 junction, 3. tumour in nasopharynx, 4. tumour in oropharynx and 5. tumour in skull base.

submucosal swelling. Oropharyngeal involvement on imaging usually refers to mucosal extension, but the anatomical boundary between the mucosa of the nasopharynx and oropharynx is controversial. Traditionally, the level of the hard palate has defined it, but this can lead to practical difficulties and now some centres use the junction of the first and second cervical vertebrae to demarcate the level of the boundary (Figure 5.5). Despite the lack of an anatomical barrier between the mucosa of the nasopharynx and oropharynx, tumour extension into the oropharynx is uncommon. When present, it is usually associated with extensive tumour spread elsewhere including to the skull base [2] (Figure 5.6).

Important imaging points for oncological management

Detection of oropharyngeal involvement, especially, if it extends below the level of the tip of the uvula, affects radiation therapy planning, in that a particularly long field may need to be used in the second phase of a course of radiotherapy.

Parapharynx (stage T2b)

The pharyngobasilar fascia borders the nasopharynx (Figure 5.7); laterally, there is a deficiency in the fascia at the sinus of morgani (the gap to allow

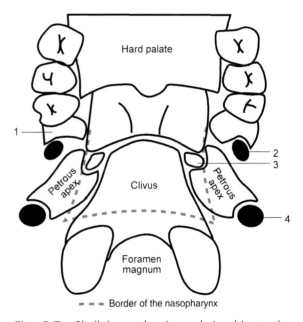

Fig. 5.7 Skull base showing relationship to the nasopharynx: 1. pterygoid plate, 2. foramen ovale, 3. foramen lacerum and 4. carotid canal.

passage of levator palatini and Eustachian tube). Parapharyngeal extension occurs when tumour spreads laterally into the parapharyngeal fat space and retrostyloid space. On CT imaging, parapharyngeal tumour invasion is defined as distortion of the

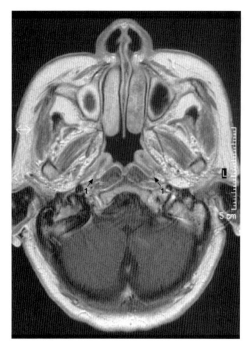

Fig. 5.8   Axial MR of the nasopharynx: 1. pharyngobasilar fascia.

parapharyngeal fat space on two or more axial slices [3]. However, the parapharyngeal fat space is asymmetrical in 30% of the normal patients [4]. Therefore, some centres diagnose parapharyngeal tumour invasion when tumour extends lateral to a line drawn from the free edge of the medial pterygoid plate to the lateral aspect of the carotid artery [4]. There is no generally agreed definition of parapharyngeal tumour extension on MR imaging. However, MR imaging has the advantage of demonstrating the pharyngobasilar fascia and the small structures that border the nasopharynx [5] (Figure 5.8, see also figures in Chapter 3). The parapharyngeal fat, extra-nasopharyngeal portion of the levator palatini muscle and Eustachian tube, the tensor palatini muscle and retrostyloid space, are within the anatomical parapharyngeal region. Tumour invasion of these structures can be depicted by MR imaging (Figure 5.9).

Compression of the Eustachian tube is more common than tumour invasion, but both may result in a middle ear and mastoid effusion (Figure 5.10).

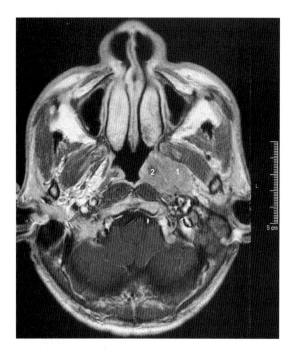

Fig. 5.9   Axial MR of tumour invading parapharynx 1. with involvement of the parapharyngeal fat, tensor palatini muscle and retrostyloid space; 2. intranasopharyngeal torus tubarius is resistant to tumour but the levator palatini is destroyed.

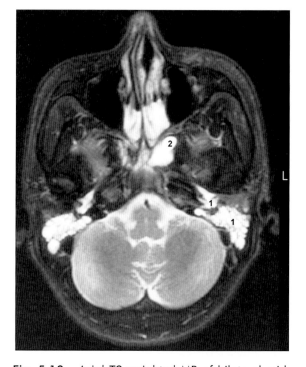

Fig. 5.10   Axial T2-weighted MR of bilateral middle ear and mastoid effusions: 1. middle ear and mastoid effusion and 2. inflammatory change in sphenoid sinus.

Important imaging points for oncological management

Detection of bulky parapharyngeal disease may require a radiation boost using conventional, stereotactic or intensity-modulated radiotherapy. It also implies more difficulty in sparing the parotid during radiotherapy planning.

Skull base (stage T3)

NPC has a propensity to invade upwards and may involve the skull base [6] without invasion elsewhere [2]. The normal anatomy of skull base and foramina are shown in the axial plane in the chapters on CT and MR imaging and in the coronal plane by CT (Figure 5.11a–c, anterior to posterior) and by MR (Figure 5.12a–c, anterior to posterior). Bony invasion occurs into the clivus, pterygoid processes and plates, body of the sphenoid and petrous temporal bones. The skull base foramina that may be involved are as follows:

1. Foramen lacerum (around the bony edge and along carotid artery rather than through the cartilage) (Figure 5.13).
2. Foramen ovale (V^3 palsy) (Figure 5.14).
3. Foramen rotundum (V^2 palsy).
4. Vidian canal (Figure 5.15).
5. Pterygomaxillary fissure (Figure 5.16).
6. Pterygopalatine fossa (Figures 5.15 and 5.16). The fossa is a major junction in the head with connections to the orbit (via the inferior orbital fissure), infratemporal fossa (via the pterygomaxillary fissure), foramen lacerum (via the vidian canal), middle cranial fossa (via the foramen rotundum), oral cavity (via the pterygopalatine canal) and nasal cavity (via the sphenopalatine foramen) (see Figure 5.17).
7. Jugular foramen (IX–XI) and hypoglossal canal (XII) involvement is unusual at presentation.

Important imaging points for oncological management

Detection of bony skull base involvement may lead to extension of the superior border of the radiation portal. However, this also increases the risk of irradiating the optic chiasm, pituitary gland and brain stem, and may lead to the use of high-precision radiotherapy techniques. T3- and T4-stage disease have a higher relapse rate than T1- and T2-stage disease and may require more intensive treatment such as an additional boost dose using stereotactic or intensity-modulated

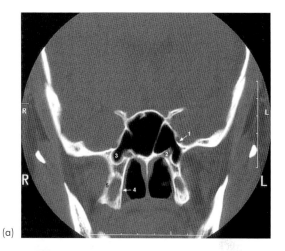

(a)

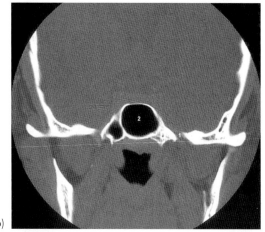

(b)

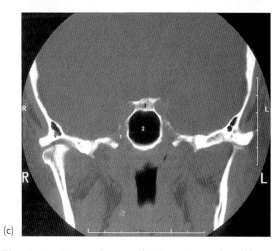

(c)

Fig. 5.11 Normal coronal CT anatomy of skull base: (a) – 1. foramen rotundum, 2. vidian canal, 3. sphenoid sinus with aerated lateral recess, 4. medial pterygoid plate and 5. lateral pterygoid plate; (b) – 1. foramen ovale and 2. sphenoid sinus; (c) – 1. foramen lacerum, 2. sphenoid sinus and 3. dorsum sella.

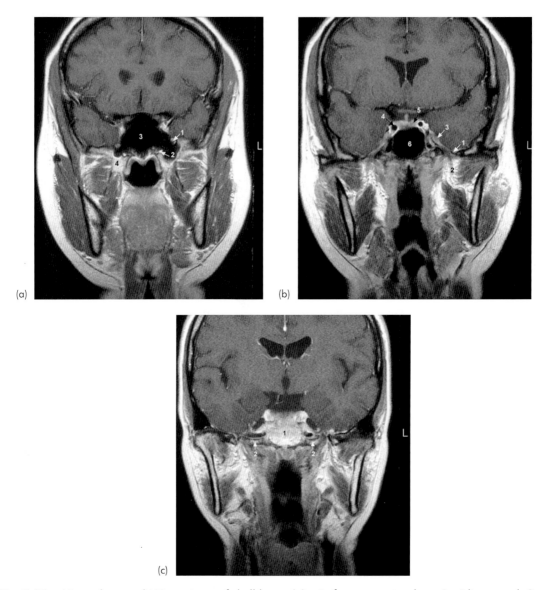

Fig. 5.12   Normal coronal MR anatomy of skull base: (a) – 1. foramen rotundum, 2. vidian canal, 3. sphenoid sinus with aerated lateral recess and 4. pterygoid bone; (b) – 1. foramen ovale, 2. V3 nerve, 3. cavernous sinus, 4. carotid artery, 5. pituitary gland and 6. sphenoid sinus; (c) – 1. clivus and 2. foramen lacerum.

radiotherapy, more radiotherapy treatment per week, or the use of concurrent chemotherapy.

Defining the exact extent of postero-lateral extension of tumour along the foramen lacerum, petro-occipital fissure and petrous temporal bone is important for guiding the posterior border of the radiation field. Cases with significant tumour extension in this region tend to pose difficulties for treatment because of the proximity to the brain stem that needs to be

avoided. More sophisticated treatment techniques such as intensity-modulated radiation therapy may be required.

Paranasal sinuses (stage T3)
The sphenoid sinus is frequently involved because of its position immediately above the roof of the nasopharynx from which it is separated by a thin plate of bone (Figures 5.18 and 5.19). The ethmoid

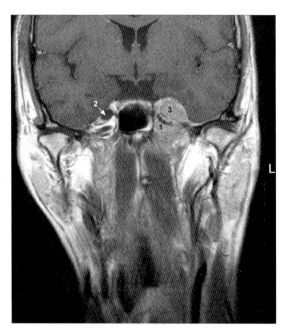

Fig. 5.13 Coronal T1-weighted MR of tumour invading foramen lacerum and cavernous sinus: 1. foramen lacerum, 2. carotid artery and 3. cavernous sinus.

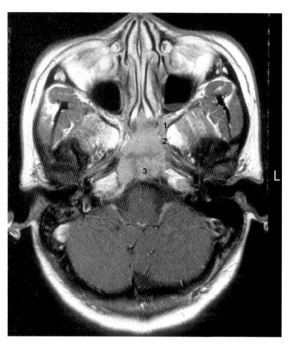

Fig. 5.15 Axial MR of tumour invading pterygopalatine fossa, vidian canal, clivus: 1. pterygoplatatine fossa, 2. vidian canal and 3. clivus.

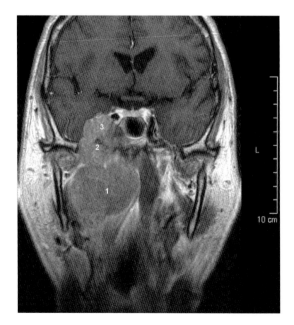

Fig. 5.14 Coronal T1-weighted MR of tumour invading sphenoid bone, foramen ovale and cavernous sinus: 1. tumour, 2. foramen ovale and 3. cavernous sinus.

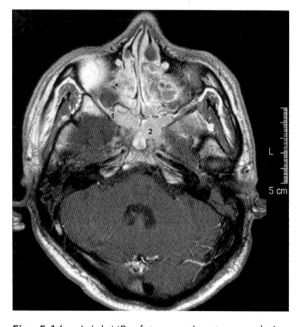

Fig. 5.16 Axial MR of tumour in pterygopalatine fossa and pterygomaxillary fissure: 1. tumour in pterygomaxillary fissure and 2. tumour in pterygopalatine fossa.

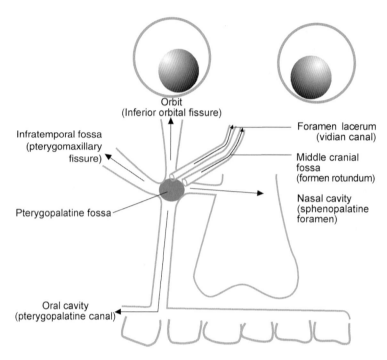

Fig. 5.17   Pterygopalatine fossa.

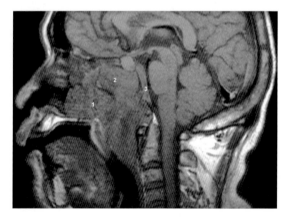

Fig. 5.18   Sagittal MR of tumour invading sphenoid sinus and clivus: 1. tumour, 2. sphenoid sinus
and 3. clivus.

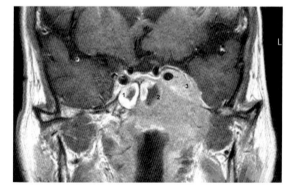

Fig. 5.19   Coronal MR of tumour invading sphenoid
sinus, skull base and cavernous sinus: 1. sphenoid
sinus (inflammatory mucosal thickening), 2. sphenoid sinus (tumour invasion) and 3. cavernous sinus.

Important imaging points for oncological management

If an opacity is found in the paranasal sinuses, the
determination of the nature of the opacity (i.e. benign
inflammatory mucosal thickening versus tumour)
has a significant impact in defining the radiation field.

sinus is secondarily invaded by tumour spreading
from the sphenoid sinus or nasal cavity (Figure 5.20).
Tumour in the maxillary sinus is a late event and a
marker of extensive disease [2].

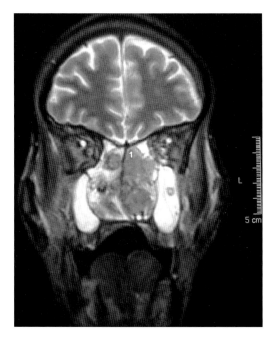

Fig. 5.20 Coronal MR image of tumour in the ethmoid sinus and nasal cavity. Note the tumour has intermediate signal and the inflammatory tissue has high signal on the T2-weighted images: 1. tumour.

This is an area where MR imaging has a major advantage over CT. In general, indeterminate cases are treated as malignant involvement and treatment morbidity is increased owing to the increased radiation coverage. This is, especially, significant for the anterior ethmoid air cells, because the adjacent ipsilateral globe and optic nerve may need to be sacrificed by inclusion into the radiation portal.

Cranium (stage T4)
NPC invades the dura and cavernous sinus (III, IV, V^1, V^2 and VI palsy) (Figures 5.13, 5.14 and 5.19) [2,7,8]. Direct invasion into the brain is rare.

Important imaging points for oncological management
See comments for skull base disease (T3) above.

Orbit (stage T4)
Invasion of the orbit at diagnosis is rare and is a marker of extensive disease. Usually, tumour invasion occurs via the orbital fissures.

Important imaging points for oncological management
The orbit would need to be sacrificed during radiotherapy treatment.

Infratemporal fossa (stage T4)
Invasion of the infratemporal fossa is a further marker of extensive disease. Invasion often occurs via lateral tumour extension along the pterygomaxillary fissure into the infratemporal fat and temporalis muscle. Some centres also include invasion of the medial and lateral pterygoid muscles (which leads to trismus and V^3 palsy) in the definition of the infratemporal fossa.

Cranial nerves (stage T4)
For the purpose of staging, cranial nerve involvement is a clinical and not a radiological diagnosis. By the nature of the position of NPC at the skull base, tumour invades the skull base foramina, and frequently surrounds the nerves causing cranial nerve palsies. True perineural tumour extension, where tumour travels along the nerve only, is not commonly found.

Imaging nodal metastases
A nodal mass in the neck is the most common presentation of NPC, 75% of patients have lymph node metastases at diagnosis. Lymph node metastases, usually, spread in an orderly fashion to involve the lateral retropharyngeal nodes (Figure 5.2), followed by the upper and then the lower deep cervical nodes [9–11] (Figure 5.21). Only 6% of patients have involvement of the cervical nodes without the evidence of retropharyngeal lymphadenopathy [11]. The lateral retropharyngeal nodes lie postero-lateral to the nasopharynx and oropharynx (down to C3) and medial to the carotid artery. The median group of retropharyngeal nodes is not identified as a discrete chain of nodes on imaging [11,12]. The cervical nodal groups that are involved are those along the internal jugular chain and posterior triangle. Involvement of the periparotid, submandibular and submental nodes are uncommon at presentation [11]. Nodal involvement down to the supraclavicular nodes is uncommon, but when present increases the risk of distant metastatic disease. Nodal metastases from NPC have a tendency to undergo necrosis (Figure 5.21).

Imaging is superior to clinical examination for the identification of neck node metastases. Imaging demonstrates those nodes in the retropharyngeal

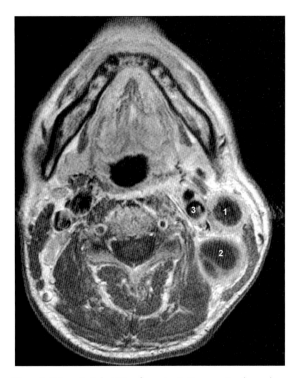

Fig. 5.21 Axial MR of metastatic cervical nodes: 1. necrotic upper internal jugular metastatic node, 2. necrotic posterior triangle metastatic node and 3. internal jugular vein.

region and superior internal jugular chain, which are not accessible to palpation, as well as those nodes that are deep to the sternocleidomastoid muscle; hence, difficult to palpate. The diagnosis of a metastatic node is based on nodal size, abnormal nodal architecture including the presence of necrosis, and extracapsular tumour extension (see Chapters 1–3). MR imaging has an advantage over CT in the detection of lateral retropharyngeal nodes and in distinguishing lateral retropharyngeal nodes from the primary tumour in the lateral nasopharynx (Figure 5.2) [5].

Important imaging points for oncological management

Currently, radiation therapy is used to treat the whole of both sides of the neck regardless of nodal staging (i.e. elective neck radiation is routinely given for N0 cases). For patients with N0 disease (apart from retropharyngeal nodes), staged by CT/MR, it is not certain whether neck irradiation could be safely withheld without leading to an increased risk of tumour relapse in the neck and a decrease in survival probability.

The definition of the location of the lowest malignant node, whether it extends down to the upper margin of the thyroid cartilage or down to the supraclavicular fossa, is important because it affects

(a) prognosis,
(b) selection of patients to be treated with concurrent chemotherapy,
(c) radiation dose delivered to the lower neck (the dose to the lower neck is reduced if the lower neck is not involved by nodal metastases).

Whether nodes are present on one side of the upper neck, both sides or absent on both sides may affect the dose to the parotid glands (and hence the side effects of mouth dryness) when intensity-modulated radiotherapy is used.

Imaging metastatic disease

Distant metastatic disease from NPC is present in about 5% of patients at diagnosis; the incidence increases with advanced nodal stage. Metastatic disease developing after treatment, usually, occurs within the first 3 years and can be found in up to 30% of patients. The sites of metastases are, in descending order of frequency, bone, liver, lung and skin. Brain metastases are very rare. A chest X-ray is performed as part of the staging investigations, but an isotope bone scan, CT thorax and liver scan are only performed if there is clinical suspicion of disease in terms of the findings on clinical examination or routine investigations, or in cases of advanced local (T4) or nodal (N3b) disease.

Important imaging points for oncological management

It has been shown that the routine screening for distant metastases is not warranted except in some high-risk groups such as N2- and N3- or T4-stage disease. If screening imaging shows distant metastases, the treatment would be changed from curative to palliative. For example, palliative chemotherapy may be used instead of radiation therapy as the initial treatment, and if radiation therapy were required to control local symptoms, a lower dose would be used.

Imaging residual and recurrent tumour

Patients should undergo regular follow-up by imaging, because tumour recurrence often occurs deep to the nasopharyngeal mucosa and cannot be detected on endoscopy. However, in many centres there are no resources for intensive follow-up with imaging. In these centres, patients are imaged either to define the extent of disease when tumour recurrence is identified on follow-up nasopharyngoscopy or to diagnose deep-seated tumour recurrence when there is strong clinical suspicion of local recurrence, such as the development of neck node metastases, cranial nerve palsies or a headache.

Imaging may be unable to differentiate tumour recurrence from radiation scarring/granulation tissue; and unfortunately, many of these abnormal areas are too deep and too difficult to biopsy. For this reason, it is important to have a post-radiation baseline study to compare the future follow-up studies. PET has the potential to improve diagnostic accuracy in these difficult cases, but as yet the role for it has not been determined and false negative results can occur, in the first 4 to 6 months.

Imaging protocol for NPC

Primary tumour and neck node metastases

CT imaging

In centres where the incidence of NPC is high, because of the limitation of resources, CT is the only examination to be performed routinely with MR reserved for selected cases. In these cases, the protocol for CT is 5 mm axial sections of the head and neck post-contrast with 3–5 mm coronal sections of the head post-contrast. Images are displayed in soft tissue windows and images through the skull base are also reconstructed into bone windows using a bone algorithm. Areas of suspicious bone invasion may be scanned using thin 1 mm sections.

MR imaging

- Where resources are available MR is the investigation of choice.
- Axial and sagittal T1-weighted images (sagittal optional).

- Axial T2-weighted images with fat saturation.
- Coronal T2-weighted images.
- Axial and coronal T1-weighted images (high resolution 512 matrix) after contrast. A post-contrast image with fat saturation can be added to detect perineural spread.

Ultrasound

Not routinely employed, but may be used in selected cases as an additional examination to CT or MR for neck nodes.

Distant metastases

- Chest X-ray (CT thorax, if lymphadenopathy or pulmonary metastases suspected on chest X-ray).
- Isotope bone scan, if clinical suspicion of bone metastases.
- Ultrasound or CT upper abdomen, if clinical suspicion of liver metastases.
- PET scanning is potentially useful and cost effective, but its role is still unclear at present.

Follow-up

Ideally, MR scans should be used for follow-up according to the following schedule:

- Scan 1–3 months after completion of treatment.
- Every 4 months for the first year.
- Every 6 months for the second year and yearly thereafter.

In many centres, where the incidence of NPC is high, there are insufficient resources for this regime of intensive follow-up imaging.

The role of PET is unclear at present.

Other tumours that arise in the nasopharynx

Lymphoma

Non-Hodgkin's lymphoma (NHL) is the second most common tumour of the nasopharynx after carcinoma, although overall lymphoma at this site is a fairly rare disease. Most NHL of the head and neck arise in the extranodal lymphatic system of Waldeyers ring (lymphoid tissue in the nasopharynx, palatine

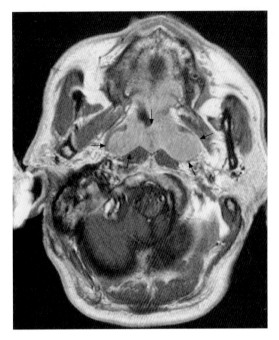

Fig. 5.22   Axial T1-weighted MR image post-contrast of a nasopharyngeal lymphoma (arrows).

tonsils, tongue base and posterior pharyngeal wall). Within Waldeyers ring, the nasopharynx is the second most common site of involvement, one-third of patients presenting with lymphoma of the nasopharynx will have other sites of Waldeyers ring involved.

Most of the patients present with a conductive hearing loss or nasal obstruction. Imaging reveals a tumour that is homogeneous and non-necrotic with moderate enhancement after contrast (Figure 5.22). Most lymphomas of the nasopharynx are well defined and exophytic rather than infiltrative in nature, although cases of invasion into the deep spaces bordering the nasopharynx and into the skull base are described. Lymphomas of the nasopharynx may be a B-cell, NK/T-cell or T-cell lymphoma. Those with a B-cell histology are more likely to have cervical lymphadenopathy, which produces homogeneous non-necrotic nodes.

MR imaging or CT is used to assess the head and neck for the primary tumour and lymphadenopathy. CT imaging of the thorax, abdomen and pelvis may also be performed to stage the extent of the disease. The main role of imaging is to provide a pretreatment assessment of tumour bulk and stage, and a post-treatment assessment of tumour response after chemotherapy and radiotherapy. NHL of Waldeyers ring has a poorer prognosis, in general, than other head and neck sites of NHL. Usually, tumour recurrence is in the first or second year after treatment and is often distant from the original site.

Rhabdomyosarcoma

Rhabdomyosarcoma is a tumour of childhood, although it rarely arises in adults also. They are invasive homogeneous or heterogeneous tumours with moderate enhancement after contrast. Rhabdomyosarcoma of the nasopharynx is classified as a parameningeal tumour. The tumour shows a tendency to invade the skull base and posterior maxillary wall. The cavernous sinus may be involved in up to one-third of cases. Lymph node metastases are found in 50% of cases and distant metastases occur to the lung and bone. Treatment is a combination of chemotherapy and radiotherapy with or without surgery. MR is the investigation of choice for demonstrating the full extent of the primary tumour and nodes.

Juvenile angiofibroma

Please refer to the chapters on the skull base and maxilla and sinuses.

Adenoid cystic carcinoma

Adenoid cystic carcinoma is a rare cancer of the nasopharynx. It may be slow growing or aggressive and has a tendency to reoccur and spread along the nerves. Patients present with cranial nerve palsies, middle ear effusions and epistaxis. It is an infiltrative disease with a marked propensity to invade the skull base. The imaging features are similar to those for NPC except that it has a higher incidence of perineural invasion and cranial nerve palsies (Figure 5.23) and lower incidence of cervical lymphadenopathy. Distant metastases occur especially to bone and lung. Treatment includes surgery and radiotherapy or radiotherapy alone.

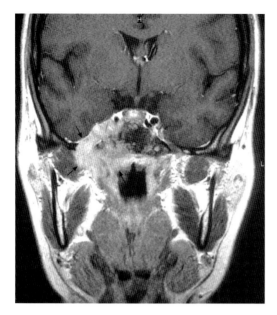

Fig. 5.23 Coronal T1-weighted MR image post-contrast of an adenoid cystic carcinoma (arrows) in the nasopharynx, skull base and cavernous sinus.

References

1. Van Hasselt CA and Leung SF. Clinical picture. In: Van Hasselt and Gibb (Eds) *Nasopharyngeal Carcinoma*, 2nd edition. The Chinese University press. Hong Kong.

2. King AD, Lam W, Leung SF, Chan YL, Teo P and Metreweli C. MR imaging of local disease in nasopharyngeal carcinoma: tumour extent vs tumour stage. *Br. J. Radiol.* 1999; **72**: 734–741.

3. Silver AJ, Mawad ME, Hilal SK, Sane P and Ganti SR. Computed tomography of the nasopharynx and related spaces. *Radiology* 1983; **147**: 725–731.

4. Cheung YK, Sham JST, Chan FL, Leong LLY and Choy D. Computed tomography of paranasopharyngeal spaces: normal variations and criteria for tumour extension. *Clin. Radiol.* 1992; **45**: 109–113.

5. King AD, Teo P, Lam WWM, Leung SF and Metreweli C. Staging of paranasopharyngeal tumor extension in nasopharyngeal carcinoma: MR vs CT imaging. *J. Clin. Oncol.* 2000; **12**: 397–402.

6. Chong VFH and Fan YF. Skull base erosion in nasopharyngeal carcinoma: detection by CT and MRI. *Clin. Radiol.* 1996; **51**: 625–631.

7. Chong VFH, Fan YF and Khoo BK. Nasopharyngeal carcinoma with intracranial spread: CT and MR characteristics. *J. Comput. Assist. Tomo.* 1996; **20**: 563–569.

8. Ng S, Chang TC, Ko SF, Yen PS, Wan YL, Tang LM *et al.* Nasopharyngeal carcinoma. MRI and CT assessment. *Neuroradiology* 1997; **39**: 741–746.

9. Sham JST, Choy D and Wei WI. Nasopharyngeal carcinoma: orderly neck node spread. *Int. J. Radiat. Oncol. Biol. Phys.* 1990; **19**: 929–933.

10. Sham JST, Cheung YK, Choy D, Chan FL and Leong L. Computed tomography evaluation of neck node metastases from nasopharyngeal carcinoma. *Int. J. Radiat. Oncol. Biol. Phys.* 1993; **26**: 787–792.

11. King AD, Ahuja AT, Leung SF, Lam WWM, Teo P, Chan YL and Metreweli C. Neck node metastases from nasopharyngeal carcinoma: MR imaging of the patterns of disease. *Head Neck* 2000; **22**: 275–281.

12. Chong VF, Fan YF and Khoo JB. Retropharyngeal lymphadenopathy in nasopharyngeal carcinoma. *Eur. J. Radiol.* 1995; **21**: 100–105.

Oral Cavity and Oropharynx

RM Evans and SC Hodder

Introduction

Squamous cell carcinoma (SCC) is the most common tumour that affects the oral cavity and oropharynx, 90% of primary tumours in this region are SCC, and these tumours account for 4–5% of all primary malignancies within the UK (Figure 6.1). In South Wales it has an incidence of 4.5 new cases per annum per 100,000 population. The two main causative factors are smoking and alcohol abuse in that order [1]. The other types of tumour that are found in the oral cavity and oropharynx are listed in Table 6.1.

The newcomer to the head and neck needs to be aware of the distinction between the oral cavity and the oropharynx – the two are not synonymous. The oral cavity refers to the vestibule of the mouth, which extends from the lips to the faucial (tonsillar) arches posteriorly. It is bounded by the hard palate superiorly and the floor of mouth and tongue inferiorly. Posteriorly the oral cavity communicates with the oropharynx through the tonsillar fauces. The oropharynx lies between the tonsillar fauces and the pharyngeal wall from the level of the soft palate to the pharyngo-epiglottic fold inferiorly. The tongue base forms its floor.

Newcomers to the head and neck must also embrace the spaces concept of the head and neck; the cervical

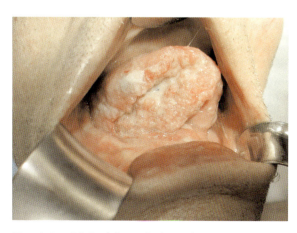

Fig. 6.1   SCC of the right lateral tongue.

Table 6.1 Primary tumours of the oral cavity and oropharynx.

SCC	90%
Adeno-carcinoma	5%
Mucoepidermoid carcinoma	
Adenoid cystic carcinoma	4%
Acinic cell carcinoma	1%
Hodgkin's and non-Hodgkin's lymphoma	<1%

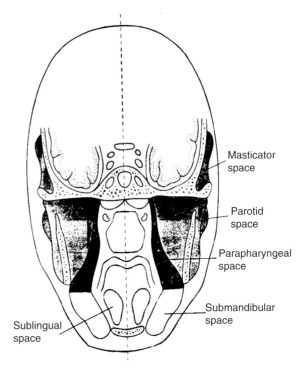

Fig. 6.3 Coronal section depicting the major head and neck spaces.

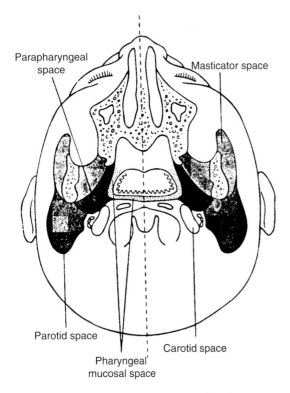

Fig. 6.2 Axial section depicting the five major spaces of the head and neck.

region is enveloped in several fascial layers. These layers outline multiple spaces within the neck; the concept of spaces allows the radiologist to offer realistic differential diagnoses for pathology within the relevant space within the neck. The cervical fascia is divided into superficial and deep layers, the more important deep layer is comprised of three layers: investing, visceral and prevertebral. There are also two minor fascia planes (namely, alar fascia and carotid sheath) which although not anatomically distinct fascial layers – they do represent fascial planes which have functional significance [2–4]. The concept of

spaces works well in the supra-hyoid neck but is less effective in the infra-hyoid neck. The major spaces are illustrated in Figures 6.2 and 6.3.

The distinction between the oral cavity and oropharynx is not a physical barrier – tumour can migrate from one region to the other. SCC does not restrict itself to one compartment, e.g. tumours of the tongue base (which is in the oropharynx) tend to spread anteriorly along the neurovascular structures into the anterior tongue, which lies in the oral cavity. One cannot, therefore, consider tumours of the oral cavity in isolation. While this chapter will deal primarily with tumours of the lips and oral cavity we will also look at the key areas of the oropharynx where tumours may migrate to, or may originate from.

Each of the following key areas will be considered: lips, floor of mouth, alveolar ridges (the tooth bearing bone ridges of the maxilla and mandible), oral tongue (anterior two thirds), the retromolar trigone (a small triangle posterior and lateral to the last molar), buccal mucosa, hard and soft palate, tonsil (which sits at the gateway to the oropharynx) and

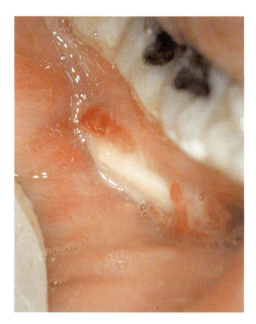

Fig. 6.4 Buccal ulcer right lower buccal sulcus, diagnosis: SCC.

the posterior third of the tongue or tongue base which is situated in the oropharynx.

Clinical presentation of SCC is usually by one of two modes:

1. A small asymptomatic lesion (ulcer or white/red patch of mucosa), which is usually picked up at a dental check up by a dentist (Figure 6.4).
2. Larger symptomatic tumours, which may be ulcerating and displacing teeth or dentures, causing pain and discomfort. This group may present to their doctor rather than their dentist (Figure 6.1).

The 5-year survival for tumours of the lip, oral cavity and oropharynx varies between 91% and 42%, depending on the site of the primary tumour [1]. The survival figures have not significantly improved over the past two decades. Imaging has a major role in the appropriate selection of patients for the various treatment options, allowing the clinician to decide whether surgery, radiotherapy, chemotherapy, brachytherapy or a combination of treatments is the best option for the patient. Imaging and more effective treatment selection has significantly decreased mobidity in patients with SCC.

The TNM classification is a clinical classification; radiologists need not become slaves to the classification. Be aware of the TNM classification, but the radiologists' role is to provide additional information that will not be provided by the TNM classification of the tumour. Tumour dimensions, tumour volumes, tumour extension and the presence of lymph node metastases will have a greater influence on treatment decisions.

Key points

TNM classification for oral cavity and oropharyngeal tumours

T Classification

Tx: Primary tumour cannot be assessed
TO: No evidence of primary tumour
Tis: Carcinoma *in situ*
T1: Tumour 2 cm or less in greatest dimension
T2: Tumour >2 cm but less than 4 cm in greatest diameter
T3: Tumour >4 cm in greatest diameter
T4 (lip): Tumour invades adjacent structures (e.g. floor of mouth, bone and inferior alveolar nerve)
T4 (oral cavity): Tumour invades adjacent structures (e.g. bone, extrinsic (deep) muscle of tongue, maxillary sinus)
T4 (oropharynx): Tumour invades adjacent structures (e.g. pterygoid muscles, mandible, hard palate, larynx, extrinsic (deep) muscles of tongue)

N Classification

Nx: Cannot assess regional lymph nodes
N0: Negative nodes *clinically*
N1: Single ipsilateral nodes <3 cm in diameter
N2a: Single ipsilateral nodes 3–6 cm diameter
N2b: Multiple ipsilateral nodes 3–6 cm diameter
N2c: Bilateral or contralateral nodes 3–6 cm diameter
N3: Ipsilateral or contralateral nodes >6 cm diameter

M Classification

Mx: Cannot assess distant metastases
M: Distant metastases

Clinicians now rely on imaging to correctly stage their patients. The TNM classification (which was originally a clinical classification) has been shown to be unreliable when used on a purely clinical basis, as a staging tool for outcome and treatment. Many authors now realise that imaging, with its ability to predict tumour volume and its mode of spread can radically alter not just the TNM classification but can dramatically influence the appropriate choice of treatment for the patient [5,6].

The concept of measuring tumour volume as an integral part of imaging is alien to most practising radiologists; however, there is increasing evidence that the current uni-dimensional TNM classification fails to define the true three-dimensional bulk of tumours in the head and neck, especially within a given T-stage [7].

As the TNM classification has been developed for prognostic purposes, adding tumour volume data may be worthwhile, e.g. allowing the patient to make a more informed decision about treatment offered (e.g. non-operative treatment options in advanced oropharyngeal carcinoma). Tumour volume measurements (on CT imaging) in advanced carcinoma have significant prognostic significance, proving more predictive than TNM staging [8,9].

Clinicians are becoming more and more aware of the information that radiologists can provide. There may be an increasing pressure to provide tumour volume as a routine part of tumour staging with imaging. Both volume acquisition using a digitally acquired cross-sectional image [8] or simply using a cuboid volume [9] using the maximum dimension in each plane on CT (both of primary and lymph node mass) have been proven to be effective prognostic indicators. When CT and MRI are compared, CT tends to over-estimate tumour volume by a factor of 1.3 as compared to MRI [10]. In the estimation of tumour volume, both intra- and interobserver error is a significant problem (89.3%) [11]. Reproducibility and reliability in tumour volume measurements may well pose a problem. Tumour volume acquisition remains a labour-intensive procedure (despite the ever increasing developments in hardware and software), which requires considerable radiological input. However, in the near future such information may well be regarded as essential by clinicians, for the effective management of head and neck tumours.

Which imaging modality is best for depicting the primary tumour? For the oral cavity and oropharynx – the evidence is sparse. Each modality has its strengths and weaknesses. Local factors, i.e. equipment and expertise will exert strong influences, as in any aspect of radiology in the UK. Leslie *et al.* [12] compared CT and MRI in staging SCC of the oral cavity and oropharynx; they found an accuracy of 77% for MRI and 57% for CT in staging primary tumours (51 tumour episodes). However, if degraded images and T1 tumours were excluded, the techniques were comparable. In the UK, the recent introduction of multi-slice CT is likely to invoke a re-appraisal of CT, its rapid acquisition time may allow CT to supplant MRI as the mainstay of imaging for head and neck cancer. While the conspicuity of tumours is currently greater with MRI than CT, with the new generation of multi-slice CT-movement degradation of the image is likely to be greatly reduced with CT.

Key points

Imaging

Conspicuity of tumour: MRI > CT
Movement degradation: Multi-slice CT > MRI
Multi-planar capabilities: MRI multi-slice CT
Marrow involvement: MRI > CT
Cortical destruction: CT > MRI
Speed: Multi-slice CT > MRI
Costs: MRI > CT

Whatever imaging method is available to the radiologist, the difficulty comes in knowing exactly what information the clinician or surgeon requires, in order to treat their patients successfully. If the radiologist is aware of the questions that need answering, radiology can play a pivotal role in the management of head and neck cancer.

This chapter will attempt to highlight the key questions that need answering for each of the main subsites where SCC occurs in the oral cavity. Primarily we will discuss assessment of the primary tumour, the problem of lymph node metastases having been dealt with in Section 1.

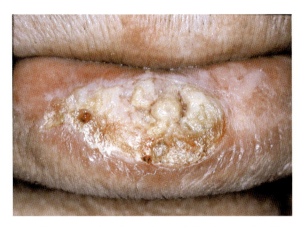

Fig. 6.5 Non-healing ulcer of the lip: early SCC (T2).

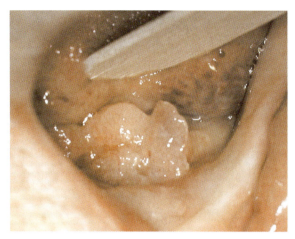

Fig. 6.6 Right floor of mouth and midline SCC.

Lip

Early presentation is the norm due to the patient's early perception of an abnormality. A non-healing ulcer is the commonest clinical presentation (Figure 6.5). On imaging tumours cannot be differentiated from the normal obicularis oris muscle; however, the role of imaging is to assess the potential spread in advanced tumours, namely: extension into mandible or maxilla. Once mandible or maxilla is involved a partial mandibulectomy or maxillectomy is required [13]. Despite early presentation however, 10% of all lip tumours will have positive lymph nodes at presentation (submental, submandibular and rarely upper cervical nodes also) [13].

> **Key points**
>
> *Lip*
>
> - Extension into mandible?
> - Lymph node metastases (submental and submandibular)

Floor of mouth

The floor of mouth refers to the half-moon-shaped area of oral mucosa between the lower attached gingival margin on the lingual side of the mandible and the undersurface or ventral surface of the anterior tongue (The oral mucosa overlies the muscles slung between the anterior mandible; namely, mylohyoid, genioglossus and geniohyoid.). The area is divided into an anterior portion, deep to the tongue, and the gutters or lateral portions of the floor of the mouth, which lie between the lateral tongue and the lateral mandible (Figure 6.6).

The key structure in the floor of mouth is the mylohyoid muscle (Figure 6.7); this is a muscular hammock which is slung between the medial bodies of the mandible and a fibrous septum forming its inferior apex. The mylohyoid muscle is thin anteriorly and thickened posteriorly with a free posterior border. It is the muscle that divides the sublingual space from the submandibular space of the neck, however, the free posterior border marks the posterior "door post" whereby the two spaces can communicate. Beneath the mylohyoid muscle the two anterior bellies of the digastric muscles delineate the boundaries of the submental triangle. The other key muscle is the hyoglossus (Figure 6.8); this is a quadrilateral-shaped muscle, which originates from the hyoid and, as an extrinsic muscle of the tongue, passes upwards into the lateral tongue. The hyoglossus and mylohyoid are the key muscles when searching for the course of the submandibular duct, submandibular gland, lingual artery and hypoglossal nerve (see Figures 6.7 and 6.8). Whatever mode of imaging used, identify these two muscles and one can then identify the major neurovascular pathways.

The sublingual gland is one of the structures that sits between the mylohyoid and the hyoglossus muscles. It can be a large structure; running from the symphysis menti to the submandibular gland posteriorly. It is

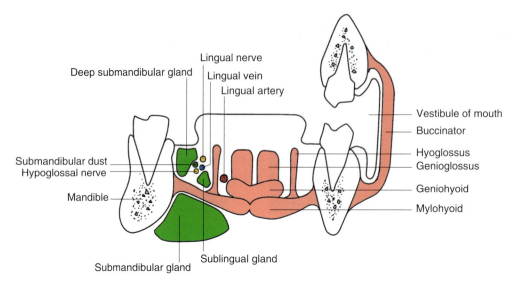

Fig. 6.7   Coronal illustration of the key structures of the floor of mouth.

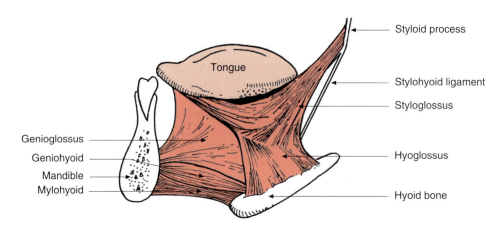

Fig. 6.8   Extrinsic muscles of the tongue.

variable in size and may merge with the submandibular gland to form one large salivary complex.

SCC of the floor of mouth usually commences as an area of leucoplakia, however, not all leucoplakia progresses to carcinoma. Tumours can extend deep into the sublingual gland, then pass posteriorly through the sublingual space to obstruct the submandibular duct and extend into the submandibular space. Extension across the midline is common, (Figures 6.9–6.10) mucosal extension up to the mucoperiosteum of the mandible presents a portal for invasion of the mandible. Take care when assessing the neck – for bilateral nodal involvement is common, particularly in midline tumours. At presentation, nodal metastases occur in 20% of patients; they tend to present first in the submandibular regions, but spread to upper cervical nodes at presentation is not uncommon.

Key points

- Look for posterior extension along neurovascular channels – between hyoglossus and mylohyoid muscles
- Does the tumour cross the midline? If so – look for bilateral cervical nodes

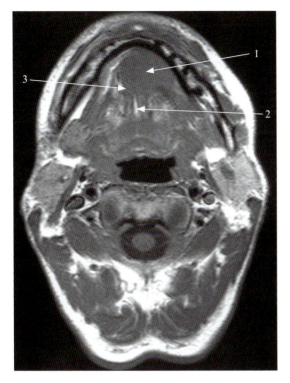

Fig. 6.9   Floor of mouth (SCC), 1. tumour, 2. fat within mid-line septum, 3. Tumour invasion contralateral bundle of genioglossus.

- Extension up to periosteum of mandible/ invasion of mandible
- Does the tumour extend into the mylohyoid, i.e. submandibular space invasion – modifies surgical approach
- Lateral floor of mouth – look for spread to submandibular space, parapharyngeal space and masticator space

Alveolar ridge of the mandible

Tumours at this site usually occur in the partially dentate or edentulous patient. Symptoms that may cause the patient to present include: pain/bleeding/ ulceration on wearing dentures, a recent change in fit of a denture or occasionally localised loosening of natural teeth. Local invasion of the mandible occurs early, by one of two routes:

- along the periodontal membrane/ligament of natural teeth or at the gingival reflection, i.e. the mucoperiosteum attachment [14] or
- in the edentulous mandible – directly through the alveolar crest [15] (Figure 6.11).

Imaging should be guided appropriately in order to try and establish the mucosal extent of the tumour, i.e. buccal or lingual extension and whether invasion of the mandible has occurred. The teeth form a natural barrier to tumour extension, however, tumour can invade along the gingival reflection at the junction of

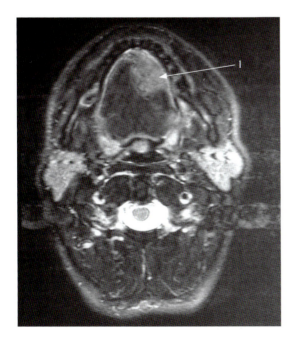

Fig. 6.10   T2 Fat saturation image, 1. Tumour extension across midline.

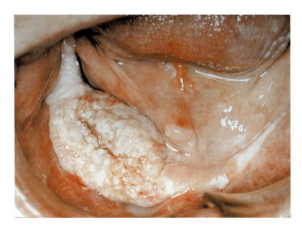

Fig. 6.11   SCC of the right alveolar edentulous crest with suspected bone involvement.

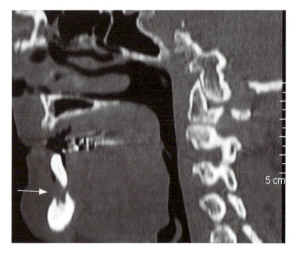

Fig. 6.12 Sagittal reconstruction SCC mandible, arrow. "floating tooth" secondary to destruction of buccal and lingual cortex.

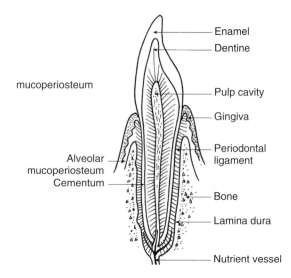

Fig. 6.14 Tooth, gingiva and socket.

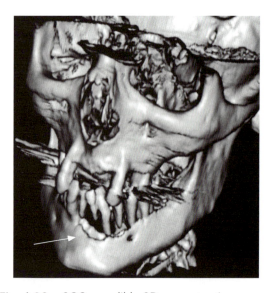

Fig. 6.13 SCC mandible-3D reconstruction, arrow. destruction of buccal and lingual plates.

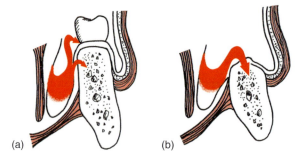

Fig. 6.15 Potential tumour spread in (a) dentate & (b) edentulous mandible.

Marrow involvement may be more easily depicted by MRI, para-sagittal or oblique tangential views to demonstrate the extent of abnormal marrow involvement are advised. The surgeon needs to know the extent of any marrow invasion and cortical invasion in order to decide how much mandible needs to be resected. This can vary from a shaving of the lingual cortex to a rim resection or a complete segment of mandible, i.e. a segmental mandibulectomy (see Figure 6.16).

Which mode of imaging to use is controversial. There is no real evidence base to favour one mode over another. As always in radiology, local resources and expertise will influence the decision. At best, most surgeons will appreciate a reasonably accurate predictor, e.g. accuracy in the 70–80% range. Many surgeons advocate periosteal stripping and direct

mucoperiosteum and periodontal membrane lining the tooth socket. MRI cannot differentiate between tumour, caries and radio-necrosis. However, if abnormal marrow signal is demonstrated, contiguous with a known tumour – this must be regarded as direct tumour extension. CT may more accurately depict cortical destruction than MRI – once bone involvement is detected fine axial sections with computed reconstructions are warranted to accurately depict the extent of cortical destruction (see Figures 6.12– 6.15).

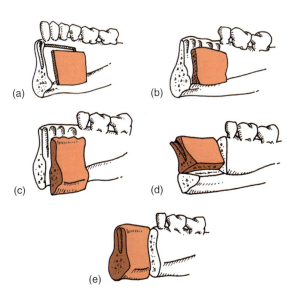

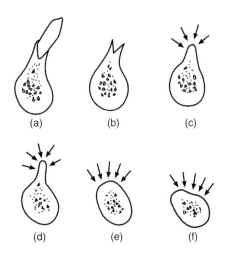

Fig. 6.17 Resorption patterns of the mandible.

Fig. 6.16 Mandibular resections: (a) shaving lingual cortex, (b) removal lingual plate to level of roots of teeth, (c) removal of entire lingual plate, (d) rim resection (leaving labial attachment) and (e) segmental resection.

examination of the underlying mandible at surgery as the best predictor of involvement. While this means the final decision is made on the operating table, imaging allows the surgeon to plan a probable course of action and allows informed consent by the patient to be obtained [14,17].

In addition to an assessment of tumour volume occupying the mandible the surgeon needs an accurate depiction of the size and configuration of the mandible, to plan his resection margins and for reconstruction planning. Radiologists need to be aware of the normal resorption patterns, which occur in the edentulous patient [16] (see Figure 6.17). This resorption follows the loss of teeth and results in significant remodelling of the mandible and maxilla. Multi-slice CT or fine section conventional CT with 3D reconstruction now allow the radiologist to provide the surgeon with a 3D display of the configuration of the mandible. This allows the surgeon to accurately calculate the size of bone graft required; allowing an accurate and correct harvest of either fibula or iliac crest for reconstruction. If titanium implants are being used the information given by CT can be used to decide where exactly the implants should be placed. The 3D reconstructions (Figure 6.18) and computer-assisted surgery considerably

assist surgeons in operation planning. Co-operation and pre-surgery discussion between surgeons, radiologists and radiographers is essential – if the relevant information is to be provided in an intelligible format e.g. allowing computer generated models to be created. This allows the Surgeon to pre-plan his resection or titanium implant/stents bar placement.

Lymph node spread is usually to the submandibular and submental nodes initially and then to the deep cervical chain, these areas all need to be assessed carefully. Incidence at presentation is 20%.

Key points

- Extent of mucosal involvement
- Cortical destruction
- Marrow involvement

Tongue

We are going to consider both the oral tongue (anterior two-thirds) and the posterior tongue or tongue base. While the oral tongue is in the oral cavity and the tongue base is in the oropharynx – tumours originating in one portion may well invade the other.

Tumours of the oral tongue usually present as a non-healing ulcer, which may be asymptomatic; pain, referred otalgia and dysarthia tend to be late symptoms. The intrinsic muscles of the tongue are a poor barrier to tumour extension, therefore, what appears to be a small lesion clinically may well be found to invade the deep tongue. Extension fore and aft along the neurovascular bundle is a common pathway for tumour spread. The term "neurovascular bundle" needs some clarification because the components are not closely related to each other but are in fact separated by the hyoglossus muscle. So take care when saying there is neurovascular bundle involvement! The components are: the lingual artery which lies medial to the hyoglossus, the hypoglossal nerve (XII-motor supply to the extrinsic muscles of the tongue) which lies lateral to the hyoglossus and inferior to the lingual vein and submandibular duct. The other major nerve is the lingual nerve (a branch of the mandibular division, i.e. V3), which lies above the hypoglossal nerve, closely related to the submandibular duct. Beyond the hyoglossus muscle this nerve is closely related to the lingual artery and hypoglossal nerve. The hyoglossus muscle is therefore a key structure to identify (see Figures 6.7 and 6.8).

The space between the mylohyoid and hyoglossus is also occupied by fat and the sublingual gland. This fat plane aids in the identification of the neurovascular pathways on both CT and MRI. The other fat plane to search for is contained in the lingual septum between the genioglossus muscles (see Figure 6.18). Whether or not the tumour crosses this septum is crucial to that patient's management and subsequent quality of life. Once a tumour extends down to the genioglossus muscle, it may then extend anteriorly into the floor of mouth. Once there is invasion of the contralateral half of the tongue, the patient is faced with the dilemma of undergoing a glossectomy rather than a hemiglossectomy if surgery is to be carried out (Figure 6.18). The impact on quality of life is immense.

If tumour has encroached on the "neurovascular bundle", i.e. probable perineural invasion – this has significant prognostic implications for the patient; clear margins may be more difficult to obtain, with reduced likelihood of local control and an increased likelihood of lymph node metastases. (Figures 6.19–6.22) On CT the features to look for are: aggressive margins, obliteration of the fat in the sublingual space and obliteration of fat surrounding lingual vessels – these findings are good predictors of perineural involvement [18]. MRI with its superior anatomical detail allows accurate assessment of the sublingual space.

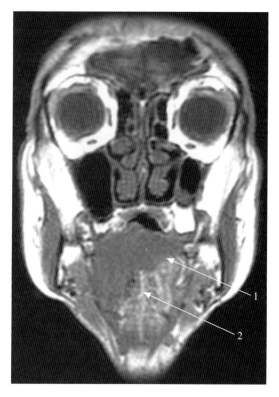

Fig. 6.18 SCC Tongue, 1. contralateral extension, unsuspected clinically, 2. fat within lingual septum.

One must not forget the neurovascular bundle when looking at the tongue base. These structures run from the tongue base into the anterior tongue. If the base of tongue is resected, the neurovascular supply of the anterior tongue is lost. Therefore, a hemiglossectomy is performed. Patients can swallow and speak despite having only half of a tongue, but once the tumour extends into the midline of the tongue base – total glossectomy is the only surgical cure due to the increased likelihood of contralateral involvement of the neurovascular bundle and the subsequent risk of an inadequate surgical clearance. Without a tongue the patient cannot form a food bolus and is, therefore, consigned to being fed through a gastrostomy tube if the surgical route is followed. In addition they have poor speech and may have problems with aspiration. At many institutions total glossectomy is rarely carried out, radiotherapy and chemotherapy are the usual modes of treatment. When assessing tumours of the tongue base, whether or not there is extension across the midline is the crucial question that imaging must answer (Figure 6.23).

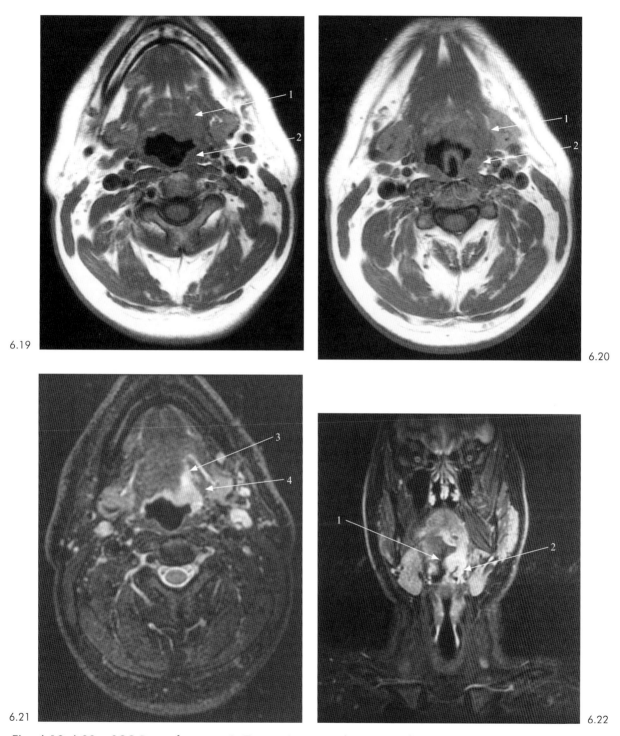

6.19

6.20

6.21

6.22

Figs 6.19–6.22 SCC Base of tongue, 1. Tumour in tongue base, extending up to mid-line, abutting left sub-mandibular gland, 2. Tumour invading lateral oro-pharyngeal wall, 3. Anterior extension along neuro-vascular bundle, 4. Hyoglossus muscle (submandibular duct seen laterally).

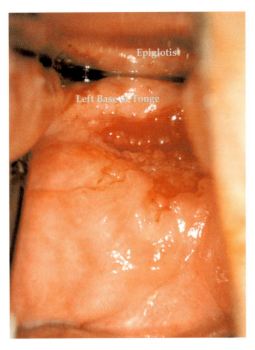

Epiglottis

Left Base of Tongue

Fig. 6.23 SCC of the posterior one-third of the tongue. This tumour has spread laterally into the retromandibular region.

Tumours in the tongue base may spread into many areas of the neck: extension into the fat containing parapharyngeal space may occur – this space communicates with the submandibular space. The palatoglossus muscle (which inserts into the postero-lateral tongue and forms the anterior tonsillar arch) can act as a pathway for tumour to extend from tongue base to tonsil and soft palate.

Nodal metastases are common at presentation (40% of T2 tumours have lymph node metastases at presentation). Skip lesions to the lower deep cervical nodes occur in 16% of cases, accounting for the high rate of neck failures in some series [19].

Key points
- Does the tumour cross the midline?
- Is there extension along the neurovascular bundle?
- Extension beyond the tongue: submandibular space, floor of mouth, parapharyngeal fat space, and mandible
- Vigilant search for lymph node metastases

Tonsil and tonsillar fossa

Small and superficial tumours of the tonsil are often not visible on imaging. This is often the case when searching for the unknown primary when a small occult carcinoma may have been found in the tonsil and even in retrospect the CT or MRI will be normal. Normal individuals may have asymmetric enlargement of their tonsils, which can also cause difficulty on imaging. Assymetric enlargement of a tonsil needs to be regarded with caution.

The normal tonsil enhances with intravenous contrast on CT and shows hyperintensity on T2 sequences on MRI, as does all the lymphoid tissue of the head and neck. One cannot rely on patterns of enhancement in assessing the tonsil. Small tumours are more likely to be picked up at endoscopy and biopsy. It is in the larger tumour group that radiology is of most benefit-in searching for deep extension. Tumour may invade the anterior faucial pillar, and hence, invade the pterygomandibular raphe, which will act as a conduit for tumour to extend into the retromolar trigone or inferiorly into the mandible. Invasion of the posterior faucial pillar can lead to inferior extension along the palatopharyngeus muscle into the pyriform sinus. Extension into and through the floor of the tonsillar fossa leads to tumour invading the pharyngeal constrictor muscles and then invasion of the parapharyngeal space. Once tumour is within this compartment it can extend freely up to the skull base, into the carotid space and extend inferiorly into the lower neck or invade the masticator space. (Figures 6.24 and 6.25) There are multiple potential routes for advanced tonsillar SCC to spread. The radiologists' role is often that of prevention of unneccesary, debilitating surgery for this group of patients with advanced disease, e.g. if extensive invasion of the parapharyngeal space is identified – surgery is not a viable option, a combination of chemotherapy and radiotherapy may be offered.

Buccal mucosa

Buccal carcinomas may arise from areas of leucoplakia; this site has the highest conversion rate from leucoplakia to carcinoma in the oral cavity. Buccal mucosa SCC tends to metastasise early and often directly extend into the parotid gland, buccinator and masseter muscles at presentation [20].

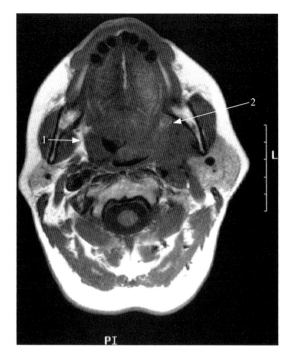

Fig. 6.24 SCC Tonsil, 1. parapharyngeal fat, 2. tumour involving parapharyngeal, masticator, parotid and carotid spaces.

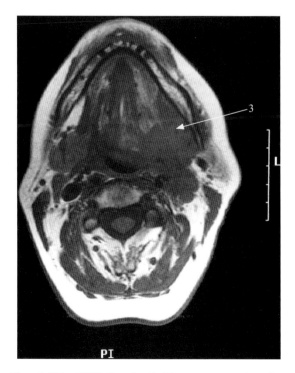

Fig. 6.25 SCC Tonsil, 3. Tumour extension into posterior tongue.

The buccal mucosa covers the inner cheek and lips; it is continuous with the gingiva of the buccal surface of both the maxillary and mandibular alveolar ridges. Posteriorly it is continuous with the retromolar trigone. The key structure is the buccinator muscle, extending from the lateral maxillary ridge to the lateral mandible (see Figure 6.7) and which posteriorly inserts into the pterygomandibular raphe. Lateral to the buccinator is the parotid space and the buccal space. The buccal space contains fat, lymph glands and the facial artery vein.

Tumours may extend submucosally or if deeper extension occurs the buccinator muscle acts as a conduit to either the maxilla, mandible or pterygomandibular raphe. Once there is bone involvement or pterygomandibular raphe involvement, local excision is no longer possible and either a wider excision or a partial maxillectomy or segmental mandibulectomy will be required for tumour clearance.

Ten per cent of buccal mucosa SCC tumours are associated with metastatic lymph nodes at presentation; these are commonly in the buccal space and submandibular regions.

Retromolar trigone

This area of the oral cavity is the small triangular pocket, which sits lateral to the last molar tooth. This area is a major junction point in the head and neck; there are many pathways from this region for tumour to travel. While small in area, a tumour that commences in the retromolar trigone can wreak havoc in the head and neck.

The pterygomandibular raphe forms a palpable ridge beneath the mucosa of the retromolar trigone; it extends from the hook of the hamulus of the medial pterygoid plate to the mylohyoid line on the medial border of the body of the mandible. The buccinator, obicularis oris and superior constrictor muscles all insert into the pterygomandibular raphe, thus tumour can extend rapidly into the buccal space, lateral floor of mouth, oropharynx (tonsillar fossa) or nasopharynx (skull base). Extension along the raphe into the hamulus of the medial pterygoid plate accesses the pterygopalatine fossa. Involvement of the medial pterygoid muscle may then lead to invasion of the pterygomandibular space (fat-filled space between medial pterygoid and

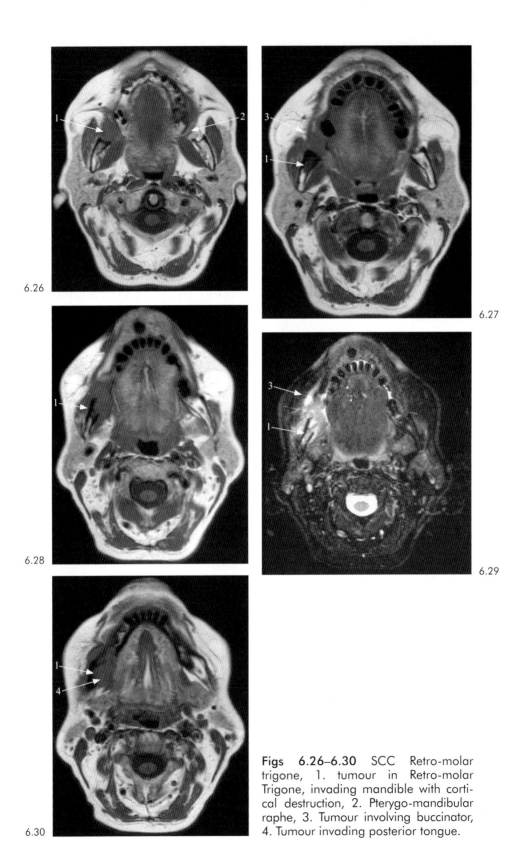

Figs 6.26–6.30 SCC Retro-molar trigone, 1. tumour in Retro-molar Trigone, invading mandible with cortical destruction, 2. Pterygo-mandibular raphe, 3. Tumour involving buccinator, 4. Tumour invading posterior tongue.

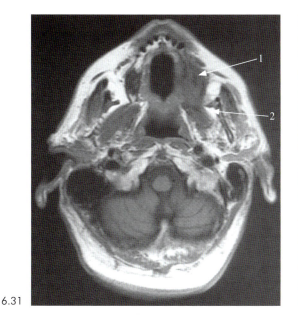
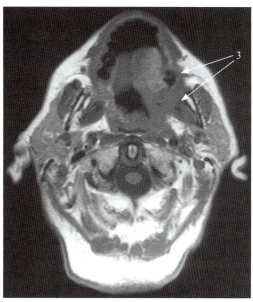

6.31

6.32

Figs 6.31–6.32 SCC Maxillary alveolus, 1. Tumour destruction of maxilla, 2. posterior extension: involving pterygoid platges, 3. involvement of medial pterygoid and buccinator muscles.

the ramus of the mandible, which contains the lingual and inferior alveolar nerves) with subsequent perineural extension. As both the anterior ramus of the mandible and the maxillary tuberosity are in close proximity, bone invasion can occur early (Figures 6.26–6.30).

The key to assessing the retromolar trigone is to regard it as a major junction, remember the many paths that emanate from this junction and search for tumour along these routes. Lymph node metastases are found in 15% of patients at presentation, take care to assess the buccal, submandibular and upper portions of the deep cervical chain (see Key points above).

Gingiva and hard palate

The upper gingiva is continuous with the mucosa of the hard palate. The gingiva is the mucous membrane that covers the alveolar bone processes and is attached to the lingual and buccal surfaces of the mandible and maxilla (Figures 6.14 and 6.31–6.32). SCC is the most common tumour to originate in the gingiva, whereas minor salivary gland carcinoma (usually adenoid cystic or mucoepidermoid types) is the most common primary malignant tumour of the

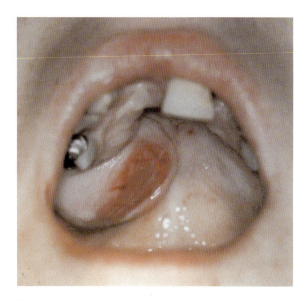

Fig. 6.33 Larger adenoid cystic carcinoma of the right palate that has now ulcerated due to local trauma to the overlying mucosa.

hard palate (Figure 6.33). However, the most common malignant tumour of the hard palate is a maxillary antral tumour that has perforated out into the mouth [21].

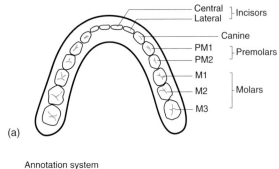

(a)

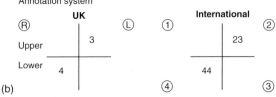

(b)

Fig. 6.34 (a) Adult dentition and (b) annotation systems (annotating left upper canine and right first lower premolar).

Primary mucosal SCC is usually assessed by direct inspection and where bone involvement is suspected – fine section CT coronal images are obligatory to look for underlying saucerisation or erosion in slow growing tumours of the maxilla, hard palate or mandible. Frank destruction is present in more aggressive tumours. When an adenoid cystic tumour is diagnosed, MRI is required to look for perineural extension. In the case of hard palate tumours the pterygopalatine fossa and foramen rotundum should be scrutinised looking for perineural extension along the greater and lesser palatine nerves (see Chapter 12).

When looking for bony involvement in gingival tumours that may be affecting either the maxillary or mandibular alveolus, the relationship of the tumour to the patient's dentition is often stated. To a radiologist, this can induce confusion. Knowledge of the location of the permanent teeth and maxillofacial surgeon's annotations will help (see Figure 6.34). In the system used in the UK, the dentition is divided into four quarters, the teeth are then numbered accordingly, the central incisor being numbered "1", the third molar (i.e. the most posterior) is numbered "8". The right and left sides are marked on the diagram. The international system differs in that the annotation reflects the side and site, thus all teeth in the right upper maxilla are prefixed "1", so the right upper canine would be annotated "13". The left

upper teeth are prefixed with the number "2", left lower with "3" and right lower with "4". Figure 6.34b shows the two annotation methods for the left upper canine and right first lower premolar.

Remember that bone involvement is the crucial information required by the surgeons for management. As discussed in the mandible section, in the dentulous patient the teeth are a relative barrier to tumour whereas in the edentulous patient tumour can infiltrate the marrow through the residual occlusal surface of maxilla or mandible (see Figure 6.15).

For primary SCC of this particular subsite of the oral cavity, lymph nodes are less common at presentation. The incidence is approximately 5% – predominantly found in the submandibular regions.

Key points

- Bone involvement
- Perineural extension – hard palate

Recurrent tumour

Imaging for tumour recurrence is fraught with difficulty in the post-surgical patient. The use of free flaps results in muscular flaps occupying the void created by tumour resection. Atrophy of this muscle rapidly occurs. This together with the associated fatty infiltration may result in confusing images. When asked to examine such patients for a tumour recurrence, trying to detect tumour can be very difficult. It is our policy that whenever a patient has undergone a significant reconstruction, particularly if a free flap has been used, then a routine post-operative baseline study is carried out at approximately 6–8 weeks post-surgery. This study is then used as a baseline if a search for a suspected tumour recurrence is needed. We use MRI for our baseline studies, our routine for oral cavity and oropharyngeal tumours, is as shown below:

Key points

Baseline MRI study

- Axial T1: Skull base to cricoid (7 mm sections)

- Axial T2 (fat sat): Skull base to cricoid (7 mm sections)
- Coronal T1: Symphysis mentis to cervical spine

In order to be able to search for lymph node metastases in the post-operative patient, the radiologist must be aware of the type of lymph node dissection carried out, if any, by the surgeon. The various types of dissection have been highlighted in Figure 6.35. Once lymph node chains have been stripped, lymph will shunt to the contralateral neck, so contralateral nodal pathways should always be diligently reviewed in the post-operative setting. In the post-radiotherapy and post-chemotherapy patient, serial measurements on comparative investigations (be it Ultrasound, MRI

Key points

Incidence of lymph node metastases according to primary subsite

Site	Incidence of positive cervical lymph nodes at presentation (%)	Post-treatment recurrence, incidence of lymph node metastases (%)
Lip	4–12	15
Floor of mouth	20	20
Tongue	40	40–60
Buccal mucosa	10	20
Maxilla	5	10
Retromolar trigone	15	30
Mandible	20	20

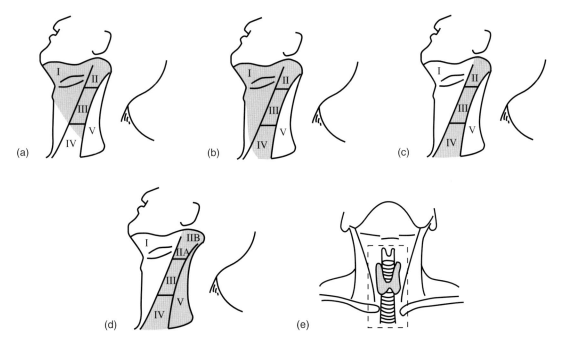

Fig. 6.35 Types of selective neck dissection: (a) supra-omohyoid, (b) extended supra-omohyoid (antero-lateral), (c) lateral, (d) postero-lateral and (e) anterior or central.

or CT) is the best indicator of tumour regression. For some tumours e.g. tongue, the incidence of lymph node metastases in patients with tumour recurrence can be as high as 40–60% (see Key points on page 85). Knowledge of the remaining lymph node territories in these post-surgical patients allows a methodical and systematic review.

Summary

Imaging is crucial to the successful management of the patient with head and neck cancer. Knowledge of the information required by the surgeon is more likely to prompt a productive report for the surgeon. Assessment of the oral cavity and oropharynx is complicated by the fact that there are a variety of subsites present and tumours behave differently according to their specific subsite. The treatment of tumours in the different subsites will vary. There is also a variety of treatment options for specific subsites e.g. for floor of mouth tumours; options include – surgery, radiotherapy, induction chemotherapy and brachytherapy. Treatment options will vary from centre to centre. The radiologist must understand what are the local practices for the treatment of head and neck cancer and direct their imaging to answering the specific needs of the surgeons, oncologists and radiotherapists. A standard imaging algorithm to cover all areas of the oral cavity and oropharynx is impossible and imaging protocols must be geared to local practice.

When imaging the primary tumour timing is crucial. Diagnostic biopsies cause oedema. A standard 10–14 days is recommended post-biopsy. Though there is no evidence base to support this definitive time period, most authors would agree that such an approach is commonsense. While the radiologist may be aware of a recent biopsy at the primary site, take care if your centre has a policy of panendoscopy to look for synchronous tumours. Multiple biopsies from multiple sites may have been taken, with its inherent potential for error. The need for panendoscopy to look for synchronous tumours is contentious; the incidence varies significantly from country to country and centre to centre. In South-West Wales the incidence of synchronous tumours is virtually zero; therefore, it is not our routine practice to carry out panendoscopy on all patients with oral cavity or oropharyngeal primary tumours.

We use MRI to stage floor of mouth, tongue, oropharyngeal and retromolar trigone tumours and in conjunction with CT to assess hard palate, maxillary or mandibular alveolar tumours where assessment of bone destruction is crucial. Assessment of lymph node metastases is by ultrasound in combination with fine needle aspiration cytology. We have shown a sensitivity of 84%, specificity of 86% and a false negative rate of 4% for this method. This multifaceted approach allows an informed decision to be made by the multi-disciplinary team regarding treatment [22].

> ## Key points
>
> *Tumour assessment*
> - Tumour dimensions
> - Tumour volume
> - Tumour extension
> - Lymph node metastases

Do not make the mistake of underestimating the importance of lymph node metastases. The patient's prognosis and treatment will depend on whether or not there are positive nodes present and, if nodal metastases are present, where they are in the neck [23]. For the oral cavity and oropharynx, the presence of an ipsilateral positive node reduces that patient's 5-year survival by 50%, if a contralateral node is found the 5-year survival is reduced by a further 50%, extracapsular spread will reduce it by a further 50%. Whether or not there are lymph node metastases present is crucial to patient management [24].

Imaging plays a pivotal role in both areas, i.e. primary tumour and lymph node secondaries. The finding of lymph node metastases has a potentially calamitous effect on survival with a massive influence on treatment options.

Clinical examination for lymph node metastases is ineffective, false negative and false positive results of as high as 40% have been reported. Yet many centres will ignore the question of lymph node metastases, often prompted by the decision to explore the neck as being a universal treatment. If the potential incidence of lymph node metastases is 40%, some surgeons will advocate a formal neck dissection (clearing levels I–III with a selective supra-omohyoid neck dissection) in all patients [25]. Yet this means that 60% of patients may have undergone unnecessary surgery with all its attendant increases in morbidity. The lymph glands are a natural barrier to cancer spread, far better to preserve rather than resect – if they are not involved.

The surgeon and radiotherapist need to know what level the disease has descended to and whether it is one or multiple nodes involved, whether there is unilateral or bilateral involvement and whether there is extracapsular spread. Extracapsular spread may manifest itself by invasion of the internal jugular vein, sternomastoid muscle or as a coalescence or matting of nodes. If this is present in the apex of the posterior triangle or at the jugulo-digastric level, the spinal accessory nerve may be involved. With the knowledge of where the lymph node metastases are in the neck, the surgeon can plan what type of neck dissection to carry out. There are many forms of neck dissection depending on which groups of nodes are to be resected (Figure 6.35). Today, most surgeons elect for selective neck dissections rather than the radical neck dissection of the past, which ended up with removal of every structure in the neck, bar the carotid artery. Which dissection is carried out will depend on tumour histology and depth, possibility of lymph node metastases and probably, more importantly, surgical preference. The way in which the N0 neck (i.e. no palpable disease) is managed in the UK will vary considerably from one centre to another. Surgical treatment is not uniform. Imaging must always be geared to the requirements of the treating surgeon or oncologist to allow informed decisions to be made by surgeon, clinician and patient alike.

With this information the surgeon can decide whether or not surgery is feasible and how aggressive or conservative that surgery should be – thus significantly decreasing morbidity without compromising survival. Limited forms of dissection for primary tumours is becoming more popular in conjunction with limited neck dissection for access of free flap reconstruction, (Figures 6.36–6.37).

The goal of imaging is to try and provide the surgeon with the information that allows the correct selection of treatment option, preventing unnecessary and disfiguring treatment which will have no or minimal

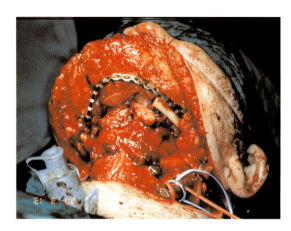

Fig. 6.36 Anterior mandibular resection via an apron flap to the mandible with bilateral functional neck dissections, the bony defect was filled with a free fibular bone graft. Radiology showed there to be lymph node involvement in the right neck only, the left was used for the flap anastamosis.

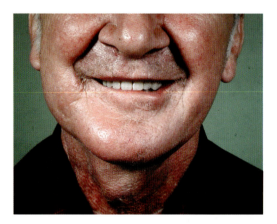

Fig. 6.37 Clinical outcome 1-year post-surgery, note the slight weakness of the mandibular branch of the facial nerve on the right.

impact on survival. A multi-disciplinary team approach is vital for the successful management of head and neck cancer. A radiologist who knows what information is needed for successful patient management will play a pivotal role in such a team.

References

1. Langdon JD and Henk JM. *Malignant Tumour of the Mouth, Jaws and Salivary Glands*, 2nd edition. Edward Arnold. 1995. London.
2. Carlson GW. Surgical anatomy of the neck. *Surg. Clin. N. Am.* 1993; **73**: 837.

3. Mukherji SK and Castillo M. A simplified approach to the spaces of the suprahyoid neck. *Radiol. Clin. N. Am.* 1998; **36**: 761.

4. Som PM and Curtin HD. Fascia and spaces. In: P Som and H Curtin (Eds) *Head and Neck Imaging*, 3rd edition. Mosby, St. Louis. 1996, 738.

5. Mukherji SK, Pilsbury H and Castillo M. Imaging squamous cell carcinoma of the upper aerodigestive tract: What the clinicians need to know. *Radiology* 1997; **205**: 629–646.

6. Mukherji SK, Castelijns J and Castillo M. Squamous cell carcinoma of the oropharynx and oral cavity: How imaging makes a difference. *Semin. Ultrasound CT MRI* 1998; **19**(6): 463–475.

7. Pameijer FA, Balm AJM, Hilgers FJ and Muller SH. Variability of tumour volumes in T3 staged head and neck tumours. *Head Neck* 1997; **19**: 6–13.

8. Johnson CR, Khandelwal SR, Schmidt-Ulrich RK, Ravalese J and Wazer D. The influence of quantitative tumour volume measurements on local control in advanced head and neck cancer using concomitant boost accelerated superfractionated irradiation. *Int. J. Radiat. Oncol. Biol. Phys.* 1995; **32**(3): 635–641.

9. Grabenbauer GG, Steininger H, Meyer M *et al.* Nodal CT density and total tumour volume as prognostic factors after radiation therapy of stage III/IV head and neck cancer. *Radiother. Oncol.* 1998; **47**: 175–183.

10. Rasch C, Kens R, Pameijer FA *et al.* The potential impact of CT/MR matching on tumour volume delineation in advanced head and neck cancer. *Int. J. Radiat. Oncol. Biol. Phys.* 1997; **39**(4): 841–848.

11. Hermans R, Feron M, Bellon E *et al.* Laryngeal tumour volume measurements determined with CT: a study of intra- and inter-observer variability. *Int. J. Radiat. Oncol. Biol. Phys.* 1998; **40**: 535–557.

12. Leslie A, Fyfe E, Guest P, Goddard P and Kaval JE. Staging of squamous cell carcinoma of the oral cavity and oropharynx: A comparison of MRI and CT in T and N staging. *J. Comput. Assist. Tomogr.* 1999; **23**(1): 43–49.

13. Kwa RR, Campana K and Moy RL. Biology of cutaneous squamous cell carcinoma. *J. Am. Acad. Dermatol.* 1992; **26**: 1–26.

14. Brown JS, Lowe D, Kalaverzos N *et al.* Patterns of invasion and routes of tumour entry into the mandible by oral squamous cell carcinoma. *Head Neck* 2002; 370–382.

15. McGregor AD and Macdonald DG. Patterns of spread of squamous cell carcinoma with the mandible. *Head Neck* 1989; **11**: 437.

16. Attwood DA. *J. Prosthet. Dent.* 1963; **13**: 811.

17. Brown JS, Griffith JF, Phelps PD and Browne RM. A comparison of different imaging modalities and direct inspection after periosteal stripping in predicting the invasion of the mandible by oral squamous cell carcinoma. *Br. J. Oral Max. Surg.* 1994; **32**(6): 347–359.

18. Mukherji SK, Weeks S, Castillo M and Krishnan LA. Squamous cell carcinomas that arise in the oral cavity and tongue base: can CT help predict perineural or vascular invasion? *Radiology* 1996; **198**: 157–162.

19. Byers RM, Weber RS, Andrews T, McGill D, Kare R and Wolf P. Frequency and therapeutic implicatons of "skip metastases" in the neck from squamous carcinoma of the oral tongue. *Head Neck* 1997; **19**: 14–19.

20. Cawson R.A. Leukoplakia and oral cancer. *Proc. Roy. Soc. Med.* 1969; **62**: 610–615.

21. Ralzer ER, Schweilzer RJ and Frazell EL. Epidermoid carcinoma of the palate. *Am. J. Surg.* 1970; **119**: 294–297.

22. Hodder SC, Evans RM, Patton DW and Silvester KC. Ultrasound and fine needle aspiration cytology in the staging of neck lymph nodes in oral squamous cell carcinoma. *Br. J. Oral Max. Surg.* 2000; **38**: 430–436.

23. Woolgar JA. Correlation of histopathologic findings with clinical and radiological assessment of cervical lymph node metastasis in oral cancer. *Int. J. Max. Surg.* 1995; **24**: 30–37.

24. Kalins IK, Loeonard AG and Sako K. Correlation between prognosis and degree of lymph node involvement in carcinoma of the oral cavity. *Am. J. Surg.* 1977; **134**: 450–454.

25. Medina JE and Byers RM. Supraomohyoid neck dissection rationale, indications and surgical technique. *Head Neck* 1989; **11**: 111–122.

Larynx and Hypopharynx

EJ Loveday and I Birchall

Clinical presentation

Laryngeal carcinoma is the commonest head and neck malignancy in most parts of the world, and comprises 30–40% of all cases. Incidence varies from 1 : 6000 in parts of Southern Europe to 1 : 12,000 in Scandinavia. There are 2,000–14,000 new cases of laryngeal cancer in the United States per annum [1,2]. Male to female ratio is 10 : 1. Distribution by subsite also varies with the population studied: in the UK, 80% occurs in the true vocal cord region, with 15% above the cords (supraglottis) and 5% below (subglottis [3,4]), with more supraglottic cancers in Southern Europe and South America. In some cases, the exact level of origin cannot be accurately defined, and the term "transglottic" is applied. Aetiological factors are smoking (relative risk 10–100) [2], alcohol consumption (relative risk 2–8) [5], male sex, low socio-economic status [6] and family history. Human papillomavirus type 16 may also be implicated [7].

Field change, as with other forms of head and neck cancer, is partly responsible for the 10% incidence of synchronous primary tumours (most commonly lung, second head and neck primary, bladder and colorectum reported) [1,6]. This must be borne in mind when interpreting images of a known primary, and increases the importance of synchronous chest imaging [8].

Ninety per cent are squamous carcinoma, with lymphoma being the second commonest diagnosis. Histological appearance characteristically includes prickle cells and keratin whorls, while cytokeratin and other immunohistochemical markers have aided diagnosis of poorly differentiated tumours [9]. Some observers have attempted to correlate radiological and histological characteristics, especially for rarer tumours [10]. Differential diagnoses of a mass in the larynx are many and readers are referred to specialist works, such as Ferlito's *Diseases of the Larynx* [11]. In particular, benign diagnoses such as tuberculosis and papillomatosis are important to differentiate as management is quite different from malignancy.

Most laryngeal carcinoma cases present with hoarseness, often of several months' duration. However, any person over the age of 40 who presents with this symptom of 3 weeks or more duration should be considered for urgent referral to an otolaryngology specialist for upper airway examination [12]. Less commonly, laryngeal carcinoma presents with a neck lump, dysphagia, stridor or haemoptysis [12]. Clearly, the co-incidence of such symptoms with risk factors such as smoking, drinking or previous smoking-related cancer increases the clinical suspicion, and these should be mentioned on the radiology referral form. Nonetheless, there is circumstantial evidence that laryngeal cancer may be increasing in persons outside traditional risk groups [13].

Carcinoma of the hypopharynx is more insidious, and commonly presents with a lump in the neck, having already metastasised to local lymph nodes. Indeed, a hypopharyngeal tumour detected radiologically would be expected to be associated with radiological evidence of regional metastasis. Other symptoms are hoarseness (due to involvement of the recurrent laryngeal nerve), dysphagia and weight loss [14]. It has the same aetiological factors as laryngeal carcinoma, but often presents in a more elderly age group. Additionally, women over the age of 65 who have

experienced iron-deficiency anaemia may develop post-cricoid (i.e. that part of the pharynx posterior to the cricoid cartilage) carcinoma as a sequel to the Plummer–Vinson syndrome [15].

Investigation

Endoscopy and biopsy are the primary investigations for laryngeal and hypopharyngeal carcinoma. This remains true despite all recent advances in imaging [16]. However, imaging remains essential for directing endoscopy, clarifying findings, improving staging and detecting metastases and second primaries. Endoscopy, in partnership with radiology, allows confirmation of diagnosis and full clinical staging, in a way not possible in the outpatients alone. Typically, endoscopy is performed under general anaesthesia, using rigid endoscopes. The larynx is best imaged by placing a rigid laryngoscope on suspension

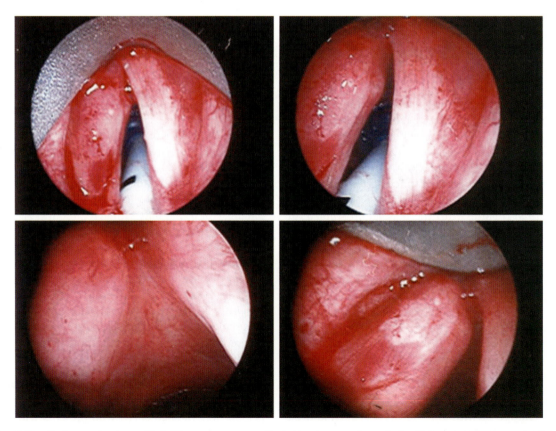

Fig. 7.1 Endoscopic view of left T1a squamous cell glottic cancer, viewed via 0° (top two images, endotracheal tube to rear) and 90° (bottom two images) Hopkins' rods under general anaesthesia. The 90° view is essential for accurate endoscopic staging and biopsy, as significant extension of tumour into the laryngeal ventricles and subglottis may be missed by one-dimensional view.

apparatus to free both of the surgeons hands. The larynx is then examined first with the naked eye, then with rigid telescopes (Hopkins' rods, 0° and 90°, Figure 7.1), and finally, with the microscope. Then, biopsies of all suspicious sites are taken [17].

Evidence is conflicting as to whether it is necessary to perform panendoscopy (to include oesophagus and bronchi) as well, the rationale being that this allows exclusion of synchronous primary tumours in 0.2–10% of patients (depending on population studied). However, radiologists need to be aware of the high incidence of other primaries in patients with head and neck cancer, the commonest site of which varies with population and may be lung (USA), second head and neck primary (Europe), lower GI (Scotland) or bladder (South of England).

Imaging

Not all laryngeal tumours require imaging. Stage I and some small stage II glottic tumours can be safely managed without need for further imaging of the primary tumour [18]. However, some centres still prefer to image all cases as part of registration protocols or trials of new treatments.

Imaging questions

Accurate TNM staging of advanced tumours has the potential to significantly enhance surgical management. In imaging it is important to consider the *site of origin* and *size* of the primary tumour, the degree of *involvement of neighbouring structures* and the *nodal staging*.

Site of origin, size

Accurate determination of *site of origin* is important because the different primary sites have different patterns of spread and staging criteria. For example, hypopharyngeal tumours have a propensity for early soft tissue spread (Figures 7.5 and 7.6) whereas tumours arising from the neighbouring aryepiglottic fold are classified as supraglottic. Another example: vocal cord fixation is of more sinister import when seen with supraglottic than with glottic tumours. The primary site is usually self-evident on endoscopic examination, but may be unclear where the tumour is large (Figure 7.6).

The *size* of the primary tumour is of obvious surgical importance and should be documented accurately for purposes of follow-up. It is possible to calculate tumour volume from CT or MRI data using various algorithms, and numerous studies have shown that pretreatment tumour volume can be used to predict response to either radiotherapy [19–23] or surgery [24].

Involvement of neighbouring structures

The staging and management then depend critically upon the involvement or otherwise of neighbouring structures. The reader should identify and examine the review areas of the larynx (pre-epiglottic space, laryngeal cartilage, paraglottis, vocal folds, laryngeal cartilage, subglottis). Interpretation depends upon understanding the characteristic patterns of spread associated with the different primary sites (see Table 7.2).

Anatomical considerations

The larynx is a complex functional unit. The *laryngeal skeleton* comprises the cricoid cartilage, paired laryngeal cartilages and hyoid bone, bound together by the cricothyroid and thyrohyoid membranes (Figure 7.2). Superficially the strap muscles are attached to the skeleton and control gross movement.

Within the larynx, the arytenoid cartilages are supported upon the posterior cricoid ring and form the posterior attachment of the vocal folds. Between the arytenoid cartilages is the *posterior commissure* (Figures 7.3 and 7.7b). The intrinsic muscles of the larynx control movement of the arytenoid cartilages and vocal folds, the key functions of which are phonation and airway protection. The vocal folds meet anteriorly in the midline at the *anterior commissure*.

Above the vocal folds the endolarynx comprises a mucosal lining beneath which is loose areolar connective tissue containing vessels and lymphatics, and forming the "false cords", parallel to and above the true vocal folds (Figure 7.4). This tissue forms the *paraglottis* or paralaryngeal space, which is deep to the laryngeal cartilage on each side (Figure 7.7a) and continuous anterosuperiorly across the midline with the *pre-epiglottic space*. This horseshoe-shaped

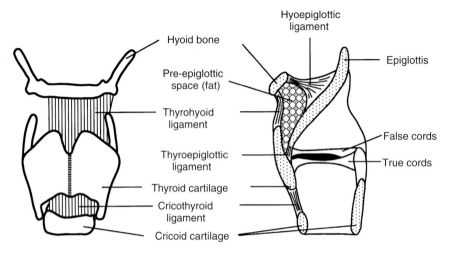

Fig. 7.2 Anterior view and midline sagittal section through the larynx, showing the principal ligaments, true and false cords and pre-epiglottic space.

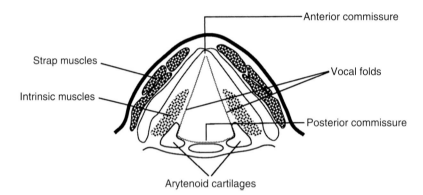

Fig. 7.3 Axial section at the level of the vocal folds.

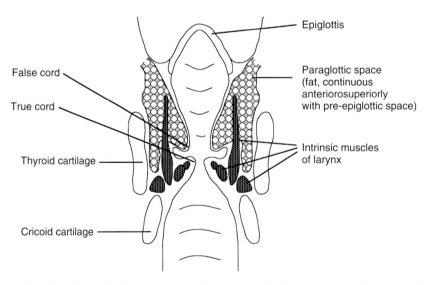

Fig. 7.4 Coronal section through the larynx showing the predominantly muscular composition of the true vocal cords, and the fatty connective tissue of the paraglottis and false cords.

space is bound anteriorly by the thyrohyoid membrane, superiorly by the hyoepiglottic membrane and posteriorly by the epiglottis itself. It is easily identified on all imaging studies due to its high fat content, but very difficult to assess clinically or endoscopically.

The upper free margin of the epiglottis, together with the aryepiglottic folds, define the superior extent of the *supraglottis*. The mucosal surfaces posterior to this margin form the anterior border of the pyriform sinus which together with the postcricoid region and posterior hypopharyngeal wall make up the *hypopharynx*. The *glottis* is comprised solely of the vocal folds with the anterior and posterior commisures, and, by convention, the 5 mm either side of the free edge, whereas the *subglottis* extends from the undersurface of the vocal folds to the inferior margin of the cricoid cartilage. *Transglottic* is a descriptive term usually used to describe tumours involving the glottis and supraglottis, with or without the subglottis, and should properly be used only when the initial site of origin is unclear Figures 7.5 and 7.6.

Tissue characteristics

The *hyoid bone* is invariably densely calcified and has a predictable appearance on all imaging studies. The *epiglottis* is made up of *elastic cartilage* and similarly presents a uniform appearance on both CT and MR imaging. The *thyroid and cricoid cartilages*, by contrast, are composed of *hyaline cartilage*, which may ossify to a variable degree and hence the appearance of these structures may vary considerably from one individual to another (Table 7.1).

Ossifying laryngeal cartilage frequently develops a marrow; although this is potentially confusing, the characteristic appearance of the marrow space facilitates the detection of tumour invasion particularly with MR imaging. The same is true of the paraglottis and pre-epiglottic space which similarly have a high fatty content, resulting in increased signal on T1-weighted (T1W) MR imaging and decreased attenuation on CT [25].

The *vocal folds* are easily distinguished from the normal false cord and paraglottis because they are mainly composed of muscle, which has clearly different signal and attenuation characteristics to the fatty connective tissue of the paraglottis and false cords.

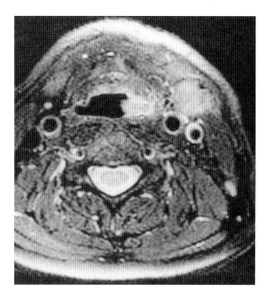

Fig. 7.5 Axial MR image (T2W FSE with fat saturation). Tumour of the left pyriform sinus with lymph node metastasis. Note characteristic obliteration of the air of the pyriform sinus and high conspicuity of the tumour on this pulse sequence. High signal extends towards the carotid sheath; this could be due to tumour or peritumoural oedema and/or inflammation. There is an adjacent metastatic lymph node with oedema of the surrounding subcutaneous fat and skin, seen as thickening with increased signal.

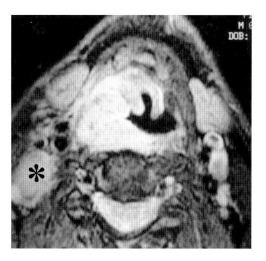

Fig. 7.6 Axial MR image (T2W FSE with fat saturation). Large right-sided tumour returning conspicuous high signal. Probable site of origin is the pyriform fossa. The tumour crosses the midline and displaces the epiglottis to the left. There is lateral soft tissue extension towards, and displacement of, the carotid vessels, and a large lymph node metastasis (asterisk).

Table 7.1 Attenuation and signal characteristics of tissues found in and around the larynx.

Tissue	CT attenuation	MR signal
Cortical bone, calcifications	High	Low
Marrow fat	Low	High
Pre-epiglottic space, paraglottis (fat)	Low	High
Noncalcified hyaline cartilage	Soft tissue	Intermediate
Muscle	Soft tissue	Intermediate/low
Air	Very low	Very low

Laryngeal *tumours* on CT are typically of soft-tissue attenuation and enhance with intravenous contrast media. Tumour tissue generally has a high unbound water content and hence has high intrinsic contrast on T2-weighted (T2W) MR imaging, particularly, if sequences are chosen which suppress signal from fat. As with CT, enhancement is usually seen following intravenous contrast media. Peritumoural oedema, however, may also display contrast enhancement, which may make it difficult to accurately define tumour margins and size.

Imaging strategy

Search pattern
Imaging should be geared to answering the key imaging questions above and may need to be tailored to the individual patient.

The search pattern should generally commence with the identification of normal anatomic landmarks, followed by the localization and description of the tumour if any. This should be followed by inspection of the review areas of the larynx.

In the *subglottis* only a mucosal layer should be seen; any soft tissue thickening is abnormal and likely to represent tumour. The same is true of the *posterior commissure*, whilst the *anterior commissure* should be no more than 2 mm thick [26].

The *vocal folds, false cords* and *cricoarytenoid joints* should be inspected for symmetry of position and signal/attenuation. The *paraglottis* and *pre-epiglottic space* should similarly be assessed for symmetry, and for the normal fatty tissue signal or attenuation (Figure 7.7a)

The *laryngeal cartilage* must be closely examined for evidence of invasion, which may be subtle if, for example, a supraglottic tumour involves the superior cornu. Replacement of the normal marrow signal or attenuation is the most reliable sign (Figure 7.8a); sclerosis may be seen on CT but is equally likely to be due to peritumoural inflammation as to tumour invasion [27].

The *aryepiglottic folds* and *pyriform sinuses* require identification and careful inspection.

The characteristic patterns of spread vary according to the primary site of the tumour, and the areas mentioned in Table 7.2 should, therefore, be systematically evaluated for tumour involvement.

The usual *nodal groups* should be inspected with particular attention to retropharyngeal adenopathy in the case of hypopharyngeal tumours of the posterior pharyngeal wall. Any *other imaging* may be reviewed; it is important to ensure that there has been a recent chest radiograph.

CT and MRI: choice of technique
Both CT and MRI perform well in imaging the larynx [28] and hypopharynx [29]. MR is generally preferred but may be poor in restless/breathless patients, and is contraindicated in some individuals. MR tends to overestimate cartilage invasion resulting in high sensitivity and lower specificity. It follows, however, that cartilage that returns a normal signal on MR is highly likely to be normal, which may be of particular value when planning conservative surgery. CT by contrast tends to underestimate cartilage invasion resulting in higher specificity. With CT small foci of mucosal tumour may be difficult to detect; with both modalities inflammatory and oedematous change may cause overestimation of tumour extent.

Helical CT has clear advantages over single-slice methods [30], including reduced motion artefact,

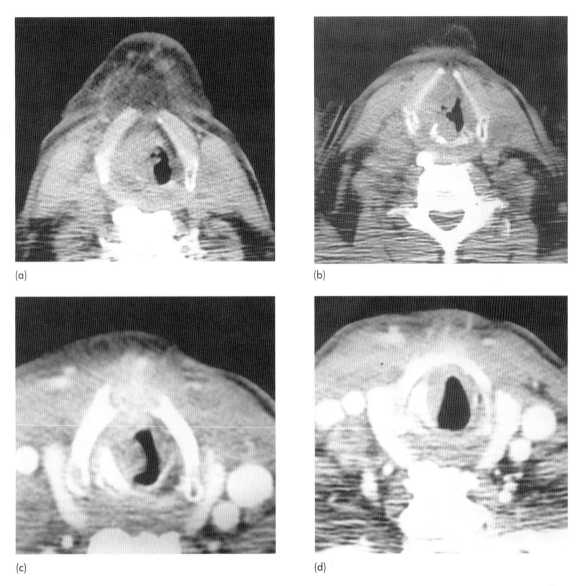

(a)

(b)

(c)

(d)

Fig. 7.7 Axial CT scans, 5.5 mm slice width. Bulky right-sided transglottic tumour demonstrating different aspects of spread: (a)–(d) are ordered from cranial to caudal; (a) and (b) are without intravenous contrast, (c) and (d) are with. (a) This demonstrates normal low attenuation paraglottic fat on the left, and replacement of paraglottic fat by tumour on the right. The air column is displaced to the left. (b) It shows tumour involving the anterior and posterior commissures. The calcified right arytenoid cartilage is displaced medially, indicating disruption of the cricoarytenoid joint. (c) There is invasion of the laryngeal cartilage anteriorly in the midline with extralaryngeal spread. Note the contrast enhancement of the tumour. (d) At the level of the cricoid cartilage subglottic spread is evident.

and improved Z-axis resolution and better multiplanar, 3D and virtual endoscopic views [31].

Each modality has its merits (Table 7.3) but since both provide acceptable results, the choice in practice may depend on other factors such as local availability,

scanning times or cost. Typical scanning protocols are listed below (Table 7.4).

Ultrasound

Ultrasound with ultrasound-guided FNA may be used in nodal staging (see elsewhere in this text).

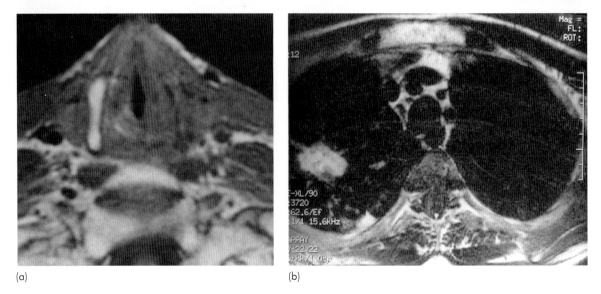

(a)   (b)

Fig. 7.8   Patient with recurrent glottic tumour. (a) Axial MR image (T1W FSE)/recurrent tumour within the left hemilarynx is seen with slight asymmetry of the air column. On the right side the marrow of the laryngeal cartilage returns normal high signal, seen here as a bright stripe. On the left this feature is absent, indicating that the cartilage has been invaded by tumour. (b) Axial MR image (T2W FSE). There is a synchronous tumour in the right lung apex.

Table 7.2   Patterns of spread by primary site.

Primary site and subsite	Look for involvement of
Supraglottic tumours	
Epiglottis	Pre-epiglottic space
Epiglottic petiole	Anterior commissure
Intralaryngeal mucosa,	Paraglottic space
false cords	Vocal fold
All	Laryngeal cartilage
Glottic tumours	
Anterior cord	Anterior commissure/contralateral cord
Posterior cord	Thyroid cartilage (Figure 7.7c) and cricothyroid membrane
All	Arytenoid cartilage/cricoarytenoid (Joint)
	posterior commissure
	Paraglottic space
	Supraglottic/subglottic spread (Figure 7.7d)
Subglottic tumours	Trachea
	Thyroid gland
	Cervical oesophagus
Hypopharyngeal tumours	
Pyriform sinus, lateral wall	Lateral soft tissues including carotid artery
Pyriform sinus, medial wall	Laryngeal cartilage (posterior aspect and superior cornua)
Posterior pharyngeal wall	Spreading involvement of oropharynx
Postcricoid	Submucosal and circumferential spread may be difficult to detect radiologically
All	Neck vessels, particularly the jugular vein
	Lymph nodes
	Thyroid cartilage

Table 7.3   Major pros and cons of CT and MRI.

Advantages	Disadvantages
CT	
Speed reduces motion artefact in breathless patients	Radiation dose
Good spatial resolution	
MRI	
Inherent tissue contrast	Movement artefact especially in breathless patients
Multiplanar imaging	
Coverage of nodal areas in coronal plane	May be contraindicated in some individuals
	Claustrophobia

Table 7.4   Scanning technique.

Typical CT technique	Typical MR technique
Patient supine, hyperextended neck, quiet nasal respiration	Patient supine, hyperextended neck, quiet nasal respiration
	Neck coil
Axial scans parallel to vocal folds	Axial scans parallel to vocal folds: T1W FSE, T2W FSE with fat saturation sequence
Helical scans, 2–2.5 mm collimated slice width	Coronal scans: T1W FSE and STIR (*)
Precontrast	Slice width 4 mm or less
Repeat sequence 30 s postcontrast (vascular anatomy)	
Optional	
Delayed post-contrast scans at 1–2 min	*Post-contrast scans*
Scans with phonation (better visualization of laryngeal ventricle and aryepiglottic fold)	(*FSE = fast spin echo; STIR = short tau inversion recovery)
Modified Valsalva: dilation of hypopharynx giving better evaluation of pyriform sinuses and postcricoid region	

Within the larynx itself excellent depiction of the pre-epiglottic space is possible, and to a lesser degree of the laryngeal cartilages, paraglottis and vocal fold movement [32,33]. Depiction of more posteriorly situated structures (arytenoid cartilage, aryepiglottic folds and pyriform fossa) is insufficiently reliable, however, to justify its routine use in staging primary laryngeal tumours.

PET

Positron emission tomography (PET) using 2-(F18) fluoro-2-deoxy-D-glucose (FDG), the so called FDG-PET can be used to evaluate laryngeal tumours [34]. This method relies upon detecting increased metabolic activity in tumour cells compared with normal tissue or mature scar tissue. It follows that increasing histological tumour grade is associated with greater uptake of FDG [35]. Spatial resolution is very low compared with other methods. PET may be useful for detection of recurrent tumour, and in initial studies has shown great promise in distinguishing tumour recurrence from postirradiation change [36–38]. Cross-sectional PET images may be matched or registered with CT or MRI images acquired in a standardised way. The superimposed images may then demonstrate where the recurrence is in relation to anatomical landmarks.

Other imaging considerations

Patients with squamous laryngeal cancers are almost invariably lifelong smokers with a high incidence of respiratory co-morbidity. A chest radiograph should form part of the routine assessment therefore. Many if not most have poor dentition, which may interfere with post-treatment swallowing and speech rehabilitation even where the teeth are not included in the radiotherapy field. An orthopantomogram (OPG) may be useful in this circumstance.

The incidence of synchronous pulmonary tumours detected by CT in patients presenting with head and neck cancers may be as high as 17% [39] (Figure 7.8b), and even higher in patients with neck node metastases [8]. In patients being staged by CT it may be tempting to include chest CT as part of the workup [39,40], since with modern equipment this adds only minutes to the total scanning time. Although UK national standards prescribe chest CT for all these patients [41], published opinion on this is conflicting [42,43], and the data for patients specifically with laryngeal cancer is limited.

Nonsquamous tumours

The great majority of laryngeal tumours are squamous carcinomas, and are readily diagnosed clinically with endoscopy and biopsy. Many nonsquamous tumours, conversely, do not involve the laryngeal mucosa and may present as a submucosal swelling or neck lump. Non-invasive imaging has a more central rôle in this situation, and fortunately many of these lesions have characteristic appearances which allow a confident diagnosis to be made [44–46] (Table 7.5).

Adenocarcinoma, adenoid cystic carcinoma and mucoepidermoid carcinoma may be indistinguishable from squamous cell carcinoma on imaging alone. Papillary carcinoma of the thyroid may arise within a thyroglossal cyst and present as a supraglottic mass in the pre-epiglottic space.

Post-treatment imaging

There are many surgical approaches to the management of laryngeal cancers, a detailed discussion of which is beyond the scope of this section [44,45,47]. Suffice to say that a close working partnership between radiologist and surgeon is an essential prerequisite in the post-treatment evaluation of these patients.

Following external beam radiation therapy a reduction in tumour volume of at least 50% can be expected by 4 months. The high doses used may lead to persistent oedema and fibrosis with thickening of glottic and supraglottic structures. Pre-epiglottic and paraglottic fat may lose its characteristic low attenuation/high T1W signal character and there may be persistent abnormal enhancement of mucosal surfaces. The detection of tumour recurrence in these circumstances, therefore, poses a considerable challenge; the radiologist may have to rely on the detection of focal masses or evidence of invasive behaviour in order to make a confident diagnosis. Co-localised PET may provide the answer here, as detailed above.

Management

Appropriate imaging as described above is a prerequisite for accurate treatment planning in most forms of laryngeal and hypopharyngeal cancer. It allows staging to progress from a certainty factor of C1 (clinical examination only, TNM staging system) to C2 (specialist diagnostic information). Subsequently,

Table 7.5 Imaging characteristics of some nonsquamous tumours.

Tumour	CT appearance	MR appearance
Chondroma/chondrosarcoma	Coarse or stippled calcifications	High signal (T2W) ± signal voids (calcifications)
Vascular tumours	Homogenous soft tissue Intense enhancement Phleboliths (diagnostic)	Homogenous high signal (T2W) Intense enhancement
Haemangioma Paraganglionoma		Conspicuous curvilinear signal voids
Lipoma	Low attenuation	High signal (T1W)

management is multidisciplinary, involving otolaryngologists and radiotherapists with a special interest in head and neck cancer, speech and language therapists, dieticians, specialist liaison nurses and others. Paramedical and psychological support is as important to outcome as the primary mode of therapy, especially since, for advanced disease, most of the improvements seen in recent decades have been in quality of life and rehabilitation rather than 5-year survival rates [48].

Curative intent

A recent Cochrane review [49] shows that the treatment of stage I/II tumours depends on which country one is treated in. Thus, in the UK and much of the USA, small field radiotherapy would be used (Figure 7.9) whilst in Europe peroral endoscopic laser or "cold steel" excision is preferred. Both seem to have comparable results based on case series and one randomised trial [50] but definitive trials, currently in the planning stage are needed.

Stage III tumours receive either surgery or radiotherapy, based on location and desire to preserve laryngeal function. Stage IV tumours receive surgery or combined treatment. For locally advanced cancers, total laryngectomy or total laryngo-pharyngectomy are the only surgical options. These lead to significant impairment of quality of life, although good specialist multidisciplinary intervention and the

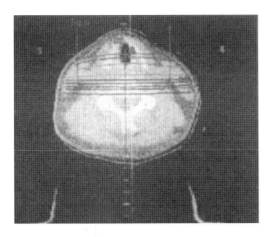
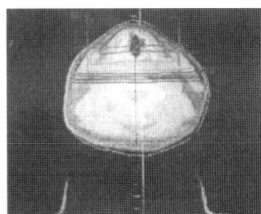
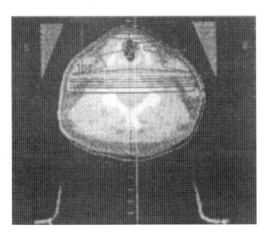
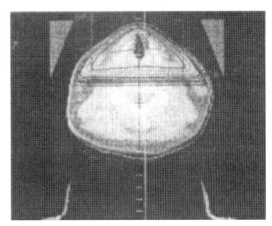

Fig. 7.9 Scans of early glottic cancer used for radiotherapy treatment planning. The triangles represent "wedges" used to prevent overdosing by overlapping of fields from opposite directions and to protect vulnerable areas, particularly the spinal cord. Each image gives isodose fields for different treatment regimens to allow comparison.

introduction of voice valves [51] have caused significant improvements.

Induction chemotherapy and synchronous chemoradiotherapy are also presently the subject of "organ-preservation" trials [52] designed to avoid the mutilation of laryngectomy. Otherwise, there is presently no good evidence for the routine use of chemotherapy with curative intent in laryngeal or hypopharyngeal cancer.

Stage	Larynx	Hypopharynx
I	Small field radiotherapy OR laser excision	Small field radiotherapy OR laser excision
II	Small field radiotherapy OR laser excision	Small field radiotherapy OR laser excision
III	Radiotherapy OR surgery (partial or total laryngectomy)	Radiotherapy OR surgery (pharyngectomy ± total laryngectomy and reconstruction)
IV	Total laryngectomy ± post-operative radiotherapy	Total laryngopharyngectomy, jejunal free flap reconstruction, postoperative radiotherapy

Palliative intent

There may be some role for chemotherapy in this setting, although radiotherapy forms the mainstay, allied to good supportive care and symptom control. Palliative care needs to take into account the possibility of airway obstruction or bleeding from neck vessels, though, in practice, such terminal events are thankfully uncommon [53].

References

1. Berg JW, Schottenfeld D and Ritter F. Incidence of multiple primary cancers. III. Cancers of the respiratory and upper digestive system as multiple primary cancers. *J. Natl. Cancer Inst.* 1970; **44**(2): 263–274.
2. Devaney KO. Pathology of malignant laryngeal tumours. In: Ferlito A (Ed.) *Diseases of the Larynx.* Arnold, London. 2000, 541–549.
3. Virtaniemi JA, Hirvikoski PP, Kumpulainen EJ, Johansson RT, Pukkala E and Kosma VM. Is the subsite distribution of laryngeal cancer related to smoking habits? *Acta Oncol.* 2000; **39**(1): 77–79

4. Cattaruzza MS, Maisonneuve P and Boyle P. Epidemiology of laryngeal cancer. *Eur. J. Cancer B Oral. Oncol.* 1996; **32B**(5): 293–305.
5. Thomas DB. Alcohol as a cause of cancer. *Environ. Health Perspect.* 1995; **103** (suppl 8): 153–160.
6. Thorne P, Etherington D and Birchall MA. Head and Neck Cancer in the South West of England: influence of socioeconomic status. *Eur. J. Surg. Oncol.* 1998; **23**: 503–508.
7. Rees L, Birchall MA and Thomas SJ. A systematic review of case control studies of human papilloma virus infection in squamous cell carcinoma of the larynx. *The First European Conference on Head and Neck Cancer*, Lille, November 16–17, 2001.
8. Houghton DJ, Hughes ML, Garvey C, Beasley NJ, Hamilton JW, Gerlinger I and Jones AS. Role of chest CT scanning in the management of patients presenting with head and neck cancer. *Head Neck* 1998; **20**(7): 614–618.
9. Listron MB and Dalton LW. Comparison of keratin monoclonal antibodies. *Am. J. Clin. Pathol.* 1987; **88**: 297–301.
10. Becker M, Moulin G, Kurt AM, Zbaren P, Dulgerov P, Marchal F, Zanaret P, Lehmann W, Rufenacht DA and Terrier F. Atypical squamous cell carcinoma of the larynx and hypopharynx: radiologic features and pathologic correlation. *Eur. J. Radiol.* 1998; **8**(9): 1541–1551.
11. Ferlito A (Ed.) *Diseases of the Larynx.* Arnold, London. 2000.
12. Department of Health Guidance Document HSC 2000/13 – Referral Guidelines for Suspected Cancer DoH, London. 2000.
13. Birchall MA and Bailey D. *SWAHN II: Head and Neck Cancer Management in the South and West of England, Quantity and Quality.* Cancer Intelligence Unit, Winchester, 2001.
14. Wight RG, Birchall MA, Stafford ND and Stanbridge RL. Management of hypopharyngeal carcinoma: a 6-year review. *J. R. Soc. Med.* 1992; **85**(9): 545–547.
15. Hoffman RM and Jaffe PE. Plummer–Vinson syndrome. A case report and literature review. *Arch. Intern. Med.* 1995; **155**(18): 2008–2011. Review.
16. Phelps PD. Carcinoma of the larynx – the role of imaging in staging and pre-treatment assessments. *Clin Radiol.* 1992; **46**(2): 77–83.
17. Benjamin B. Technique of Laryngoscopy. *Int. J. Pediatr. Otorhinolaryngol.* 1987; **13**(3): 299–313.
18. Curtin HD. Larynx. In: Som PM and Curtin HD (Eds.) *Head and Neck Imaging* 3rd edition Mosby, St. Louis. 1996, 612–707.
19. Hermans R, Van den Bogaert W, Rijnders A and Baert AL. Value of computed tomography as outcome predictor of supraglottic squamous cell carcinoma treated by definitive radiation therapy. *Int. J. Radiat. Oncol. Biol. Phys.* 1999; **44**: 755–765.
20. Hermans R, Van den Bogaert W, Rijnders A, Doornaert P and Baert AL. Predicting the local outcome of glottic squamous cell carcinoma after definitive radiation therapy: value of computed tomography-determined tumour parameters. *Radiother. Oncol.* 1999; **50**: 39–46.
21. Parmeijer FA, Hermans R, Mancuso AA et al. Pre- and post-radiotherapy computed tomography in laryngeal cancer: imaging-based prediction of local failure. *Int. J. Radiat. Oncol. Biol. Phys.* 1999; **45**: 359–366.
22. Mancuso AA, Mukherji SK, Schmalfuss I et al. Preradiotherapy computed tomography as a predictor of local control in supraglottic carcinoma. *J. Clin. Oncol.* 1999; **17**: 631–637.
23. Lo SM, Venkatesan V, Matthews TW and Rogers J. Tumour volume: implications in T2/T3 glottic/supraglottic squamous cell carcinoma. *J. Otolaryngol.* 1998; **27**: 247–251.
24. Mukherji SK, O'Brien SM, Gerstle RJ, Weissler M, Shockley W and Castillo M. Tumour volume: an independent predictor of outcome for laryngeal cancer. *J. Comput. Assis. Tomogr.* 1999; **23**: 50–54.

25. Sakai F, Gamsu G, Dillon WP, Lynch DA and Gilbert TJ. MR imaging of the Larynx at 1.5T. *J. Comput. Assist. Tomogr.* 1990; **14**: 60–71.

26. Kallmes DF and Phillips CD. The normal anterior commissure of the glottis. *AJR* 1997; **168**: 1317–1319.

27. Becker M, Zbären P, Delavelle J et al. Neoplastic invasion of the laryngeal cartilage: reassessment of criteria for diagnosis at CT. *Radiology* 1997; **203**: 521–532.

28. Zbären P, Becker M and Läng H. Pretherapeutic staging of laryngeal carcinoma. *Cancer* 1996; **77**: 1263–1273.

29. Zbären P, Becker M and Läng H. Pretherapeutic staging of hypopharyngeal carcinoma. *Arch. Otolaryngol. Head Neck Surg.* 1997; **123**: 908–913.

30. Korkmaz H, Cerezci NG, Akmansu H and Dursun E. A comparison of spiral and conventional computerized tomography methods in diagnosing various laryngeal lesions. *Eur. Arch. Otorhinolaryngol.* 1998; **255**: 149–154.

31. Rodenwaldt J, Kopka L, Roedel R, Margas A and Grabbe E. 3D virtual endoscopy of the upper airway: optimization of the scan parameters in a cadaver phantom and clinical assessment. *J. Comput. Assist. Tomogr.* 1997; **21**: 405–411.

32. Loveday EJ, Bleach NR, Van Hasselt CA and Metreweli C. Ultrasound imaging in laryngeal cancer: a preliminary study. *Clin Radiol* 1994; **49**: 676–682.

33. Loveday E. The larynx. In: Ahuja AT and Evans RM (Eds.) *Practical Head and Neck Ultrasound.* Greenwich Medical Media, London. 2000, 107–120.

34. Lowe VJ, Kim H, Boyd JH, Eisenbeis JF, Dunphy FR and Fletcher JW. Primary and recurrent early stage laryngeal cancer: preliminary results of 2-(fluorine 18)fluoro-2-deoxy-D-glucose PET imaging. *Radiology* 1999; **212**: 799–802.

35. Slevin NJ, Collins CD, Hastings DL et al. The diagnostic value of positron emission tomography (PET) with radiolabelled fluorodeoxyglucose (18F-FDG) in head and neck cancer. *J. Laryngol. Otol.* 1999; **113**: 548–554.

36. Stokkel MP, Terhaard CH, Hordijk GJ and van-Rijk PP. The detection of local recurrent head and neck cancer with fluorine-18 fluorodeoxyglucose dual-head positron emission tomography. *Eur. J. Nucl. Med.* 1999; **26**: 767–773.

37. Greven KM, Williams DW, Keyes JW, McGuirt WF, Watson NE and Case LD. Can positron emission tomography distinguish tumor recurrence from irradiation sequelae in patients treated for larynx cancer? *Cancer J. Sci. Am.* 1997; **3**: 353–357.

38. McGuirt WF, Greven KM, Keyes JW, Williams DW and Watson N. Laryngeal radionecrosis versus recurrent cancer: a clinical approach. *Ann. Otol. Rhinol. Laryngol.* 1998; **107**: 293–296.

39. Houghton DJ, McGarry G, Stewart I, Wilson JA and MacKenzie K. Chest computerized tomography scanning in patients presenting with head and neck cancer. *Clin. Otolaryngol.* 1998; **23**: 348–350.

40. Halpern J. The value of chest CT scan in the work-up of head and neck cancers. *J. Med.* 1997; **28**: 191–198.

41. Wilson JA (Ed.). *Effective Head and Neck Cancer Management. Consensus Document*, 2nd edition. British Association of Otorhinolaryngologists, Head and Neck Surgeons, London. 2000.

42. Nilssen EL, Murthy P, McClymont L and Denholm S. Radiological staging of the chest and abdomen in head and neck squamous cell carcinoma – are computed tomography and ultrasound necessary? *J. Laryngol. Otol.* 1999; **113**: 152–154.

43. Tan L, Greener CC, Seikaly H, Rassekh CH and Calhoun KH. Role of screening chest computed tomography in patients with advanced head and neck cancer. *Otolaryngol. Head Neck Surg.* 1999; **120**: 689–692.

44. Becker M. Larynx and Hypopharynx. *Radiol. Clin. N. Am.* 1998; **36**: 891–920.

45. Becker M, Moulin G, Kurt AM et al. Non-squamous cell neoplasms of the larynx: radiologic–pathologic correlation. *Radiographics* 1998; **18**: 1189–1209.

46. De Foer B, Hermans R, Van der Goten A, Delaere PR and Baert AL. Imaging features in 35 cases of submucosal laryngeal mass lesions. *Eur. Radiol.* 1996; **6**: 913–919.

47. Castelijns JA, Hermans R, van den Brekel MWM and Mukherji SK. Imaging of laryngeal cancer. *Semin. Ultrasound CT MR* 1998; **19**: 492–504.

48. Groome PA, O'Sullivan B, Irish JC et al. Glottic cancer in Ontario, Canada and the SEER areas of the United States: do different management philosophies produce different outcome profiles? *J. Clin. Epidemol.* 2001; **54**: 301–315.

49. Dey P, Arnold D, Wight R, MacKenzie K, Kelly C and Wilson J. Radiotherapy versus open surgery versus endolaryngeal surgery (with or without laser) for early laryngeal squamous cell cancer. Systematic Review. Cochrane Database Review, March 2002.

50. Ogoltsova ES, Paches AI, Matyakin EG et al. Comparative evaluation of the efficacy of radiotherapy, surgery and combined treatment of stage I–II laryngeal cancer (T1–2N0M0) on the basis of co-operative studies. *J. Otorhinolaryngol.* (Moscow) 1990; **3**: 3–7.

51. Singer MI and Blom ED. An endoscopic technique for restoration of voice after laryngectomy. *Ann. Otol. Rhinol. Laryngol.* 1980; **89**: (6 Pt 1): 529–533.

52. Nishioka T, Shirato H, Fukuda S, Arimoto T, Kamada T, Furuta Y, Nishino S, Hosokawa Y, Kitahara T, Kagei K, Inuyama Y and Miyasaka K. A phase II study of concomitant chemoradiotherapy for laryngeal carcinoma using carboplatin. *Oncology* 1999; **56**(1): 36–42.

53. Forbes K. Palliative care in patients with cancer of the head and neck. *Clin Otolaryngol.* 1997; **22**(2): 117–122.

Oesophageal Carcinoma

JF Griffith and ACW Chan

Introduction

Oesophageal carcinoma is relevant to imaging of head and neck tumours in three respects:

(a) The cervical oesophagus is not an uncommon site of primary oesophageal tumours.
(b) Cervical or thoracic oesophageal tumours frequently metastasise to the neck lymph nodes.
(c) Synchronous tumours can occur in the cervical oesophagus with a second primary tumour elsewhere in the head or neck or thoracic oesophagus.

This chapter deals in turn with each of these three aspects.

> **Key points**
> - Primary tumours not uncommonly arise in the cervical oesophagus
> - Synchronous head and neck tumours not uncommonly involve the cervical oesophagus

> - Cervical or thoracic oesophageal tumours commonly metastasise to neck nodes

Cervical oesophageal carcinoma
Background

Both the diagnosis and staging of oesophageal carcinoma has changed considerably over the past two decades. In the 1970s, oesophageal carcinoma was investigated solely by barium studies supplemented, if necessary, by rigid oesophagoscopy. Accurate staging with respect to perioesophageal spread and regional metastases was only possible at the time of exploratory surgery. This led to surgery being performed for tumours too advanced for curative resection. There was little opportunity for tailoring different treatments according to tumour extent and making objective comparisons of different

Table 8.1 Conventional divisions of the oesophagus.

Cervical	Lower border of cricopharyngeus to sternal notch
Upper thoracic	Sternal notch to carina
Mid-thoracic	Carina to midway to gastro-oesophageal junction
Lower thoracic	Midway to gastro-oesophageal junction to gastro-oesophageal junction

treatment protocols. This situation has changed significantly following the emergence of flexible oesophagoscopy, computed tomography (CT), high-resolution percutaneous and endoscopic ultrasound (EUS), thoracoscopy and laparoscopy.

Key points

- The staging of oesophageal carcinoma has improved dramatically over the past two decades

Relevant anatomy

The oesophagus extends from the lower border of the cricopharyngeus muscle (at the level of C6) to the gastro-oesophageal junction (about 1 cm below the oesophageal diaphragmatic hiatus). For descriptive purposes, it is convenient to arbitrarily divide the oesophagus into five regions: the cervical oesophagus, the upper-, mid- and lower-thoracic oesophagus and the gastro-esphageal junction (Table 8.1).

The oesophagus is composed of a stratified squamous mucosa, a lamina propria, a submucosa, an inner circular and an outer longitudinal muscle layer. It does not possess a serosa. A dense meshwork of lymphatics surrounds the oesophagus, which connects perioesophageal nodes to the mediastinal nodes, the neck nodes and the upper abdominal nodes.

Key points

- The oesophagus does not possess a serosa.
- It is surrounded by a dense mesh of lymphatics

Location of oesophageal carcinomas

Less than 10% of oesophageal carcinoma involves the cervical oesophagus [1,2], a prevalence that seems to be fairly consistent throughout the world. The incidence of non-cervical oesophageal carcinoma varies considerably. In the East, only about 15% of oesophageal carcinomas involve the gastro-oesophageal junction [2]; while in the West, about 65% of oesophageal carcinomas involve the gastro-oesophageal junction [3,4].

Key points

- Less than 10% of oesophageal carcinoma arise within the cervical oesophagus

Histology of oesophageal carcinoma

Nearly all tumours arising within the cervical or thoracic oesophagus are squamous in origin. Tumours arising at or close to the gastro-oesophageal junction are adenocarcinoma in type. Over the past two decades, there has been a declining or static incidence of squamous cell carcinoma, while that of adenocarcinoma is rising. Regardless of cell type, oesophageal cancer is a disease of the middle-aged or elderly with a moderate male predominance. Tobacco and alcohol consumption are recognised risk factors for squamous oesophageal carcinoma.

Key points

- Cervical oesophageal tumours are squamous in type

Spread of oesophageal carcinoma

Oesophageal carcinoma, as per definition, arises in the epithelium from where it spreads progressively through the walls of the oesophagus (T1/T2), to the perioesophageal fat (T3) to invade adjacent structures (T4) (Table 8.2). The significance of spread to adjacent structures depends heavily on whether the

Table 8.2 Staging of oesophageal carcinoma.

T0 – carcinoma *in situ*
T1 – submucosal invasion
T2 – muscle invasion
T3 – perioesophageal fat invasion
T4 – adjacent organ invasion
Tx – unknown stage
N0 – no nodal metastases
N1 – local nodal metastases
M0 – no distal metastases
M1 – distal nodal or non-nodal metastases

invaded structure can be surgically resected or not. For example, if involved, the thyroid could be resected along with a primary cervical oesophageal carcinoma, though the same may not be true for the common carotid artery or brachial plexus. Tumours of the upper cervical oesophagus may spread vertically across the cricopharyngeus to involve the hypopharynx. If this is the case or if the proximal border of the tumour is too close to the hypopharynx to allow a clear dissection margin, then much more extensive surgery (e.g. pharyngolaryngo-oesophagectomy (PLO) rather than oesophagectomy) may be required [1]. Squamous oesophageal carcinoma spreads early to regional nodes with 50% of T1/2 tumours and 70% of T3/4 tumours reported to have nodal metastases evident at operation [5]. Metastases to the neck nodes are found in 30% of cases undergoing surgical neck dissection [6,7].

Key points

• Cervical oesophageal tumours may spread horizontally to adjacent structures in the neck or vertically to the hypopharynx
• Oesophageal tumours metastasise early to the extensive lymphatic meshwork surrounding the oesophagus

Imaging modalities currently used to diagnose oesophageal carcinoma

Endoscopy

"Ignore dysphagia at your peril" is a wise dictum, especially in the middle-aged or elderly. Endoscopy is a very effective means of diagnosing oesophageal carcinoma and should be the first line investigation in patients with dysphagia. It allows a direct inspection of the oesophageal mucosa and enables suspicious areas to be biopsied. The location and length of tumours are assessed relative to the incisors. Nowadays, endoscopy can be performed with little or no sedation. Very early tumours, i.e. carcinoma *in situ* or epithelium dysplasia can be revealed by spraying Lugol's iodine onto the mucosa. Non-stained mucosa indicates dysplastic epithelium, which can be biopsied for histological confirmation. This dye technique is, particularly, important when endoscopy is performed for surveillance of synchronous or metachronous oesophageal cancers in high-risk patients, such as those with the concurrent head and neck cancers.

Key points

• Lugol's dye technique is useful at detecting early oesophageal carcinomas

Double-contrast barium oesophagography ("barium swallow")

Double-contrast barium oesophagography is a sensitive test for the diagnosis of oesophageal carcinoma, allowing a clear delineation of the mucosal extent of the tumour (Figure 8.1). Barium studies are disadvantageous in three respects. First, the sensitivity and specificity of diagnosing early oesophageal carcinoma is slightly less than endoscopy. Second, barium aspiration may potentially occur in patients with severe swallowing difficulty. Third, barium, as it passes through the bowel, may impede the quality of a staging thoraco-abdominal CT examination, if performed within 1 week of the barium examination. Barium studies are, particularly, useful in those patients with clinically suspected oesophageal motility disorders.

Key points

• Barium studies are useful at investigating motility disorders of the oesophagus

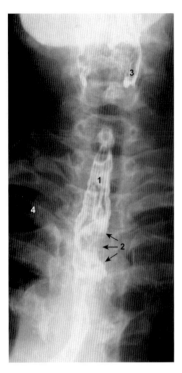

Fig. 8.1 Barium swallow examination: 1. cervical oesophagus, 2. filling defect indicating tumour of lower cervical oesophagus, 3. left pyriform fossa and 4. right clavicle.

Staging of oesophageal carcinoma

Tumour staging involves determining the extent (i.e. spread) of the tumour both locally and systemically. As it is an expensive and time-consuming practice, one should be able to justify tumour staging in terms of improved management and patient care.

Pre-treatment staging of oesophageal carcinoma is currently justified in that it allows

(i) allocation of patients to appropriate treatment regimes, i.e. palliative or curative intent;
(ii) individualisation of tumour treatment, e.g. radiation therapy fields can be tailored precisely to the tumour margins allowing administration of larger does of radiotherapy (up to 60 Gy) to tighter fields without increase in morbidity;
(iii) a more informed prediction of prognosis and
(iv) in the research setting, a truer comparison of different treatment regimes.

Key points

Staging allows

- allocation of patients to appropriate treatment regimes
- individualisation of tumour treatment
- prediction of prognosis
- comparison of different treatment regimes

Modalities currently used to stage oesophageal carcinoma

For all tumours, the imaging modalities used to stage the disease is tailored according to the most common method of spread of that tumour. Staging of oesophageal carcinoma focuses primarily on establishing as accurately as possible the local extent of the tumour and the locoregional nodal and non-nodal (lungs, adrenals and liver) metastatic spread.

Computed tomography

CT is one of the main imaging modalities used to establish local, nodal and non-nodal locoregional spread of oesophageal carcinoma.

Key points

Single detector CT protocol

- Patient fasting for 4 h
- No barium study during the previous week
- Effervescent granules per-oral
- Intravenous antispasmodic agent
- Intravenous contrast, pitch 10
- Contiguous 5 mm acquisitions from larynx to sternal notch
- Contiguous 10 mm acquisitions from sternal notch to lower border of kidneys

CT is useful for assessing the

(i) size and extent of the primary tumour,
(ii) presence of nodal metastases,
(iii) presence of non-nodal metastatic disease and providing a roadmap to the endoscopist prior to EUS examination.

(i) As the oesophagus is vertically aligned, it is ideally suited to cross-sectional imaging in the axial

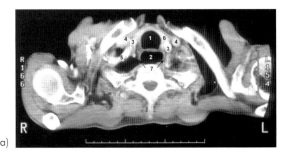

(a)

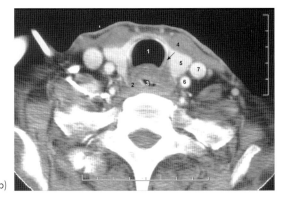

(b)

Fig. 8.2   Axial CT of lower neck with intravenous contrast: (a) – 1. tracheal lumen, 2. oesophageal lumen distended with gas, 3. common carotid artery, 4. internal jugular vein, 5. right subclavian artery, 6. thyroid and 7. normal thickness of oesophageal wall; (b) – 1. tracheal lumen, 2. oesophageal tumour, 3. oesophageal lumen, 4. infiltration of oesophageal tumour between left lateral wall of trachea and left lobe of thyroid, 5. left lobe of thyroid, 6. common carotid artery and 7. internal jugular vein.

plane by CT. This is in contrast to other regions of the gastrointestinal tract, which are not aligned in a vertical plane, and where partial volume averaging may hamper interpretation. If the oesophagus is distended (by prior administration of gas granules orally and an intravenous antispasmodic agent), thickening of the oesophageal wall calibre can be readily appreciated (Figures 8.2a and b). This allows the proximal and distal extent of oesophageal tumours to be accurately delineated in most of the cases. Delineating the tumour length is useful in two respects. First, in less than 10% of oesophageal tumours, there may be complete or almost complete occlusion of the oesophageal lumen, such that even a small endoscope cannot be passed through to assess the lower limit of the tumour. Second, a minority of tumours may have appreciable submucosal spread

beyond the mucosal aspect of the tumour evident on standard endoscopy or barium studies.

Delineation of the tumour margins also allows one to estimate the tumour volume through tracing out the tumour margins on serial CT images. Serial volume measurements pre- and post-chemotherapy can allow one to objectively assess any change in tumour volume (with chemotherapy or chemoirradiation) though as yet there is no evidence that change in tumour volume has any bearing on patient outcome [8] (Figures 8.3a and b). While CT estimation of tumour volume is accurate when compared to gross tumour volume estimation on resected specimens, neither method can reliably separate tumour from peritumoural oedema. CT can predict the likelihood of tumour spread beyond the oesophageal wall into adjacent neck or mediastinal structures (Figure 8.2b). The relative frequency of extraoesophageal spread and the accuracy of the CT parameters used in predicting this spread are shown in Table 8.3.

If, as is ideally the case, both CT and EUS are included in the work-up of oesophageal carcinoma, it is preferable to perform CT prior to EUS, as CT is a useful roadmap to focus the endoscopists' attention on those areas of suspected invasion or lymphadenopathy.

Key points

CT of primary tumour size and extent
- CT is less accurate than EUS at predicting local tumour invasion
- CT is a useful roadmap for the endoscopist to define areas of suspected invasion
- CT is better at depicting change in tumour volume with chemotherapy
- Less than 10% of oesophageal tumours are too stenosed to allow full endoscopic assessment

(ii) Detection of enlarged nodes in the mediastinum by CT is facilitated by the presence of easily recognisable nodal stations and the conspicuity of most of the enlarged nodes. Though tumour enlargement occurs primarily in the immediate vicinity of the primary tumour, all the cervical, mediastinal and upper abdominal nodes should be routinely assessed (irrespective of the primary tumour location), as it is not

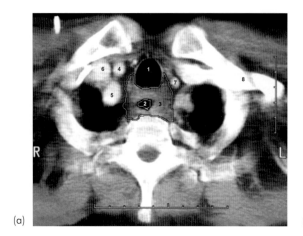
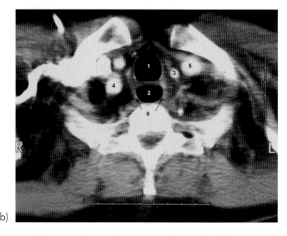

(a)   (b)

Fig. 8.3 Axial CT of lower neck with intravenous contrast: (a) pre-chemotherapy – 1. tracheal lumen, 2. oesophageal lumen, 3. oesophageal tumour; the tumour volume is being measured by outlining the tumour margins and the margin of the oesophageal lumen, 4. right common carotid artery, 5. right subclavian artery, 6. internal jugular vein, 7. left common carotid artery and 8. left subclavian artery; (b) post-chemotherapy – 1. tracheal lumen, 2. oesophageal lumen, 3. common carotid artery, 4. right subclavian artery, 5. internal jugular vein and 6. oesophageal tumour volume has decreased dramatically after chemotherapy.

Table 8.3 CT criteria applied to diagnose infiltration of perioesophageal structures.

T-stage	Resectability	Site of tumour spread	Frequency	CT imaging criteria used	Accuracy
T3	Resectable	Perioesophgeal fat	Common	Tumour spreading into perioesphageal fat Obtuse tumour angles	Reasonable
T4	Unresectable	Aortic adventitia	Uncommon	Tumour contacting >100° of aortic circumference	Good
T4	Unresectable	Tracheobronchial	Common	Tumour displacing or indenting main bronchi Tumour displacing or indenting trachea or extending around the sidewall(s) of the trachea	Poor
T4	Resectable	Pericardium	Uncommon	Tumour pressing up against pericardium in three consecutive images, pericardial effusion	Fair
T4	Resectable	Diaphragmatic crus	Common	Tumour thickening of diaphragmatic crus	Good
T4	Resectable	Parietal pleura	Uncommon	Localised thickening of pleura with normal lung	Good
	Unresectable	Visceral pleura and lung	Uncommon	Localised thickening of pleura with abnormal lung	Good
T4	Resectable	Thyroid	Uncommon	Visible tumour infiltration to thyroid	Good
T4	Unresectable	Liver	Uncommon	Visible tumour infiltration to liver	Good

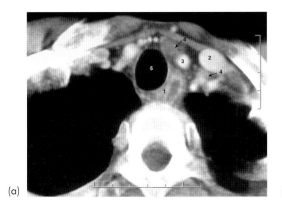 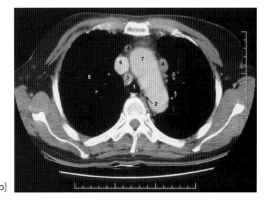

(a)   (b)

Fig. 8.4   Contrast axial CT of (a) lower neck – 1. oesophagus tumour, 2. left internal jugular vein, 3. left common carotid artery, 4. metastatic lymph nodes and 5. tracheal lumen; (b) superior mediastinum – 1. tracheal lumen, 2. oesophagus, 3. enlarged para-tracheal lymph node, 4. Enlarged para-aortic lymph nodes, 5. right lung, 6. superior vena cava and 7. aortic arch.

uncommon to find nodal metastases removed from the primary tumour with apparent non-involvement of intervening nodal stations (Figures 8.4a and b).

(iii) A contrast CT of the thorax and abdomen is the most accurate means of screening for metastatic disease in the lungs, liver and adrenal glands preoperatively. Pulmonary metastases are usually seen as small rounded opacities (akin to small cherries) typically located peripherally and at the bases (reflecting relatively increased perfusion of the lung bases) (Figure 8.5a) Oesophageal liver metastases are seen as discrete hypodense foci (reflecting relative hypovascularity) within the liver (Figure 8.5b) though not as well defined and hypodense as simple liver cysts (Figure 8.5c). Adrenals metastases are seen as discrete masses, usually greater than 1 cm in diameter, within the adrenals glands. Even in the presence of oesophageal malignancy, it is unwise to assume that accompanying lung, liver or adrenal nodules are necessarily metastatic. Each lesion should be judged on its own merits with clarification, when appropriate, either through other imaging modalities (e.g. MRI for adrenal masses) or percutaneous biopsy. With improving CT technology, the virtual barium swallow (Figure 8.6) and endoscopic capabilities of CT are likely to improve.

Key points

- Irrespective of the location of the primary tumour, all nodal stations in the mid to lower neck, the mediastinal and upper abdomen should be routinely assessed
- CT is accurate at depicting regional metastatic disease in oesophageal carcinoma

Endoscopic ultrasound

EUS is performed using a flexible endoscope incorporating an ultrasound transducer at its tip. Usually, the transducers are either 7.5 MHz (7–10 cm depth penetration, 0.2 mm axial resolution) or 12.5 MHz (3 cm depth penetration, 0.12 mm axial resolution) in type. EUS provides a detailed display of the oesophageal wall comprising five layers of altering echogenicity. Oesophageal carcinoma is seen as a hypoechoic mass disrupting the normal layered pattern of the oesophageal wall (Figure 8.7). EUS is currently the most accurate means available to assess T-stage and N-stage. Sensitivities and specificities of over 90% have been reported for T-stage with slightly less for N-stage. Limiting features are operator experience, stenosing tumours (less than 10% of oesophageal tumour do not allow passage of the endoscope) and differentiation of peritumoural inflammation from tumour infiltration.

Overstaging may occur with ulcerated tumours with a large inflammatory component. Some nodes may be hidden from the endoscopists view by the trachea. In this situation, the combination of CT and EUS allows a full assessment of nodal involvement.

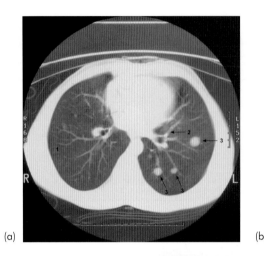

(a)

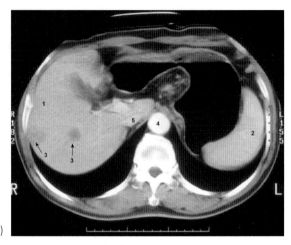

(b)

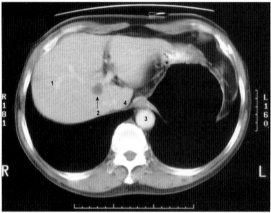

(c)

Fig. 8.5 (a) Axial CT of thorax: 1. right lung, 2. pulmonary vessels and 3. pulmonary metastatic deposits; (b) – contrast axial CT of upper abdomen: 1. right lobe of liver, 2. spleen, 3. metastatic deposits right lobe of liver (the lesions are of higher attenuation than a simple hepatic cyst), 4. aorta and 5. inferior vena cava; (c) – 1. right lobe of liver, 2. simple hepatic cyst (cf. b), 3. aorta and 4. inferior vena cava.

Key points

- EUS is very accurate at local staging of oesophageal carcinoma and at identifying locoregional nodes though some nodes may be hidden from the operator's view

Neck ultrasound

Neck ultrasound coupled with fine needle aspiration for cytology is recommended as a routine investigation when staging squamous oesophageal carcinoma. Neck ultrasound will detect malignant neck nodes in about 30% of patients presenting with squamous oesophageal carcinoma and 5–10% of patients with adenocarcinoma [8, 9]. Most of these nodes will not be palpable. Abdominal ultrasound is useful at detecting upper abdominal adenopathy and confirming the absence of liver metastases (as very occasionally, ultrasound will detect liver metastases not apparent on CT).

Key points

- Neck ultrasound helps to detect and characterise impalpable neck nodes
- Abdominal ultrasound helps detect and characterise upper abdominal nodes, liver and adrenal metastases

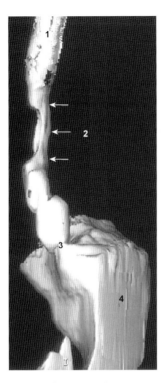

Fig. 8.6 3DCT of lower thoracic oesophageal cancer: 1. trachea, 2. oesophageal tumour with underdistension of lumen as a result of oesophageal carcinoma, 3. gastro-oesophageal junction and 4. stomach.

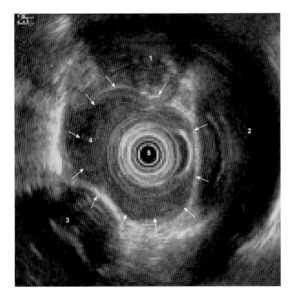

Fig. 8.7 EUS: 1. trachea, 2. aorta, 3. spine, 4. oesophageal tumour and 5. EUS transducer.

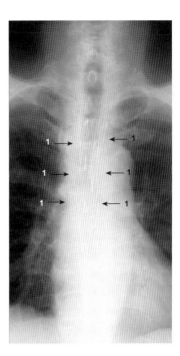

Fig. 8.8 Coned frontal chest radiograph: 1. oesophageal stent located in upper thoracic oesophagus.

Management and prognosis of oesophageal carcinoma

Oesophageal carcinoma is treated in a variety of ways depending on the extent of the tumour at presentation, the age and general condition of the patient. Means of treatment include oesophageal stenting (Figure 8.8), radiotherapy, chemotherapy and surgery either alone or in combination.

Patients with oesophageal carcinoma often present late and have a poor prognosis. The two most important prognostic factors are the local extent (T-stage) of the primary tumour at presentation and the presence of lymph node metastases (N-stage). The majority of tumours are T3 or T4 at presentation and most of them will have lymph node metastases. However, even earlier tumours (T1/T2) are associated with lymph node metastases in 30% of cases. Overall, distant non-nodal spread (to the lungs, liver or adrenal) of oesophageal carcinoma at presentation is not common; and when it does occur, it is seen most frequently with adenocarcinoma (i.e. liver metastases) rather than squamous cell carcinoma.

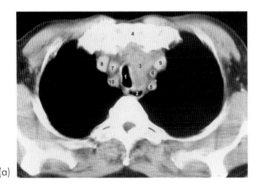 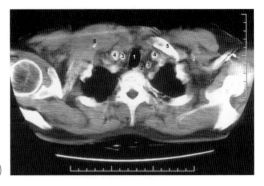

(a) (b)

Fig. 8.9 Contrast axial CT of (a) upper thorax: 1. tracheal lumen, 2. oesophageal lumen, 3. local tumour recurrence in left paratracheal region from cervical oesophageal carcinoma, 4. manubrium, 5. left common carotid artery, 6. left subclavian artery, 7. innominate artery, 8. right subclavian vein, 9. left brachiocephalic vein and 10. superior vena cava; (b) lower neck: 1. tracheal lumen, 2. oesophagus, 3. common carotid artery, 4. internal jugular vein, 5. left clavicle and 6. large metastatic deposit infiltrating right clavicle and surrounding tissues (from oesophageal carcinoma treated by chemoirradiation with good response).

Although the prognosis of oesophageal carcinoma has improved slightly in recently years (with the use of combination therapy comprising chemotherapy, radiotherapy and or surgery), it still remains poor. The 2-year survival is approximately 50%, while the 5-year survival is 10% [3]. While the prognosis is worse for those with more extensive tumours (T3/T4 and/or N1, M1), it is also poor in so-called early disease (T1/T2, N0, M0).

Even in those patients who undergo complete surgical resection of all macroscopic tumour, locoregional and, to lesser extent, distal recurrences occurring within 1–2 years remain the rule (Figure 8.9a and b).

> **Key points**
>
> • Despite advances in diagnosis and treatment, oesophageal carcinoma continues to have a poor prognosis

Neck nodal metastases from infraclavicular oesophageal or other tumours

Neck node metastases may also be found as a result of a primary oesophageal tumour located in the thoracic as opposed to the cervical oesophagus. While neck node metastases from cervical oesophageal carcinoma may be located in any of the neck nodal stations, the vast majority of metastatic neck nodes from infraclavicular oesophageal tumours are located in the lower jugular chains or in the tracheo-oesophageal grooves. Overall, 75% of cervical oesophageal tumours have neck node metastases detectable on ultrasound at presentation (Figure 8.10). This decreases to 50% for tumours located in the upper thoracic oesophagus, 30% for the mid-thoracic oesophagus and 5% for the lower thoracic oesophagus [8]. Squamous neck nodal metastases may also occur as a result of other intra-thoracic tumours, the main one being lung carcinoma. In a retrospective study of 352 patients with undifferentiated neck nodal metastases and no known primary over 20 years, the emergence of the occult primary was observed in one-fifth of patients. Half of the emerging primaries were within the head and neck region with oropharynx, hypopharynx and oral cavity being the most common sites. Emerging primaries outside the head and neck region were primarily located in the lung and oesophagus [10].

> **Key points**
>
> • Metastatic neck nodes from cervical oesophageal tumours can occur almost anywhere in the neck region
> • Metastatic neck nodes from infraclavicular oesophageal and lung tumours are principally located in the lower jugular chains or the tracheo-oesophageal grooves

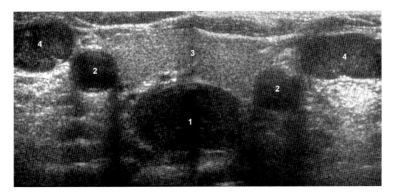

Fig. 8.10   Composite transverse ultrasound of lower neck: 1. cervical oesophageal tumour, 2. common carotid arteries, 3. thyroid gland and 4. metastatic cervical lymph nodes.

Key points

The incidence of (oesophageal) neck nodal metastases is
- 75% – when the primary tumour is in the *cervical* oesophagus
- 50% – when the primary tumour is in the *upper thoracic* oesophagus
- 30% – when the primary tumour is in the *mid-thoracic* oesophagus
- 5% – when the primary tumour is in for the *lower thoracic* oesophagus

Synchronous tumours (of the cervical oesophagus)

Tumours of the cervical oesophagus may arise synchronously with other squamous cell carcinomas of the head and neck (such as the pharynx or the larynx). This probably reflects the similar predisposing factors (such as smoking, diet, age, etc.) for both tumours. For similar reasons, patients with a prior head and neck cancer are at increased risk of oesophageal carcinoma and vice versa (i.e. metachronous tumours not arising at the same time).

The poor prognosis of the two primary tumours individually and their anatomic proximity limits and complicates the treatment choices for each tumour. Most of the oesophageal synchronous tumours are located in the hypopharynx. About 3%

of patients with oesophageal carcinoma will have a synchronous tumours of the hypopharynx [1].

Treatment usually aims to either

(a) first cure the head and neck cancer (with radiotherapy) and then proceed to oesophagectomy to treat the cervical carcinoma or
(b) PLO to simultaneously treat both tumours.

The increasing operative difficulty leads to an appreciable mortality (about 10%) and morbidity from anastomotic leaks or pulmonary infection [1].

Key points

- Tumours of the cervical oesophagus may occur synchronously (or metachronously) with other head and neck squamous cell carcinomas (most commonly hypopharyngeal tumours)

Conclusion

Endoscopy is the preferred means of diagnosing oesophageal carcinoma, while barium studies are of most benefit in patients with suspected oesophageal motility disorders. In staging oesophageal carcinoma, CT, EUS and ultrasound of the neck and abdomen are complimentary in defining locoregional spread. Only when the true extent of the tumour is known, can the appropriate treatment be administered (Figure 8.11).

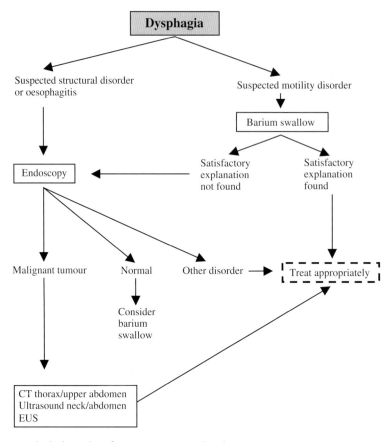

Fig. 8.11   Recommended algorithm for investigating dysphagia.

References

1. Bottger T, Bumb P, Dutkowski P, Schlick T and Junginger T. Carcinoma of the hypopharynx and the cervical oesophagus: a surgical challenge. *Eur. J. Surg.* 1999; **65**: 940–946.
2. Griffith JF, Chan AC, Ahuja AT, Leung SF, Chow LT, Chung SC and Metreweli C. Neck ultrasound in staging squamous oesophageal carcinoma – a high yield technique. *Clin. Radiol.* 2000; **55**: 696–701.
3. Dresner SM and Griffin SM. Pattern of recurrence following radical oesophagectomy with two-field lymphadenectomy. *Br. J. Surg.* 2000; **87**: 1426–1433.
4. Dresner SM, Lamb PJ, Bennett MK, Hayes N and Griffin SM. The pattern of metastatic lymph node dissemination from adenocarcinoma of the esophagogastric junction. *Surgery* 2001; **129**: 103–139.
5. Nishimaki T, Tanaka O, Suzuki T, Aizawa K, Hatakeyama K and Muto T. Patterns of lymphatic spread in thoracic esophageal cancer. *Cancer* 1994; **74**: 4–11.

6. Akiyama H, Tsurumaru M, Udagawa H and Kajiyama Y. Radical lymph node dissection for cancer of the thoracic esophagus. *Ann. Surg.* 1994; **220**: 364–372.
7. Okuma T, Kaneko H, Yoshioka M, Torigoe Y and Miyauchi Y. Prognosis in esophageal carcinoma with cervical lymph node metastases. *Surgery* 1993; **114**: 513–518.
8. Griffith JF, Chan ACW, Chow LTC, Leung SF, Lam YH, Liang EY, Chung SCS and Metreweli C. Assessing chemotherapy response of squamous cell oesophageal carcinoma with spiral CT. *Br. J. Radiol.* 1999; **859**: 678–684.
9. Van Overhagen H, Lameris JS, Berger MY *et al.* Supraclavicular lymph node metastases in carcinoma of the esophagus and gastro-oesophageal junction: assessment with CT, US, and US-guided fine-needle aspiration biopsy. *Radiology* 1991; **179**: 155–158.
10. Grau C, Johansen LV, Jakobsen J, Geertsen P, Andersen E and Jensen BB. Cervical lymph node metastases from unknown primary tumours. Results from a national survey by the Danish Society for Head and Neck Oncology. *Radiother. Oncol.* 2000; **55**: 121–129.

Salivary Gland Cancer

AT Ahuja, RM Evans and AC Vlantis

Introduction

Salivary gland neoplasms represent <3% of all tumours [1]. The majority of tumours are benign and so malignant tumours are rare; 70–80% of parotid tumours, 40–55% of submandibular tumours, 15–30% of sublingual tumours and 20–51% of minor salivary gland tumours (located in the submucosa throughout the oral cavity) are benign. In general, the smaller the salivary gland involved, the greater the likelihood that the tumour is malignant [2–4].

Key points

- Majority of salivary gland tumours are benign

- The smaller the salivary gland, the greater the likelihood that the tumour is malignant

Management of malignant tumours remain a challenge for the head and neck surgeon as

- the relative rarity makes it difficult to study their biological behaviour and response to treatment,
- they are unpredictable and have a prolonged risk of recurrence.

Clinical presentation of salivary gland cancers

- Asymptomatic slow growing masses: one should, therefore, view these tumours with a high degree of clinical suspicion.

- Duration of symptoms is generally shorter in malignant tumours than benign lesions.
- Constant pain is more suggestive of a malignant lesion. Pain is experienced in 10–29% of patients with parotid cancers and 6.5% in patients with submandibular cancers [5].
- Rapidly progressive facial nerve paralysis is seen in 10–15% of parotid malignancies [6].
- Ulceration within the oral cavity or denture discomfort may be the presenting features of a minor salivary gland cancer of the hard palate.
- Trismus in cancers of parotid and minor salivary glands suggests extension into the infratemporal fossa.
- Cranial nerve palsies:
  - hoarseness (X);
  - aspiration (IX and X);
  - shoulder dysfunction (XI);
  - atrophy of hemitongue (XII).

Clinical evaluation of submandibular tumours should include assessment of adjacent structures, such as the floor of the mouth, the tongue and mandible.

Intraoral examination is indicated to assess oropharyngeal bulging that is suggestive of deep parotid lobe involvement or of a primary parapharyngeal tumour.

The palate and intraoral mucosa should be evaluated for the presence of a subtle submucosal cancer of the minor salivary glands.

The ears, nasopharynx, cranial nerves, skin and neck should be examined to detect spread.

Prognostic indicators
Facial nerve paralysis

- Facial nerve paralysis indicates an adverse prognosis and an increased rate of nodal metastases of 66–77%, with a 5-year survival rate of between 9% and 14% [7].
- Frequency of facial nerve paralysis with parotid tumours:
  - undifferentiated carcinoma: 24%,
  - squamous cell carcinoma: 19%,
  - adenoid cystic carcinoma: 17%,
  - adenocarcinoma: 11%,
  - mucoepidermoid carcinoma: 9%,
  - carcinoma-ex-pleomorphic adenoma: 7%,
  - acinic cell carcinoma: 1%.

Pain

- Not a definite criterion for malignancy, since 5.1% of benign tumours and 6.5% of malignant tumours present with pain.
- In a patient with known cancer it suggests a poorer prognosis with a 5-year survival of 35% compared to 68% for patients with no pain [7].

Location

- Location of cancers within the gland have no bearing on prognosis (i.e. superficial or deep for parotid tumours).

Histopathologic diagnosis

- High-grade cancers have a worse prognosis than low-grade cancers [8].

Lymph node metastases

- Adversely affects prognosis, 10-year-specific survival for patients without nodal metastases is 63% compared to 33% for patients with neck node involvement.
- Frequency of nodal metastases [7]
  - Parotid:
    - Clinically apparent: high-grade mucoepidermoid: 44%, squamous cell carcinoma: 37%, adenocarcinoma: 25%, undifferentiated carcinoma: 23%, carcinoma-ex-pleomorphic adenoma: 21%, acinic cell carcinoma: 13% and adenoid cystic carcinoma: 5%.
    - Occult: squamous cell carcinoma: 40%, high-grade mucoepidermoid: 16%, adenocarcinoma: 9%, acinic cell carcinoma: 6%.
  - Submandibular, sublingual and minor salivary gland cancers:
    - Carcinoma-ex-pleomorphic adenoma: 42%, all grades mucoepidermoid: 33%, squamous cell carcinoma: 33%, adenoid cystic carcinoma: 13%.

Distant metastases [7]

- The presence of distant metastases is a predictor of poor prognosis.
- Overall 20% of all parotid cancers have distant metastases:
  - adenoid cystic carcinoma: 42%,
  - undifferentiated carcinoma: 36%,
  - adenocarcinoma: 27%,
  - squamous cell carcinoma: 15%,
  - acinic cell carcinoma: 14%,
  - mucoepidermoid: 8%.

Recurrence

- The overall recurrence rate for salivary gland tumours is between 27% and 38% [9] and is related to tumour grade and adequacy of resection.
- Recurrence adversely affects prognosis with a 5-year survival rate of 37% for recurrent parotid malignancies [10].

Key points

Prognostic factors

- Facial nerve paralysis
- Pain
- Tumour histology
- Nodal metastases
- Distant metastases
- Tumour recurrence

Imaging for salivary gland tumours

Why image at all?

Most salivary gland tumours arise in the parotid gland, 90% are in the superficial lobe [11] and 80% of all parotid tumours are benign. These are readily amenable to surgical excision, so why image?

The rationale behind imaging is the fact that although these tumours are common and a large proportion benign, malignant tumour, although rare, does occur. Imaging helps to identify the small proportion of patients with cancer who require aggressive treatment and to reassure and avoid unnecessary investigations and treatment for the majority with benign disease.

It is commonly accepted that as the proportional incidence of cancer in submandibular, sublingual and minor salivary glands is high, imaging is routinely indicated.

Which imaging modality to use?

The modalities often involved in imaging the salivary glands include CT, MRI and ultrasound (US). Nuclear medicine and PET scans currently do not appear to have any role in the imaging of parotid masses [5].

In our experience, MRI should preferably be the initial investigation in all patients who have clinical signs suggestive of malignancy, tumours that appear to arise from the deep lobe of the parotid, large tumours, and tumours that bulge into the oral cavity or oropharynx (Figure 9.1).

US with a guided FNAC is used as the first investigation for tumours arising in the superficial lobe of the parotid (the bulk of all salivary gland masses) and for submandibular tumours (Figure 9.2). This often provides the surgeon with the information to plan surgery and counsel the patient [12].

Irrespective of the modality used, radiological studies should not be considered specific enough to preclude a tissue diagnosis.

Key points

- US + FNAC – first investigation for superficial parotid and submandibular lesions
- MR – first investigation in patients with clinical signs of malignancy, deep lobe parotid tumours and tumours that bulge into oral cavity or oropharynx

Computed tomography

- Advantages:
  - readily available,
  - salivary glands are easily visualised,
  - relationship of parotid tumour to facial nerve can be identified,

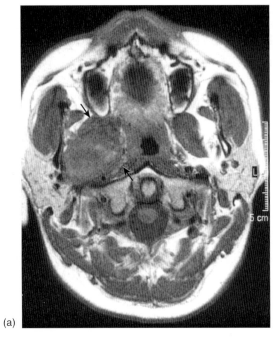

(a)

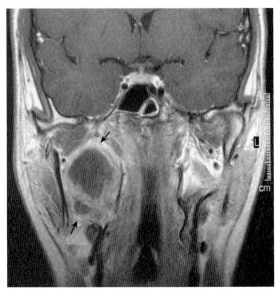

(b)

Fig. 9.1 (a) Axial T1W MR and (b) post-gadolinium coronal T1W MR showing a tumour (arrows) in the parapharyngeal soft tissues with heterogeneous enhancement. Surgery confirmed it to be a malignant tumour arising from a minor salivary gland. Tumours in such locations cannot be evaluated/visualised by US. Such tumours cause a bulge in the oral cavity and CT/MR are the investigations of choice.

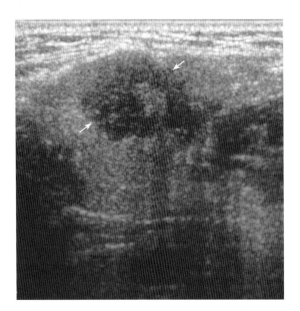

Fig. 9.2 Transverse grey-scale sonogram of the submandibular gland showing a ill-defined, hypoechoic, heterogeneous mass (arrows). The US appearances are of a malignant lesion and surgery confirmed a adenoid cystic carcinoma.

    – following contrast, major vasculature of the tumour identified,
    – evaluates associated nodal pathology.
- Disadvantages:
    – involves ionising radiation,
    – involves injection of intravenous contrast,
    – relatively expensive (compared to US),
    – dental artefacts may degrade image quality.

CT sialography is not routinely indicated as it is unable to distinguish benign from malignant lesions. Its role is fairly restricted to the evaluation of the ductal system.

Magnetic resonance imaging

- Advantages:
    – does not involve ionising radiation,
    – superior soft tissue detail,
    – images in multiple planes,
    – relationship of parotid tumour to facial nerve can be identified,
    – clearly evaluates extraglandular tumour extent,
    – evaluates nodal pathology.

- Disadvantages:
  - not readily available at all centres,
  - expensive modality,
  - may require injection of contrast,
  - more sensitive to motion artefact,
  - poor cortical detail of adjacent mandible.

Ultrasound

- Advantages:
  - relatively inexpensive,
  - readily available,
  - does not involve ionising radiation,
  - does not routinely involve contrast injection,
  - easily images the superficial parotid and submandibular glands,
  - real-time, multiplanar information available,
  - Doppler evaluates tumour vascularity,
  - readily combined with FNAC/biopsy,
  - partially evaluates nodal pathology,
  - relationship of parotid tumour to facial nerve can be inferred.
- Disadvantages:
  - requires specialist expertise,
  - does not evaluate the deep lobe of parotid gland,
  - cannot evaluate minor salivary gland tumours,
  - cannot clearly evaluate deep soft tissue, bone and peri-neural spread,
  - does not evaluate oropharyngeal/retropharyngeal nodes.

The role of FNAC for salivary gland tumours

Although FNAC is routinely used in the evaluation of salivary gland tumours, some controversy exists as the results may not be consistent in every centre. The reported sensitivity and specificity for FNA has been between 88–93% and 75–99%, respectively [13–15].

The diagnosis of cancer on FNAC aids in the counselling of patients about the chances of facial nerve sacrifice and reconstruction as well as the possibility of neck dissection.

FNAC is useful in avoiding surgery when a diagnosis of metastases, lymphoma, sialadenosis, and benign salivary gland tumour (particularly in patients who are poor surgical risks) is suggested.

It has been reported that cytology and imaging are comparable in their ability to identify malignant lesions pre-operatively [16]. MRI has sensitivity of 88%, specificity of 77% and an accuracy of 83%. CT has a sensitivity of 100%, specificity 42% and accuracy 69%. FNAC has a sensitivity of 83%, specificity 86% and accuracy of 85%.

> ### Key points
>
> *Role of FNAC*
>
> - Counselling patients regarding risk of facial nerve palsy
> - Counselling for possibility of neck dissection
> - Avoid surgery in metastases, lymphoma, sialadenosis and some benign lesions

Staging system for major salivary gland cancers (AJCC, UICC)

Tx: Primary tumour cannot be assessed.

T0: No evidence of primary tumour.

T1: Tumour 2 cm or less in greatest dimension.

T2: Tumour >2 cm, but <4 cm in greatest dimension.

T3: Tumour >4 cm, but <6 cm in greatest dimension.

T4: Tumour >6 cm in dimension.

All categories of AJCC and UICC are subdivided into

- no local extension,
- local extension (clinical or macroscopic evidence of invasion into skin, soft tissues, bone or nerve).

Imaging characteristics

The following paragraphs will broadly discuss imaging features that help in distinguishing benign from malignant tumours.

Malignant salivary tumours often have similar appearances and imaging cannot differentiate between the various cancers. Any specific characteristics of the tumour will be highlighted during the course of the discussion.

Key points

Malignant salivary tumours often have similar appearances and imaging cannot differentiate between various cancers.

Computed tomography/magnetic resonance imaging

Imaging patterns on CT and MRI [17,18] include the following:

- Encapsulated rounded, homogeneous soft tissue density on CT or mild hyperintensity on

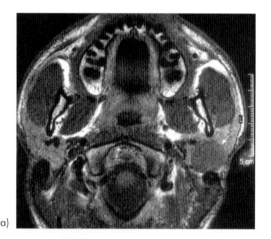

(a)

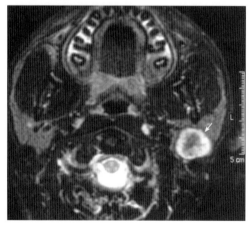

(b)

Fig. 9.3 (a) Axial T1W and (b) fat suppressed T2W MR of a parotid tumour (arrow). Note its low-signal intensity on T1W scans (a) and high signal on T2W scans (b). This feature is often seen in benign lesion. Biopsy of the tumor revealed a pleomorphic adenoma.

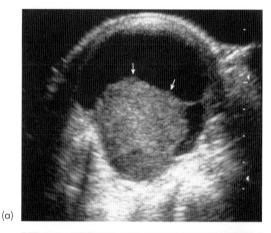

(a)

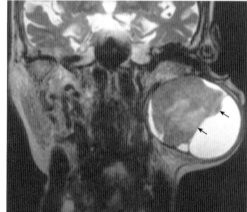

(b)

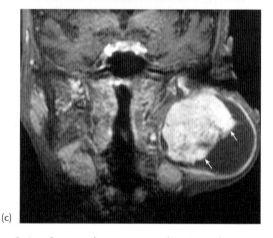

(c)

Fig. 9.4 Grey-scale sonogram showing a large parotid tumour with solid (arrows) and cystic elements. The T2W coronal MR clearly demonstrates a large solid portion (arrows) which shows heterogeneous enhancement (arrows) on a post-gadolinium fat suppressed, coronal, T1W MR. Biopsy of the solid portion confirmed a malignant tumour. A previous blind FNAC was non-diagnostic and yielded only haemorrhagic fluid.

T2-weighted (T2W) images is more consistent with a benign tumour (Figure 9.3).

• Lobulated pattern of encapsulation with mixed signal, internal cystic change/necrosis may represent intermediate pathology (Figure 9.4).

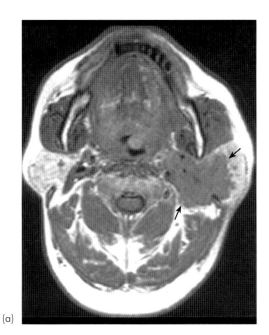

(a)

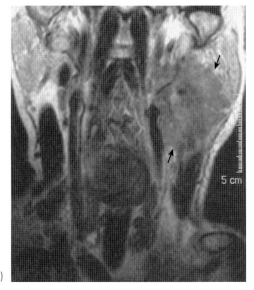

(b)

Fig. 9.5 (a) Axial T1W and (b) coronal T2W MRI showing a large ill-defined tumour (arrows). Note it is of low-signal intensity on both T1W and T2W scans, features often seen in malignant lesions.

• Infiltrative edges (Figure 9.5), cystic change and necrosis indicate aggressive pathology. Identification of a capsule on MRI is a useful sign in predicting pleomorphic adenoma.

• High-grade cancer has low-signal intensity on T1-weighted (T1W) and T2W images (Figure 9.5), whereas less aggressive cancers and benign lesions have low-T1W and high-T2W signal intensities (Figure 9.3). This is attributed to the higher amounts of serous and mucoid material in low-grade and benign tumours compared to high-grade aggressive tumours [7].

• Cancers generally enhance with gadolinium contrast compared to the relatively poor enhancement seen in benign tumours [18]. However, in the authors experience, both benign and malignant tumours show variable degree of enhancement. This is best appreciated on fat suppressed, post-gadolinium T1W sequences. Malignant tumours show a heterogeneous enhancement and benign tumours such as a pleomorphic adenoma demonstrate homogeneous enhancement (Figures 9.6 and 9.7). The larger pleomorphic adenomas where there is intratumoral necrosis or haemorrhage the enhancement pattern may also be heterogeneous. Warthins tumours also have a variable but predominantly heterogeneous enhancement pattern.

• Soft tissue involvement and enlargement of the facial nerve indicates malignant tumour (Figure 9.8).

• Using two phase helical CT, one may be able to differentiate between a pleomorphic adenoma and Warthin's tumour but differentiation between malignant tumours is not possible [19].

Although CT and MRI have the same diagnostic potential in salivary gland neoplasms [20], MRI better delineates parapharyngeal involvement and the relationship to the facial nerve. Minor salivary gland cancers are also better delineated by MRI and these tumours are more hyperintense compared to surrounding tissue [21].

Peri-neural spread of the tumour can be a diagnostic challenge and the nerves commonly involved are the facial and trigeminal nerves in patients with adenoid cystic carcinoma. Neural involvement predicts poor prognosis and tumour recurrence. Although both MRI and CT can demonstrate peri-neural spread, CT is less sensitive and detects involvement near the neural foramina that are enlarged due to nerve expansion. However, this occurs late in the course of the disease and early changes may be missed. MRI is better able to detect peri-neural involvement as it better evaluates soft tissues and detects signal changes surrounding the nerves involved by cancer.

Ultrasound

US is unable to differentiate between the various malignant salivary gland tumours.

US features that help in differentiating benign from malignant tumours:

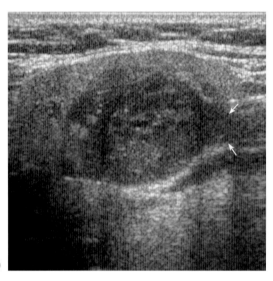
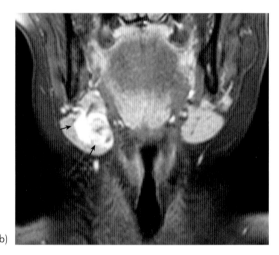

(a)   (b)

Fig. 9.6   (a) Grey-scale sonogram of the submandibular gland shows an ill-defined (arrows) hypoechoic mass within the submandibular gland. (b) Its location in the submandibular gland, ill-defined edges and heterogeneous enhancement (arrows) on a post-gadolinium coronal fat suppressed T1W MR suggest a malignant lesion. Histology confirmed an adenoid cystic carcinoma.

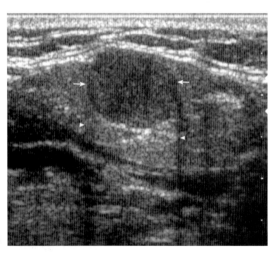
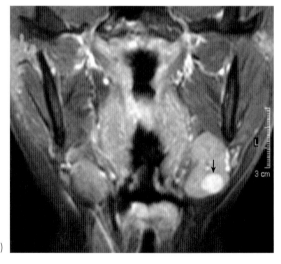

(a)   (b)

Fig. 9.7   (a) Grey-scale sonogram showing a well-defined, homogeneous submandibular pleomorphic adenoma (arrow) with posterior enhancement (arrowheads). (b) Well-defined edges and intense homogeneous enhancement (arrow) on the post-gadolinium fat suppressed coronal T1W MR.

- Edge
  - Malignant tumours have ill-defined edges compared to benign lesions (Figures 9.8, 9.9 and 9.10).
  - This is better appreciated on magnified images.
- Internal architecture
  - Malignant tumours have a heterogeneous internal architecture (Figure 9.11a), whereas benign tumours are more homogeneous (Figure 9.12a and c). This heterogeneity represents necrosis or haemorrhage within the tumour.
- Colour flow imaging
  - Malignant tumours are more likely to show pronounced vascularity (Figure 9.11a), a resistive index (RI) > 0.8 and a pulsatility index (PI) > 2 [22]. Pleomorphic adenomas demonstrate peripheral vascularity (Figure 9.12b) compared to malignant tumours that demonstrate a hilar vascular pattern [23] (Figure 9.11b).
- Associated lymphadenopathy
  - Adjacent abnormal malignant nodes help to identify malignant salivary gland tumours.

The following paragraphs briefly discuss individual salivary gland tumours, including imaging, clinical presentation and pathologic characteristics specific to various lesions.

Cancer of the salivary glands is rare and a large number of tumours encountered in routine clinical practice are benign. We will describe the more common benign lesions (pleomorphic adenoma, Warthins tumour/adenolymphoma) first before discussing malignancies.

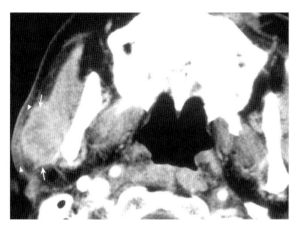

Fig. 9.8 Contrast enhanced axial CT scan shows heterogeneous enhancement in a malignant parotid mass (arrows). Note the overlying skin and subcutaneous involvement (arrowheads).

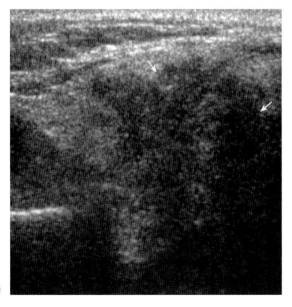

(a)

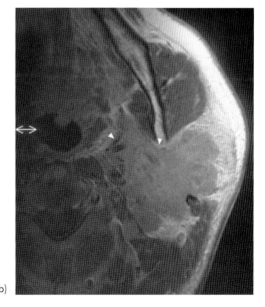

(b)

Fig. 9.9 (a) Transverse grey-scale sonogram showing a ill-defined, hypoechoic malignant parotid mass (arrows) involving superficial and deep lobes. (b) The entire extent of deep lobe involvement (arrowheads) and the poor definition of the tumour are better seen on a contrast enhanced axial T1W MR.

Pleomorphic adenoma (benign mixed tumour)

Pleomorphic adenoma (benign mixed tumour) is the commonest salivary gland tumour and represents 70–80% of all benign tumours of major salivary glands [24]. Although 50% of all minor salivary gland tumours are malignant, pleomorphic adenoma is still the single most common tumour of these glands.

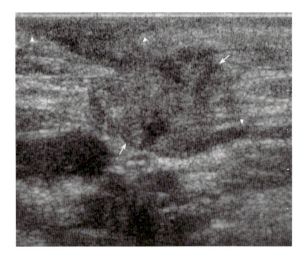

Fig. 9.10 Transverse grey-scale sonogram of the submandibular gland showing an ill-defined, hypoechoic, solid, heterogeneous malignant mass (arrows). Note its extension into the subcutaneous tissue, skin and adjacent soft tissue (arrowheads).

There is a slight female predominance usually occurring over the age of 40. They are commonly solitary and a primary multicentric origin is seen in 0.5% of pleomorphic adenomas [24].

These tumours are benign but if left untreated, nearly 25% of pleomorphic adenomas will turn malignant [25,26]. The longer the tumour remains untreated the greater the chance is that it will become malignant. Three types of malignancies are commonly associated with pleomorphic adenomas:

- carcinoma-ex-pleomorphic adenoma (malignant mixed tumour),
- carcinosarcoma,
- metastasising benign mixed tumour [27,28].

Imaging features of benign pleomorphic adenoma (Figures 9.3, 9.7, 9.12 and 9.13) are as follows.

Computed tomography

- Smoothly marginated spherical tumours.
- Higher attenuation than the parotid gland.
- Small tumours have homogeneous internal architecture and the larger lesions may have a non-uniform attenuation representing haemorrhage, necrosis and cystic change.
- Do not enhance significantly after contrast.
- Larger tumours may have lobulated outlines.
- Dystrophic calcification or ossification may be seen occasionally.

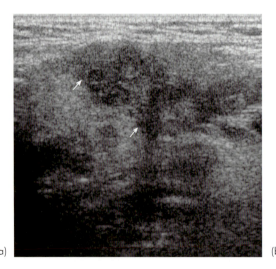
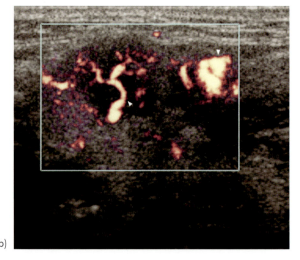

(a)   (b)

Fig. 9.11 (a) Transverse grey-scale sonogram of the submandibular gland showing an ill-defined, hypoechoic, heterogeneous mass (arrows). (b) Note prominent vessels (arrowheads) within the mass on power Doppler examination. The appearances are of a malignant mass, confirmed at surgery.

Magnetic resonance imaging

- Small lesions have a fairly homogeneous low-T1W and high-T2W signal intensity [24].
- Larger tumours may have a non-homogeneous low- to intermediate-T1W and intermediate-to-high-T2W signal intensity.
- Regions of necrosis within the tumour have low-T1W and high-T2W signal intensity.
- Areas of haemorrhage appear as regions of high-signal intensity on both T1W and T2W sequences.
- The presence of a capsule on MRI.

- Small tumours show homogeneous enhancement after gadolinium, whereas larger lesions demonstrate heterogeneous enhancement.

Ultrasound (specificity 87% and accuracy 89% [12])

- Well defined, round or lobulated.
- Homogeneous internal architecture in smaller lesions.
- Areas of cystic change and necrosis in larger tumours.

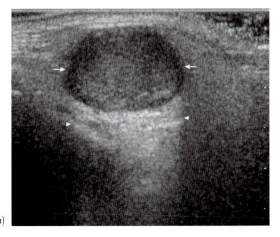

(a)

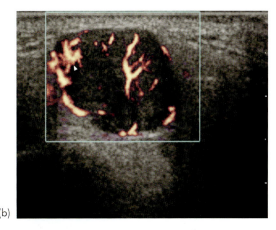

(b)

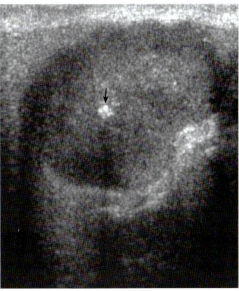

(c)

Fig. 9.12 (a) Grey-scale sonogram shows a well-defined, hypoechoic, solid mass (arrows) with homogeneous internal echoes and posterior enhancement (arrowheads). (b) Power Doppler demonstrates some vessels (arrowhead) within the mass which reportedly demonstrate low resistance. Note the perinodular vascularity. (c) Calcification (arrow) may be seen in long-standing lesions.

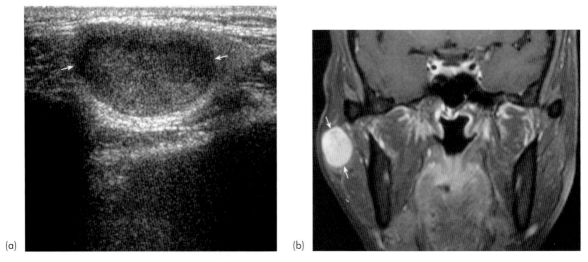

Fig. 9.13 (a) Grey-scale sonogram showing a well-defined parotid pleomorphic adenoma (arrows) with homogeneous, intense enhancement (arrows) on a post-gadolinium fat suppressed coronal T1W MR (b).

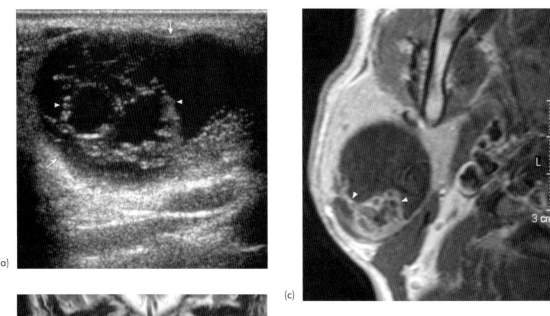

Fig. 9.14 (a) Grey-scale sonogram showing a predominantly cystic mass (arrows) with septation (arrowhead) in the superficial lobe of the parotid gland. (b) A coronal T2W MR showing the cystic component as a bright signal (arrows) and (c) a post-gadolinium T1W axial MR showing heterogeneous enhancement and septation (arrowhead). FNAC confirmed a Warthins tumour.

- Poorly reflective, homogenous echopattern with posterior enhancement/through transmission.
- Peripheral vascularity, low-resistance vessels on colour Doppler.

Warthins tumour (adenolymphoma)

Warthins tumour (adenolymphoma) is the second most common tumour of the parotid glands representing 2–10% of all parotid tumours [24]. This tumour selectively involves the parotid gland and may arise in heterotopic salivary tissue in periparotid lymph nodes. It may be multifocal or bilateral (10%), has a male preponderance and is commonly

seen in patients between 40 and 70 years of age. This tumour is benign and may undergo surveillance without resorting to surgery. It is commonly located in the apex/tail of the superficial lobe of the parotid gland.

Imaging features of a Warthins tumour (Figures 9.14–9.17) are as follows.

Computed tomography

- Smoothly marginated and ovoid lesions.
- Homogeneous, non-calcified and soft tissue density.

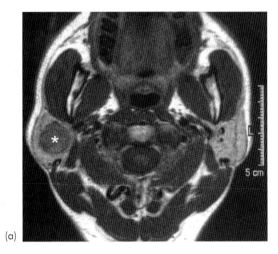
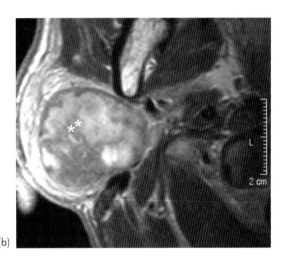

Fig. 9.15 (a) Axial T1W MR and (b) post-gadolinium T1W MR showing a tumour with low-signal intensity (*) and heterogeneous enhancement following gadolinium (**). Biopsy confirmed a Warthins tumour.

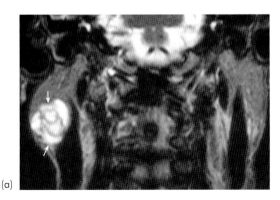
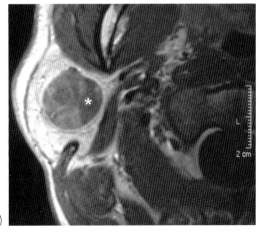

Fig. 9.16 (a) Coronal T2W MR and (b) post-gadolinium T1W MR showing a tumour with high-signal intensity on T2W (arrows) and heterogeneous enhancement following gadolinium (*). Biopsy confirmed a Warthins tumour.

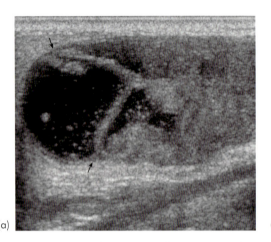

(a)

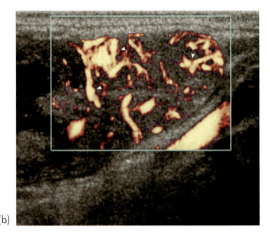

(b)

Fig. 9.17   (a) Longitudinal grey-scale sonogram showing a mass (arrows) in the superficial lobe of the parotid with cystic change, septation and solid elements. (b) A power Doppler reveals multiple peripheral vessels (arrowheads) within the solid portion which reportedly demonstrate low intravascular resistance, a sign of benignity.

- Cyst formation is common, being either thin or thick walled. Focal tumour nodules may be present within the "cyst".

Magnetic resonance imaging [24]

- When solid, they are similar to pleomorphic adenomas (low-T1W and high-T2W signal intensities).
- Large tumours are more heterogenous because of cystic change within.
- Demonstrate a heterogeneous enhancement after gadolinium.

Ultrasound (specificity 91% and accuracy 89% [12])

- Well defined, non-calcified.
- Hypoechoic and heterogeneous internal architecture.
- Multiseptated cystic mass with thick walls.
- Low-resistance vessels in the septa on colour Doppler.

Malignant salivary tumours

Mucoepidermoid carcinoma

Mucoepidermoid carcinoma accounts for <10% of all salivary gland tumours but 30% of all salivary gland cancers. Nearly 50% of these lesions arise in the parotid gland and 45% in minor salivary glands in the palate and buccal mucosa [4,25].

In adults, mucoepidermoid carcinoma is the most common malignancy of the parotid gland and the second most common malignancy of the submandibular gland after adenoid cystic carcinoma. Most patients are in their third to fifth decades and there is no sex bias.

They can be classified as low- (Grade 1), intermediate- (Grade 2) and high-grade tumours (Grade 3), and the grade correlates well with prognosis [29]. The low-grade lesions almost behave like benign lesions and may be well defined, contain cysts with blood and mucus, and may haemorrhage and undergo necrosis. They may infiltrate locally but metastases are rare. Intermediate-grade tumours have a greater tendency to recur and metastasize. High-grade lesions are predominantly solid, poorly circumscribed with infiltrative edges and have a high incidence of recurrence and metastases. They metastasize primarily to subcutaneous tissue, lymph nodes, the lungs and bones.

Their imaging appearances are related to the grade with low-grade tumours mimicking benign salivary gland lesions.

Adenoid cystic carcinoma

Adenoid cystic carcinoma accounts for 2–6% of parotid gland tumours, 12% of submandibular gland tumours, 15% of sublingual gland tumours and 30% of minor salivary gland tumours [25,30,31].

They occur commonly in the parotid gland, sub-mandibular gland and in the minor salivary glands of the palate. Most patients are in their fifth and sixth decades of life and the tumour is uncommon in patients <20 years of age. These tumours are only partially encapsulated and have little tendency for cyst formation and haemorrhage. Nodal metastases are uncommon but haematogenous spread to lungs and bones occurs in 20–50% of cases [2,25]. Peri-neural invasion is the hallmark of this tumour and accounts for the relatively frequent associated pain.

On imaging, parotid tumours may appear either as benign or malignant lesion, whereas minor salivary gland tumours have infiltrative margins. Retrograde skull base invasion occurs via the facial or mandibular nerves and is best demonstrated by contrast MRI.

Acinic cell carcinoma

Acinic cell carcinoma represents only 2–4% of all major salivary gland tumours, occurring almost exclusively in the parotid glands. They account for 15–17% of all malignant parotid tumours. Bilateral parotid tumours occur in 3% making these second only to Warthins tumour to have bilateral involvement [2,25]. The patients are commonly in their fifth or sixth decades of life. Metastases to regional nodes occur in 10–19% of patients and distant metastases to the lung and bones in 15% [32,25].

The imaging appearances of this tumour are non-specific with most lesions appearing to have similar features to pleomorphic adenoma on CT and MRI .

Carcinoma-ex-pleomorphic adenoma

Carcinoma-ex-pleomorphic adenoma is either a malignant change in a benign mixed tumour or is the development of a malignant tumour in a patient having previously undergone resection of a pleomorphic adenoma. Usually, the malignant component is an adenocarcinoma.

The patient often has a long history of a benign mixed tumour with recent rapid enlargement. Pain and facial paralysis are often present.

The main sites of metastases are regional nodes, lungs, bones and brain [3].

Salivary duct carcinoma

Salivary duct carcinoma is an uncommon and aggressive tumour which affects males and has a predilection for parotid glands [24]. These tumours are aggressive and are capable of both haematogenous (lung, bone and brain) and lymphatic dissemination and survival is usually poor. Peri-neural spread is common and cervical lymph node involvement is seen in 70% of cases [24].

Imaging patterns of malignant tumours (Figures 9.4, 9.5, 9.8–9.11, 9.18–9.25)

Computed tomography and magnetic resonance imaging [17,18]

- Infiltrative edges, involvement of overlying skin and soft tissues, poorly defined mass, cystic change and necrosis indicate aggressive pathology.
- High-grade cancer has a low-signal intensity on T1W and T2W images, whereas less aggressive cancers and benign lesions have low-T1W and high-T2W signal intensities. This is attributed to the higher amounts of serous and mucoid material in low-grade and benign tumours compared to high-grade aggressive tumours [7].
- Malignant tumours generally show heterogeneous enhancement with gadolinium contrast.
- Soft tissue involvement (subcutaneous metastases in mucoepidermoid carcinoma) and enlargement of the facial nerve indicates malignant tumour (adenoid cystic carcinoma and salivary duct carcinoma). Contrast MRI is the imaging modality of choice to evaluate peri-neural spread.
- Associated adjacent malignant nodes, or evidence of disseminated disease.

Ultrasound

- Malignant tumours have ill-defined edges compared to benign lesions.
- Malignant tumours have a heterogeneous internal architecture, whereas benign tumours have a more homogeneous internal architecture. This

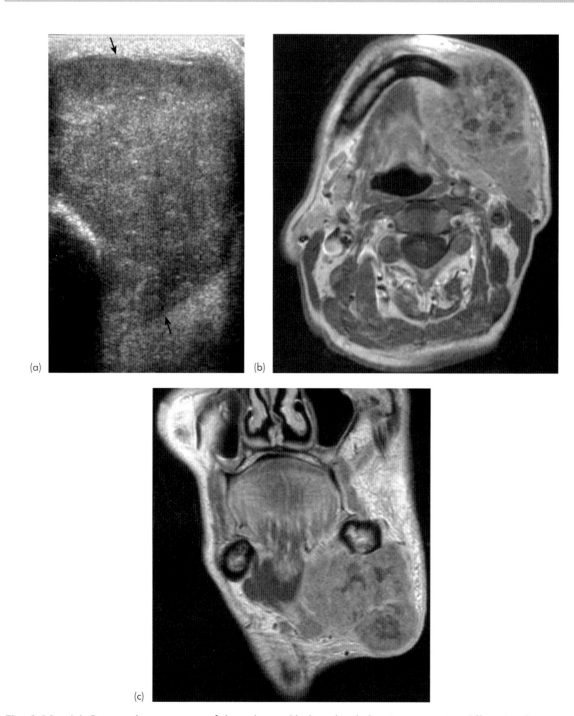

Fig. 9.18 (a) Grey-scale sonogram of the submandibular gland showing extensive diffuse involvement of the gland by tumour (arrows). Note the entire extent and anatomical relationships of the tumour cannot be defined by US. (b) Post-gadolinium T1W axial and (c) coronal MR showing the large tumour involving the submandibular gland. Note the heterogeneous enhancement. The extent of the tumour is better defined and allows for better surgical planning. Surgery confirmed an undifferentiated carcinoma.

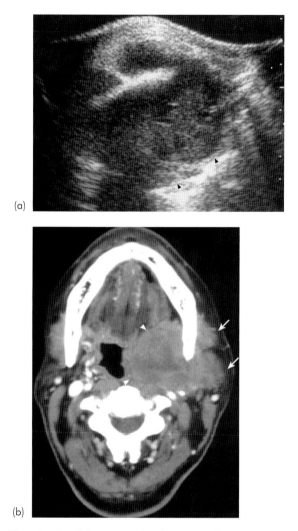

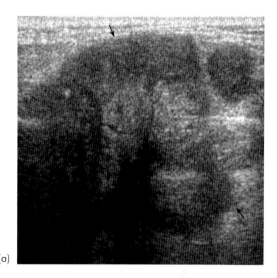

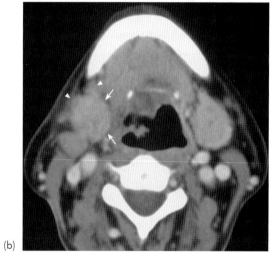

Fig. 9.19 (a) Longitudinal grey-scale sonogram showing a large parotid tumour with superficial and a large deep lobe (arrowheads) component. (b) Although US identified the mass, it is unable to define its entire extent which is clearly seen on a contrast CT (arrowheads). Note the ill-defined edges on CT (arrows). Surgery confirmed a leiomyosarcoma.

Fig. 9.20 (a) Grey-scale sonogram showing a hypoechoic, solid, lobulated, ill-defined mass arising from the submandibular gland (arrows). (b) A contrast enhanced CT demonstrating the mass (arrows) and its ill-defined infiltrative edges (arrowheads). Surgery confirmed a high grade muco-epidermoid carcinoma.

heterogeneity represents necrosis or haemorrhage within the tumour.
- Malignant tumours are more likely to show pronounced vascularity and have a RI > 0.8 and a PI > 2 [22].
- Involvement of overlying skin and subcutaneous tissue is indicative of a malignant process.
- Adjacent abnormal malignant nodes also help to identify malignant salivary gland tumours.

Lymphoma

Both primary and secondary lymphomas of the salivary glands are rare. The diagnosis of primary lymphoma can be suggested only after there is histological involvement of lymphoma of the salivary parenchyma with no intraglandular or extraglandular nodal involvement. Primary lymphomas are considered as MALT (mucosal associated lymphoid tissue) lymphomas. The parotid gland is involved in

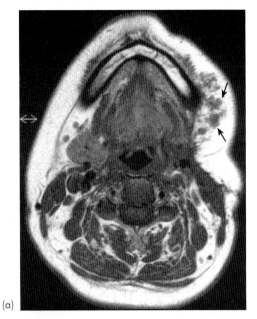

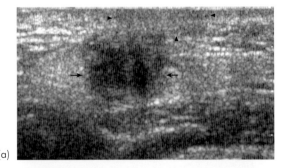

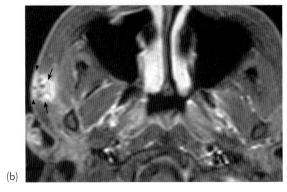

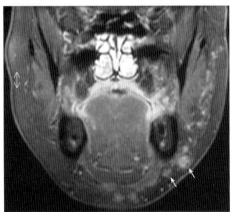

Fig. 9.21   (a) T1W axial and (b) post-gadolinium, fat suppressed T1W coronal showing multiple, small, soft tissue deposits (arrows) in a patient with malignant salivary tumor. Such soft tissue involvement is better detected/demonstrated by MR rather than US.

Fig. 9.22   (a) Longitudinal grey-scale sonogram and (b) post-gadolinium, fat suppressed T1W axial scan showing an ill-defined, solid, hypoechoic mass (arrows) on US. Note the subtle infiltration into the overlying skin and subcutaneous tissues on US (arrowheads). The tumour shows intense, heterogeneous enhancement on MR (arrows) and obvious subcutaneous involvement (arrowheads). Histology confirmed a malignant tumour.

80% of reported cases and the submandibular gland in 20% [24].

Secondary lymphomas are also rare with 80% of cases involving the parotid glands. The overall incidence of salivary gland involvement is 1–8% of all cases of lymphoma. As there is disseminated disease outside the gland, the prognosis of these patients is poor.

Imaging appearances of lymphoma (Figures 9.26 and 9.27) are as follows.

Computed tomography

- If confined to parotid nodes, the nodes are homogeneous and may slightly enhance with contrast.
- If the parenchyma is involved, there may be diffuse infiltration of the gland or focal lesions with poorly defined margins.
- Extraparotid nodal disease helps in the diagnosis.

Magnetic resonance imaging [24]

- Homogeneous intermediate signal intensity on all sequences.
- Adjacent nodal involvement.
- Heterogeneous enhancement following gadolinium.

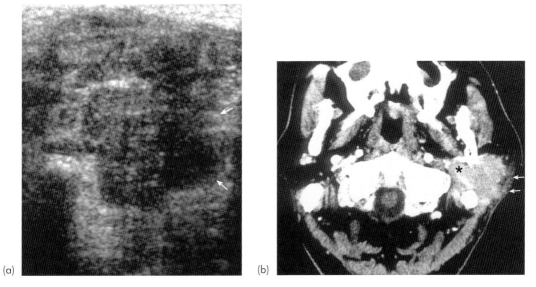

Fig. 9.23 (a) Transverse grey-scale sonogram and (b) an axial contrast CT showing an ill-defined, solid, hypoechoic, heterogeneous mass in the parotid (arrows) on US. Note on CT the deep lobe extension (*) and extra-parotid extension (small arrows) is better demonstrated. Histology confirmed a malignant tumour.

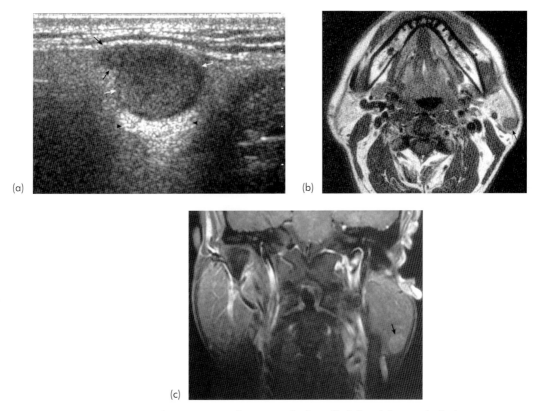

Fig. 9.24 (a) Transverse grey-scale sonogram showing a fairly well-defined, hypoechoic, homogeneous mass (white arrows) with posterior enhancement (arrowheads) in the superficial lobe. The sonographic features are suggestive of a non-aggressive lesion such as a pleomorphic adenoma. However, a small segment of the mass is ill-defined (black arrows) and worrying on US. (b) T1W axial and (c) coronal T1W fat suppressed, post-gadolinium MR showing a fairly well-defined mass (arrow) with smooth outlines and enhancement (arrow). Although appearances mimic a benign lesion, histology confirmed a malignant tumour.

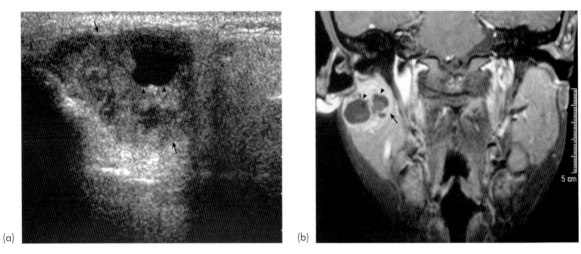

Fig. 9.25 (a) Transverse grey-scale sonogram showing an ill-defined, hypoechoic mass (arrows) with heterogeneous internal echoes and a cystic component (arrowheads). (b) A coronal, fat suppressed, post-gadolinium T1W MR shows the mass (arrow) with diffuse heterogeneous enhancement and cystic areas (arrowheads). Histology confirmed a malignant tumour.

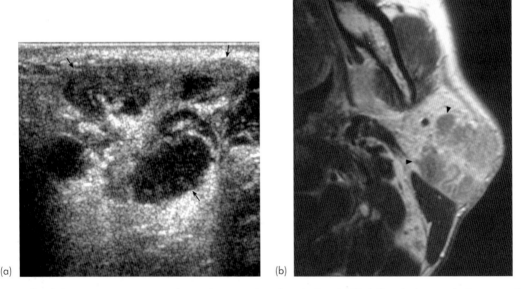

Fig. 9.26 (a) Transverse grey-scale sonogram showing a focal, ill-defined, hypoechoic mass (arrows). (b) The involvement of the superficial lobe and extent (arrowheads) is better demonstrated on a post-gadolinium T1W axial MR. Patient had evidence of disseminated lymphoma.

Ultrasound

- The nodes are usually hypoechoic, predominantly solid with a "pseudosolid" or "reticulated" echo-pattern.

- Multiple nodes scattered within the parotid gland with adjacent extraglandular nodal involvement.
- Exaggerated hilar vascularity on Doppler, intermediate intravascular resistance.

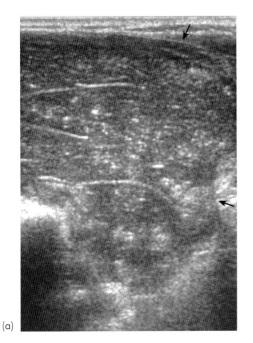

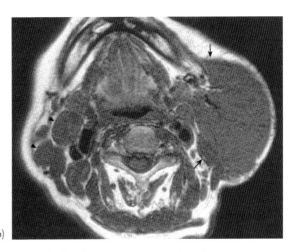

(a)   (b)

Fig. 9.27 (a) Transverse grey-scale sonogram of the parotid gland showing rounded outlines and complete replacement of parenchyma by diffusely hypoechoic tumour tissue (arrows). (b) A T1W axial MR clearly demonstrates the entire parotid involvement (arrows). Note abnormal lymphomatous nodes on the contralateral side (arrowheads), evidence of disseminated disease.

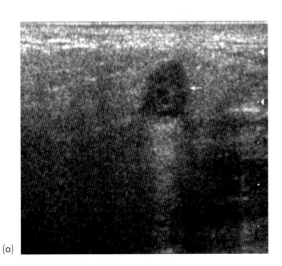

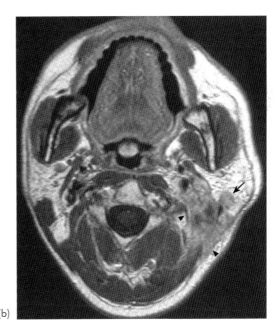

(a)   (b)

Fig. 9.28 (a) Grey-scale sonogram of the parotid in a patient with recurrent nasopharyngeal carcinoma showing a solid, hypoechoic, fairly well-defined nodule in the left parotid gland (arrow). FNAC confirmed a metastatic lesion from the NPC. (b) A T1W axial MR also identifies the lesion (arrow). Also note recurrent tumour in the adjacent soft tissues of the posterior triangle (arrowheads).

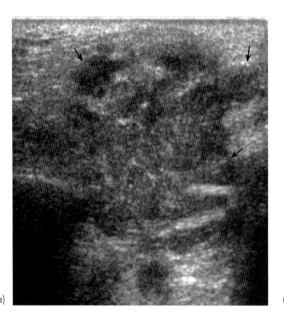
(a)

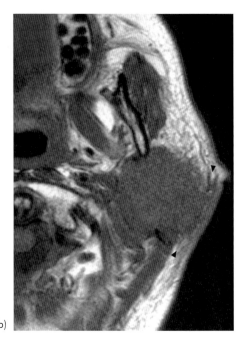
(b)

Fig. 9.29 (a) Another metastatic lesion (again from recurrent NPC) in the parotid gland with ill-defined edges (arrows) on US. (b) Note the invasion into skin and subcutaneous tissue (arrowheads) seen on an axial T1W MR.

Metastases to the salivary glands

The presence of multiple intraparotid nodes makes it susceptible to involvement by metastatic disease. These nodes are predominantly located in the superficial lobe and drain lymphatics from the scalp, external auditory canal and deep fascial spaces. Melanoma of the scalp is the commonest tumour to metastasise to the parotid. The other primary tumours that metastasise to the parotid include, nasopharyngeal carcinoma (Figures 9.28 and 9.29), squamous cell carcinoma of the mouth, ear, base of tongue, pyriform fossa and sinuses.

Masseter muscle lesions mimicking a parotid tumour

Masseter muscle hypertrophy

Masseter muscle hypertrophy may be unilateral or bilateral and is commonly seen in the second and third decades of life, with no sex predeliction. The aetiology is obscure, however, most patients have habitual clenching of the jaw or grind their teeth particularly at night.

Although US is an ideal imaging modality, it can readily compare the two sides and rule out a mass lesion within the masseter muscle. MR demonstrates the anatomy and comparison better (Figure 9.30). No further imaging is necessary for the diagnosis.

Haemangiomas

Haemangiomas are uncommon in the head and neck (15% of all haemangiomas), the masseter muscle being the most common site (36%) [33–35]. The role of imaging is to identify the anatomic location and extent of the mass. These lesions present as painless masses of several months duration. Reddish or bluish discolouration of the overlying skin is a typical feature, and on auscultation a bruit may be heard.

The diagnosis is readily made by US, but MRI best depicts the exact anatomic location and extent (CT has been largely replaced by MRI).

Ultrasound [36] (Figure 9.31a)

• Hypoechoic mass with a heterogeneous echo-pattern.

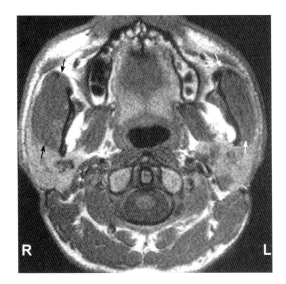

Fig. 9.30 T1W axial MR showing unilateral hypertrophy of the masseter muscle on the right (black arrows) compared to the left (white arrows).

- Multiple sinusoidal spaces are seen within the mass.
- Slow flow is seen within the mass on grey-scale sonography or Doppler.
- The presence of phleboliths is diagnostic.

Magnetic resonance imaging

(Figures 9.31b and 9.31c)

- On T1W sequences haemangiomas appear well circumscribed and are isointense or slightly hypointense compared to skeletal muscle.
- Hyperintense on T2W sequences.
- Variable post-gadolinium enhancement.
- Circular signal voids within the lesion may represent phleboliths and curvilinear flow voids may denote arterial or venous channels.

Metastases

Metastases to skeletal muscle are rare and represent <1% of all haematogenous metastases. Metastases to the masseter muscle are even rarer. The common tumours that metastasise to skeletal muscle are breast, colon and lung, whereas the reported metastases to the masseter originated from cancers in the cervix, breast and kidney [37–39].

Due to the superficial location of the masseter, US is the ideal initial investigation of choice, however, CT

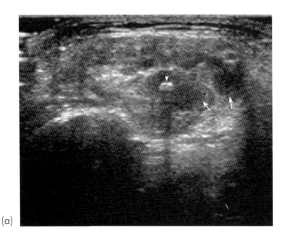

(a)

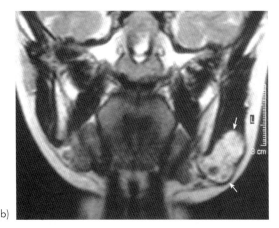

(b)

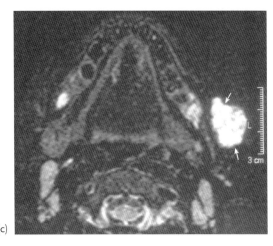

(c)

Fig. 9.31 (a) Grey-scale sonogram showing a masseter muscle haemangioma with phlebolith (arrowhead) and vascular spaces (arrows). (b) A coronal T2W MR and (c) a fat suppressed axial T2W MR show the typical high signal of a haemangioma (arrows).

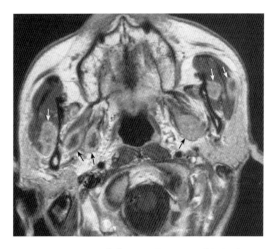

Fig. 9.32   Post-gadolinium T1W axial MR showing metastatic deposits in both masseters (white arrows). Also note the metastatic lesions in the pterygoid muscles (black arrows).

or MRI help to identify other sites of tumour deposits in the head and neck.

Ultrasound [40]

- The metastases are ill defined, hypoechoic with heterogeneous internal architecture.
- Lesions are aligned along the long axis of the muscles.

Magnetic resonance imaging [41]

(Figure 9.32)

- Isointense to muscle on T1W and hyperintense on T2W sequences.
- Intense heterogeneous enhancement after gadolinium injection.
- Evidence of other lesions in the head and neck is readily evaluated.

Imaging of recurrent tumours

This section discusses the imaging of recurrent tumours in patients who have had previous surgery for benign and malignant tumours.

Benign tumours

Pleomorphic adenomas are the tumours that may recur. The recurrence rates vary between 1% and 50%, and is directly related to the initial surgical procedure [24].

Higher recurrence rates are seen in patients

- who are treated by enucleation alone rather than a parotidectomy,
- patients who had capsular rupture at the time of initial surgery.

When recurrences occur, they are often multiple and clustered at the site of previous surgery.

Due to the superficial location of these recurrences, US is an ideal initial investigation and the diagnosis is readily confirmed by FNAC. However, post-operative scarring and altered anatomy may make US a slightly more difficult procedure.

Malignant tumours

The overall recurrence rate for salivary gland tumours is between 27% and 38% [9] and is related to tumour grade and adequacy of resection.

In any patient who has undergone previous surgery for a malignant nodule, CT or preferably MRI (Figure 9.33) is the investigation of choice for evaluating recurrent disease. Despite the altered anatomy, recurrences and adjacent extent of invasion can be readily evaluated. The extent of nodal involvement, if any, can also be assessed.

Management of salivary gland tumours

Surgery is the primary treatment for benign and malignant tumours of the salivary glands. Post-operative radiotherapy is given when indicated to improve local control and survival. Radiotherapy is used as the treatment modality for inoperable tumours and in those patients unfit for surgery [42].

A mass in a major salivary gland that has not been proven to be malignant is treated surgically with an *en bloc* procedure. If in the parotid gland and depending on its location, the mass will require either a superficial or a total parotidectomy together with an adequate margin of normal gland. A complete submandibular gland excision is undertaken for a mass situated within this gland [43].

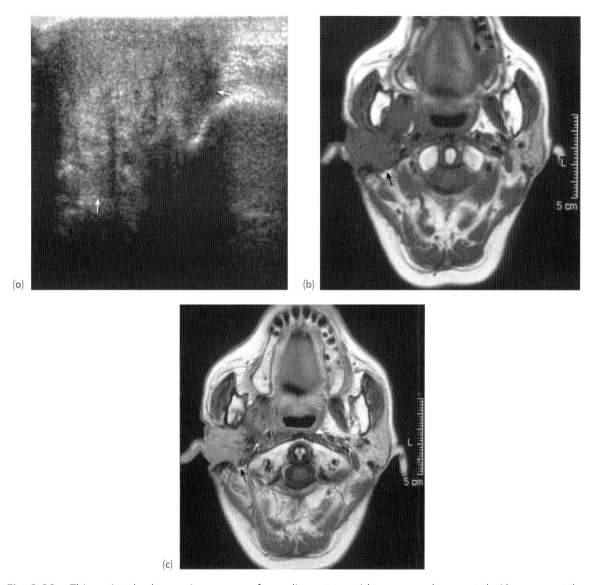

(a)

(b)

(c)

Fig. 9.33 This patient had a previous surgery for malignant parotid tumour and presented with a mass at the surgical site. (a) Grey-scale sonogram showing a solid, ill-defined, hypoechoic mass (arrows) consistent with recurrent disease. (b) An axial non-contrast and (c) post-gadolinium enhanced T1W MR showing a tumour (arrow) with low-signal intensity and enhancement at the surgical site. Biopsy confirmed tumour recurrence.

A malignant mass in the parotid gland requires a total parotidectomy, and in the submandibular gland a submandibular gland excision. Wide excision and gross total removal of all tumour must be ensured [44].

The facial nerve should always be preserved where possible. If the nerve is close to the tumour, it should be carefully dissected free of the mass. If the nerve is surrounded by tumour, the involved part of the nerve is resected followed by immediate reconstruction.

A neck dissection is performed when there are proven lymph node metastases either pre-operatively, or peroperatively on frozen-section examination of suspicious regional lymph nodes.

Recurrence of any salivary gland tumour is treated aggressively with radical surgery and post-operative radiotherapy, if no previous radiotherapy has been given. A facial nerve monitor may be used to locate and preserve the facial nerve during dissection.

Conclusion

Most salivary gland masses are seen in the parotid glands where 80% are benign and 90% are located in the superficial lobe. US is, therefore, the most cost-effective investigation for such cases and can be readily combined with FNAC. It has a high sensitivity and specificity. However, whenever deep lobe extension is suspected, even for benign masses, a CT or preferably MRI should be performed.

In our experience CT, or preferably MRI should be the initial investigation in all patients who have clinical signs suggestive of malignancy, tumours that appear to arise from the deep lobe of parotid, large tumours, tumours with submucosal intraoral presentation and all recurrent tumours.

References

1. Eneroth CM. Salivary gland tumors in the parotid gland, submandibular gland and the palate region. *Cancer* 1971; **27**: 1415–1418.
2. Rabinov K and Weber AL. *Radiology of the Salivary Glands.* GK Hall & Co, Boston, MA. 1985, 292–367.
3. Rankow RM and Polayes IM. Surgical treatment of salivary gland tumors. In: RM Rankow and IM Polayes (Eds) *Diseases of the Salivary Glands.* WB Saunders Co, Philadelphia, PA. 1976, 239–283.
4. Audair PL, Ellis GL, Gnepp DR *et al.* Salivary gland neoplasms. General considerations. In: G Ellis, P Audair, D Gnepp (Eds) *Surgical Pathology of the Salivary Glands.* WB Saunders Co, Philadelphia, PA. 1991.
5. Alvi A, Myers EN and Carrau RL. Malignant tumors of the salivary glands. In: EN Myers and JY Suen (Eds) *Cancer of the Head and Neck,* 3rd edition. WB Saunders Co, Philadelphia, PA. 1996, 525–561.
6. Eneroth CM. Facial paralysis: a criterion of malignancy in parotid tumors. *Arch. Otol.* 1972; **95**: 300–304.
7. Thackray AC and Sobin LH. Histological typing of salivary gland tumors. In: *International Histological Classification of Tumours,* No. 7. World Health Organization, Geneva. 1972.
8. Johns ME and Coulthard SW. Survival and follow up in malignant tumors of the salivary glands. *Orol. Clin. N. Am.* 1977; **10**: 510–516.
9. Kaplan MJ and Hohns ME. Malignant neoplasms. In: CW Cummings, JM Frederickson, LA Harker *et al.* (Eds) *Otolaryngology, Head and Neck Surgery.* Mosby-Year Book, St Louis. 1993, 1043–1078.
10. Hanna DC, Dickason WL, Richardson GS *et al.* Management of recurrent salivary gland tumors. *Am. J. Surg.* 1976; **132**: 453–458.
11. Ariyoshi Y and Shimahara M. Determining whether a parotid tumor is in the superficial or deep lobe using magnetic resonance imaging. *J. Oral. Max. Surg.* 1998; **56**: 23–26.
12. Evans RM. Salivary glands. *Bull. Br. Med. Ultrasound Soc.* 2001; **9**: 20–25.
13. Frable MS and Frable WJ. Fine needle aspiration biopsy of salivary glands. *Laryngoscope* 1991; **101**: 245–249.
14. Cohen MB, Resnicek MJ and Miller TR. Fine needle aspiration of the salivary glands. *Pathol. Ann.* 1992; **27**: 213–245.
15. Jayaram G, Verman AK, Sood N *et al.* Fine needle aspiration cytology of salivary gland lesions. *J. Oral. Pathol. Med.* 1994; **23**: 256–261.
16. Bartels S, Talbot J, DiTomasso J *et al.* The relative value of fine needle aspiration and imaging in the preoperative evaluation of parotid masses. *Head Neck* 2000; **22**(8): 781–786.
17. Kassel EE. CT sialography, Part II. Parotid masses. *J. Orolaryngol.* 1982; **12**: 11–24.
18. Som PM and Biller HF. The MR identification of high grade parotid tumors. *Radiology* 1989; **173**: 823–826.
19. Choi D, Na D, Brun H *et al.* Salivary gland tumours: evaluation with two phase Helical CT. *Radiology* 2000; **214**: 231–236.
20. Lack EE and Upton MP. Histopathologic review of salivary gland tumors in children. *Arch. Otolaryngol. Head Neck Surg.* 1988; **114**: 898–906.
21. Snyderman Nl and Suen JY. Neoplasms. In: Cummings CW, Fredrickson JM, Harker LA *et al.* (Eds) *Otolaryngology – Head and Neck Surgery,* 2, Chapter 58. Mosby-Year Book, St Louis. 1986, 1027–1069.
22. Bradley MJ. Colour flow Doppler in the investigation of salivary gland tumours. *Abs/Eu J U/S,* 1998; **7**(suppl 2): S16.
23. Martinoli C, Derchi L, Solbiati L *et al.* Color Doppler sonography of salivary glands. *Am. J. Roentgenol.* 1994; **163**: 933–941.
24. Som PM and Brandwein M. Salivary glands. In: Som PM and Curtin HD (Eds) *Head and Neck Imaging,* 3rd edition, 2, Chapter 17. Mosby-Year Book, St. Louis. 1996, 823–914.
25. Peel RZ and Gnepp DR. Diseases of the salivary glans. In: Barnes L. (Ed.) *Surgical Pathology of the Head and Neck,* 1. Marcel Dekker Inc., New York, NY. 1985, 533–645.
26. Som PM, Shugar JMA, Sacher M *et al.* Benign and malignant parotid pleomorphic adenomas: CT and MR studies. *J. Comput. Assist. Tomogr.* 1988; **12**: 65–69.
27. Batsakis JG. *Tumors of the Head and Neck, Clinical and Pathological Considerations,* 2nd edition. Williams & Wilkins Baltimore, MD. 1979, 1–20.
28. Gnepp DR. Malignant mixed tumors of the salivary glands: a review. *Pathol. Ann.* 1993; **28**: 279–328.
29. Healey WV, Perzin KH and Smith L. Mucoepidermoid carcinoma of salivary gland origin. *Cancer* 1970; **26**: 368–388.
30. Conley J and Dingman DL. Adenoid cystic carcinoma in the head and neck (cylindroma). *Arch. Otolaryngol.* 1974; **100**: 81–90.
31. Auclair PL, Ellis GL, Gnepp DR *et al.* Salivary gland neoplasms: general considerations. In: GL Elli, PL Auclair and DR Gnepp (Eds.) *Surgical Pathology of the Salivary Glands.* WB Saunders Co., Philadelphia, PA. 1991.
32. Andersen LJ, Therkildsen MH, Ockelmann HH *et al.* Malignant epithelial tumors in the minor salivary glands, the submandibular gland and the sublingual gland. *Cancer* 1991; **68**: 2431–2437.
33. Rossiter JL, Hendrix RA, Tom LWC *et al.* Intramuscular hemangioma of the head and neck. *Otolaryngol. Head Neck Surg.* 1993; **108**: 18.
34. Batsakis JG. Vasoformative tumors. In: JG Batsakis (Ed.) *Tumors of the Head and Neck: Clinical and Pathological Consideration,* 2nd edition. Williams & Wilkins, Baltimore, MD. 1979, 294.
35. Shallow TA, Eger SA and Wagner FB. Primary hemangiomatous tumours of skeletal muscle. *Ann. Surg.* 1944; **119**: 700.
36. Yang WT, Ahuja A and Metreweli C. Sonographic features of head and neck hemangiomas and vascular malformations: review of 23 patients. *J. Ultrasound Med.* 1997; **16**: 39–44.
37. Wong BJF, Passy V and DiSaia P. Metastatic small cell carcinoma to the masseter muscle originating from the uterine cervix. *Ear Nose Throat J.* 1995; **74**: 118.

38. Tosios K, Vasilas A and Arsenopoulos A. Metastatic breast carcinoma of the masseter: case report. *J. Oral. Max. Surg.* 1999; **50**: 304.

39. Nekagawa H, Mizukami Y, Kimura H *et al*. Metastatic masseter muscle tumour: a report of a case. *Laryngo. Otol.* 1996; **110**: 172.

40. Ahuja At, King Ad, Bradley MJ, Yeo W, Mok TSK and Metreweli C. Sonographic findings in masseter muscle metastases. *J. Clin. Ultrasound* 2000; **28**: 299–302.

41. Chan NPH, Yeo W, Ahuja AT and King AD. Multiple skeletal muscle metastases: the apperances on MR imaging. *HK Med. J.* 1999; **5**: 410.

42. Leverstein H, Van Der Wal JE, Tiwari RM *et al*. Malignant epithelial parotid gland tumours: analysis and results in 65 previously untreated patients. *Br. J. Surg.* 1998; **85**(9): 1267–1272.

43. Rice DH. Salivary gland disorders. *Med. Clin. N. Am.* 1999; **83**(1): 197–217.

44. Rice DH. Malignant salivary gland neoplasms. *Otolarygol. Clin. N. Am.* 1999; **32**(5): 875–886.

CHAPTER 10

Thyroid Cancer

AT Ahuja, RM Evans and AC Vlantis

Introduction

A solitary thyroid nodule is defined as a palpable discrete swelling in an otherwise normal thyroid gland. They are common and most are benign. The incidence of solitary thyroid nodules is approximately 3.2% of the population in the UK and 4.2% of the population in the USA. They are four times more common in women than in men and their prevalence increases with age [1–4]. Clinical palpation is poor at detecting small thyroid nodules, highlighted by the fact that approximately 70% of normal thyroid glands contain nodules of <1 cm when examined sonographically [5–9]. The risk of malignancy in a euthyroid patient with a solitary thyroid nodule is estimated to be 5–10% with a range of 3.4–29% [10–15]. Although thyroid cancer is relatively uncommon, 0.5% of all malignancies, it remains a significant clinical problem because of the:

- unpredictable nature of malignant thyroid tumours,
- difficulty in differentiating a malignant nodule from a more common benign thyroid nodule or of identifying a malignant nodule in a nodular goitre,

- management of a solitary nodule is often contentious [16].

Clinicians evaluate all thyroid nodules carefully and have developed rational approaches to their diagnosis and management. The main aim in the management of a thyroid nodule is to identify the small group of patients in whom the nodule is malignant while avoiding unnecessary investigations and treatment in the majority of patients who have a benign nodule.

Clinical presentation of thyroid carcinoma

The most common presentation of a thyroid carcinoma is the presence of a thyroid nodule, noticed either by the patient or physician. Clinical features that are suspicious of thyroid cancer include:

- firm, non-tender nodule;
- cervical lymph node enlargement;
- recent onset of hoarseness;
- vocal cord paralysis;
- haemoptysis;
- dysphagia;

- previous history of exposure to radiation;
- family history of thyroid cancer.

Clinical examination of the thyroid gland may reveal a solitary or multiple thyroid nodules. The physical examination must include a careful evaluation of the larynx, tongue and the neck for lymphadenopathy. Most patients will have no overt signs of thyroid cancer and so the clinical examination is limited mainly to distinguish a benign from a malignant lesion and to detect small nodes.

The aetiology, epidemiology, surgical pathology and various staging classifications for thyroid cancer are beyond the scope of this chapter. However, this chapter will discuss the role of imaging and fine needle aspiration cytology (FNAC) in the identification of thyroid malignancies.

Management protocol

The vast majority of patients with thyroid malignancy will be euthyroid. Although of limited value, it is commonly agreed that most patients should have a baseline thyroid function test. A hyperfunctioning or hot nodule and hence suppressed TSH is associated with a low risk of malignancy [17]. Thyroid antibodies may be positive in both benign and malignant conditions and are unhelpful in the diagnosis of malignancy [17].

The investigation of a thyroid nodule will vary among different centres, and is based on local expertise and the availability of investigations. The mainstay of the initial evaluation of thyroid nodules has been ultrasound (US), FNA and thyroid scintigraphy. All three have been used in various combinations with little consensus in the literature about their respective values [18]. It is now commonly believed that only FNAC and US have a role in the routine work-up of thyroid nodules. The main aim of these investigations is to accurately identify those patients with malignant thyroid nodules so that appropriate surgery is offered to patients with the correct indication.

We will mainly discuss the role of FNAC and sonography in the identification of thyroid malignancies. The CT and MR characteristics of various thyroid cancers will be briefly described.

Fine needle aspiration cytology

FNAC is an inexpensive, widely available and easy to perform examination that is commonly regarded as the initial investigation of choice for a thyroid nodule. Acute complications are rare and there are no reported cases of cutaneous implantation of malignancy following a thyroid FNAC [19]. It has a pre-operative predictive accuracy of >90% [19] and helps the surgeon to select the most appropriate procedure pre-operatively. It has reduced the cost of work-up since in many centres an FNAC with cytological analysis is less expensive than either US or scintigraphy [14]. However, its success depends on the skill of the person doing the procedure and on the experience of the cytopathologist [19]. FNAC has an overall false negative rate of between 0.5% and 11.8% (pooled rate of 2.4%) and a false positive rate ranging from 0% to 7.1% (pooled rate of 1.2%) [14,20]. The false negative rates can be reduced by better sampling techniques, meticulous follow-up and serial FNAC examinations [19]. Acceptable diagnostic results can be obtained by clinicians who perform at least 20–35 FNAs per year [21].

While the non-diagnostic rate of FNAC may vary among different centres depending on the level of local expertise, 15% non-diagnosis is the maximum acceptable limit recommended by the Papanicolaou Society Guidelines [22].

Conventional FNAC or US-guided FNAC?

Despite the general acceptance of FNAC as a standard diagnostic tool, the role of US-guided FNAC has been a source of controversy in the literature, and therefore, its use may vary among different centres.

In an ideal situation, US-guided FNAC would be the diagnostic procedure of choice as it clearly directs and identifies the position of the needle at all times, in routine practice, however, a conventional FNAC is the most cost-effective initial procedure [23].

A US-guided FNAC is recommended for [24–26]:

- impalpable or poorly palpable nodules (<2 cm),
- non-diagnostic or failed previous conventional FNAC.

Tumour staging

Tumour-node-metastasis (TNM) classification for papillary and follicular carcinoma.

T0	No tumour
T1	Tumour <1 cm
T2	Tumour 1–4 cm
T3	Tumour >4 cm
T4	Tumour invades beyond thyroid capsule
N0	No nodes
N1a	Ipsilateral cervical nodes
N1b	Bilateral, midline, contralateral or mediastinal nodes
M0	No distant metastases
M1	Distant metastases

Thyroid imaging
Ultrasound

As US routinely identifies small nodules in about 70% of patients, we feel that its main role is to pick out a malignant nodule from the vast number of benign nodules. The following paragraphs will briefly discuss the features elucidated by US and identify those that help to identify malignancy (alone or in combination).

Any sonographic examination of the thyroid must include a detailed examination of the neck for nodal disease. Metastatic nodes are frequently seen in many thyroid cancers and may alter the surgical management of patients. When an elective neck dissection is performed for palpable lymph nodes, up to 90% of patients with papillary carcinoma will have regional nodal metastases. If no neck dissection is performed when no nodes are palpable, nodes later develop in 7–15% of patients, with a mean delay of 4.5 years [27]. Medullary carcinoma is associated with palpable nodes in 25% of patients at presentation and 50–75% of patients will have positive nodes at surgery.

Echogenicity
It is reported that the incidence of malignancy is 4% when a solid lesion is hyperechoic. If the lesion is hypoechoic (Figure 10.1) the incidence of malignancy rises to 26% [28]. Hypoechogenicity alone is inaccurate in predicting malignancy and as a sole

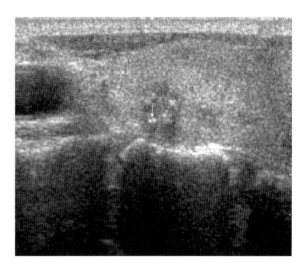

Fig. 10.1 Longitudinal sonogram showing punctate calcification (arrow) in an ill-defined, hypoechoic nodule. Such calcification is typically seen in papillary carcinoma of thyroid.

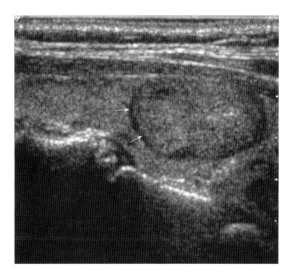

Fig. 10.2 Longitudinal sonogram of an isoechoic thyroid nodule with a well-defined perinodular halo (arrows). Surgery confirmed a follicular adenoma.

predictive sign has poor specificity (49%) and poor positive predictive value 40% [29].

Margins
A peripheral halo (Figure 10.2) of decreased echogenicity is seen around hypoechoic and iso-echoic nodules and is caused by either the capsule of the nodule or compressed thyroid tissue and vessels [30].

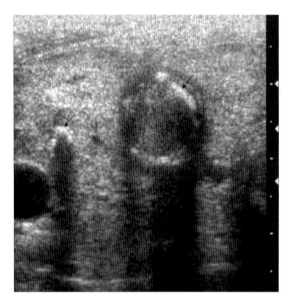

Fig. 10.3 Transverse sonogram showing curvilinear calcification (arrows) with dense posterior shadowing. The appearances are suggestive of benign calcification in nodular goitre.

The absence of a halo (Figure 10.1) has a specificity of 77% and sensitivity of 67% in predicting malignancy [31].

Calcification

Fine punctate calcification (Figure 10.1) due to calcified psammoma bodies within the nodule is seen in papillary carcinoma in 25–40% of cases [32]. As a sole predictive sign of malignancy, microcalcification is the most reliable sign with an accuracy of 76%, specificity of 93% and a positive predictive value of 70% [29]. Coarse, dysmorphic curvilinear calcification commonly indicates benignity (Figure 10.3).

Comet tail sign

The presence of a comet tail (Figure 10.4) sign in a thyroid nodule indicates a benign colloid nodule [33]. In the authors experience, this sign has never been detected in malignant nodules.

Multinodularity (Figure 10.5)

The fact that multinodularity implies benignity is a myth as approximately 10–20% of papillary carcinomas may be multicentric [30,34]. In those with true solitary nodules confirmed at surgery, the risk of cancer is the same as in those with multinodular goitres [35].

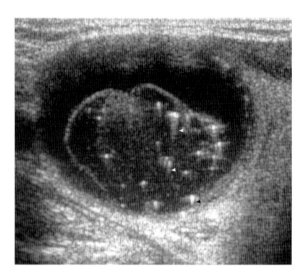

Fig. 10.4 Transverse sonogram showing comet tail artefact (arrowheads) in a cystic colloid nodule.

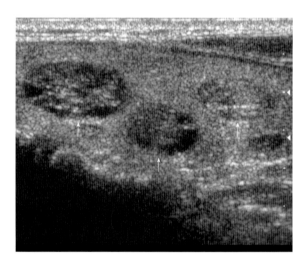

Fig. 10.5 Longitudinal sonogram showing multiple nodules (arrows). Note the cystic change and septation, which are commonly seen in hyperplastic nodules.

Colour flow patterns

There are three general patterns of vascular distribution of a thyroid nodule [36]:

- Type I: Complete absence of flow signal within the nodule.
- Type II: Exclusive perinodular flow signals (Figure 10.6).

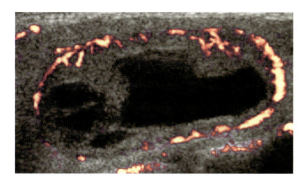

Fig. 10.6 Longitudinal power Doppler sonogram showing benign, perinodular type II vascularity.

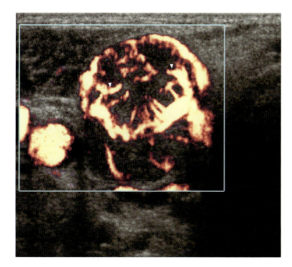

Fig. 10.7 Transverse, power Doppler sonogram showing large intranodular (arrowheads) type III vascularity, suggestive of a malignant thyroid nodule.

- Type III: Intranodular flow with multiple vascular poles chaotically arranged, with or without significant perinodular vessels (Figure 10.7).

Type III pattern is, generally, associated with malignancy and types I and II are seen in benign hyperplastic nodules [36,37]. However, with the use of newer high-resolution transducers, in the authors experience type I vascularity is quite uncommon.

However, as a sole predictor of malignancy, colour flow characteristics are not accurate [31]. It is well recognised that the predictive ability of US for malignancy is effective only when multiple signs are present in the same nodule. Although their predictive value increases in summation, it is at the cost of sensitivity [31].

Of the various combinations of US criteria used to determine malignancy:

- microcalcification and a solid nature [29] showed the highest accuracy (77%), specificity (96%), positive predictive value (75%) but a low sensitivity (30%);
- absent halo and the presence of microcalcification had a specificity of 93% and sensitivity of 27% [31];
- a combination of an absent halo, intranodular flow and the presence of microcalcification had a specificity of 97% and sensitivity of 16% [31].

	Benign	Malignant
Echogenicity		
Hyper	+++	
Iso	++	
Hypo		++
Halo		
Absent		++
Present	++	
Calcification		
Micro		+++
Curvilinear/coarse	+++	
Comet tail sign		
Present	+++	
Multiplicity		
Solitary		+
Multiple	++	
Colour flow		
Peripheral	+	
Intranodular		++

+++ High probability.
++ Intermediate probability.
+ Low probability.

Other imaging modalities

Scintigraphy

Although thyroid scintigraphy is often used, our experience has been similar to other recent reports that state that scintigraphy has no place in routine clinical practice as it is unable to accurately differentiate a benign from a malignant nodule [16,19,23,

38,39]. We believe that the role of scintigraphy should be used for:

- a palpable nodule in a patient with hyperthyroidism to rule out an autonomously functioning nodule;
- a hyperthyroid patient with possible thyroiditis.

CT and MRI

CT and MRI have virtually no role in the routine investigation of a thyroid nodule. In invasive thyroid malignancy they evaluate the extrathyroid spread of tumour to the larynx, trachea and adjacent vessels [19,40] and provide evidence of regional or distant metastases.

The CT and MR appearances of malignant lesions are generally non-specific, and in our experience only useful in three specific instances:

- Detection of calcification: The presence of fine punctate calcification within a nodule or adjacent metastatic node on CT would suggest papillary carcinoma.
- Cystic papillary carcinoma: Benign cystic thyroid lesions (simple serous cysts, end-stage degenerative cysts) display low attenuation on CT. They are hypointense on T1W and hyperintense on T2W MR sequences. Due to the presence of thyro-globulin within a cystic papillary carcinoma these tumours may appear isointense (to muscle) on CT and maybe hyperintense on T1W as well as on T2W sequences on MR. Similar features are seen in cystic nodal metastases from papillary carcinoma.
- Recurrent thyroid cancer (post-operative).

Common thyroid carcinomas

Papillary carcinoma

Papillary carcinoma accounts for 60–70% of all thyroid malignancies [41], with a peak incidence in the third and fourth decades. The majority of patients are female. It has an excellent prognosis with the 20-year survival rate as high as 90% [32].

Poor prognostic factors include:

- male sex,
- increased age (>45 years),
- large size, >3 cm,
- vascular invasion,
- extraglandular extension,
- poor differentiation on pathology.

Papillary carcinomas are firm, non- or partially encapsulated tumours that may be located anywhere within the thyroid gland.

The tumour commonly invades regional lymphatics accounting for the multifocal nature of the tumour within the thyroid gland and its spread to regional lymph nodes. Venous invasion occurs in 7% of papillary carcinomas and distant metastases to bone and lung are seen in 5–7%. Survival may be improved with radio-iodine treatment [42].

Ultrasound features of papillary carcinoma

- Predominantly solid (70%) and hypoechoic (77–90%) [32,37] (Figure 10.8).
- 20–30% may have a cystic component (Figure 10.9).
- 10–20% are multifocal on US [30].

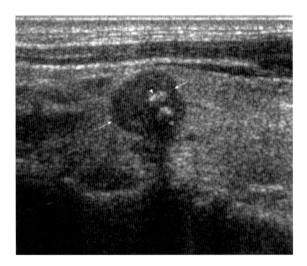

Fig. 10.8 Longitudinal sonogram of the thyroid showing the typical appearances of a papillary carcinoma (arrows). It is solid, hypoechoic, with ill-defined edges posteriorly and punctate calcification (arrowhead).

- Punctate microcalcification (25–90%) [32,37] (Figure 10.8).
- 15–30% are well-defined and haloed [43–46] (Figure 10.10).
- Chaotic intranodular vascularity on colour flow imaging [37] (Figures 10.9 and 10.10).
- Adjacent characteristic lymph nodes [47]: cystic necrosis in 25%, microcalcification in 50% (Figure 10.11), located in the pre/paratracheal regions and along the cervical chain.

CT in papillary carcinoma

- Identification of microcalcification.
- Define tumour extent (involvement of larynx, trachea and adjacent vessels).
- Lung metastases.

MRI in papillary carcinoma

- Define tumour extent (involvement of larynx, trachea and adjacent vessels) (Figures 10.12–10.14).

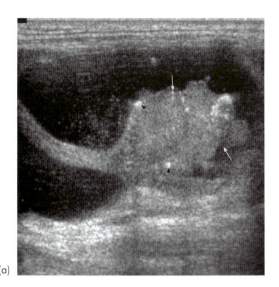

(a)

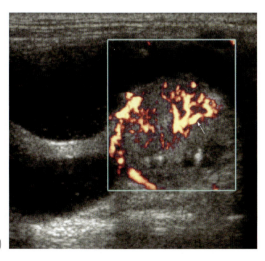

(b)

Fig. 10.9 Transverse sonogram (a) of the thyroid shows a predominantly cystic mass with a solid mural nodule (arrows). Note the punctate calcification (arrowheads) and vascularity (b) (small arrows) within the mural nodule. FNAC of the solid portion confirmed a papillary carcinoma.

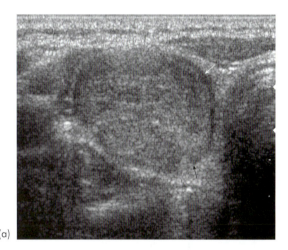

(a)

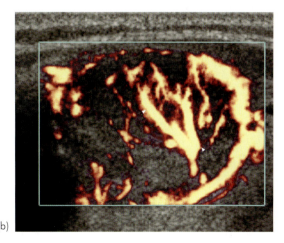

(b)

Fig. 10.10 Transverse sonogram of the thyroid (a) showing a fairly well-defined, hypoechoic mass (arrows). The large intranodular vessels (arrowheads) on power Doppler (b) suggested the malignant nature of the mass. FNAC confirmed a papillary carcinoma.

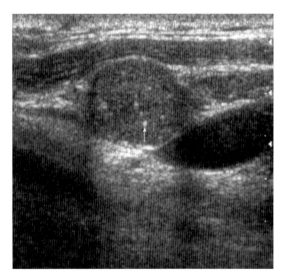

Fig. 10.11 Grey scale sonogram showing a nodal metastasis from a papillary carcinoma of the thyroid. The punctate echogenic foci (arrow) is the clue to the origin of the metastases.

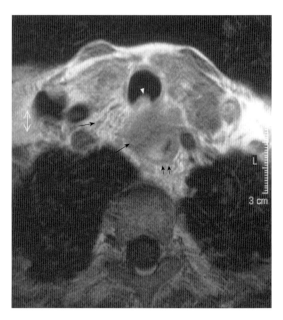

Fig. 10.13 Post-gadolinum T1W MRI showing a papillary carcinoma invading the soft tissues posteriorly (large arrows). Note the involvement of the trachea (arrowhead) and oesophagus (small arrows).

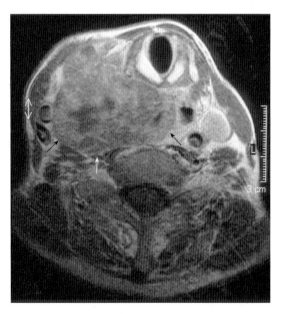

Fig. 10.12 Post-gadolinum T1W MRI showing a large papillary carcinoma in the right lobe with extensive involvement of extrathyroid soft tissues (arrows).

- Cystic metastatic nodes can be correctly identified by MR. Due to the presence of thyroglobulin within cystic nodes, they maybe hyperintense on both T1W and T2W sequences on MR (Figure 10.15).

Key points

Papillary carcinoma

- Predominantly solid, ill defined, hypoechoic
- Punctate calcification
- Chaotic vascular pattern on colour flow imaging
- Associated characteristic lymphadenopathy

Anaplastic carcinoma

Anaplastic carcinoma is one of the most aggressive head and neck cancers and is associated with a poor prognosis and accounts for 15–20% of all thyroid cancers [41]. The diagnosis is often clinical with rapid growth in a long-standing thyroid nodule. Patients frequently present with signs and symptoms of airway compression.

Ultrasound features

- Hypoechoic tumour diffusely involving the entire lobe or gland (Figure 10.16).

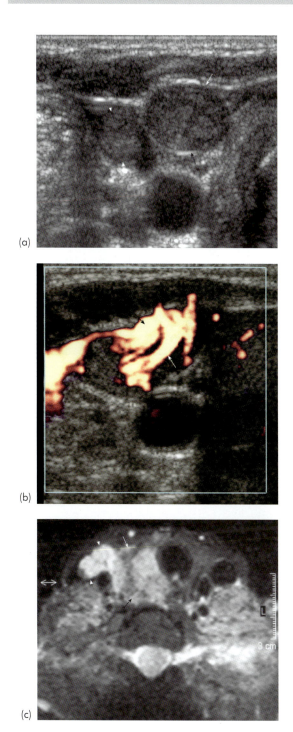

(a)

(b)

(c)

Fig. 10.14 Transverse sonogram of the thyroid (a) showing a solid, hypoechoic, malignant-looking nodule (arrows). Note the thrombus in adjacent internal jugular vein (arrowheads), which shows tumour vascularity (arrows) on power Doppler. (b) A T2W MRI with fat saturation (c) shows the malignant thyroid nodule (arrows) and adjacent thrombus in IJV (arrowheads).

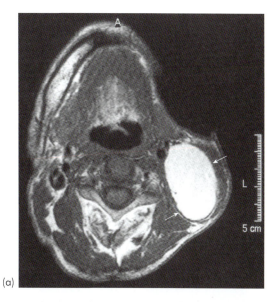

(a)

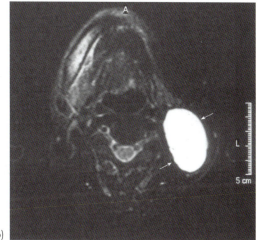

(b)

Fig. 10.15 Axial T1W (a) and T2W (b) MRI images showing a large cystic mass in the left neck (arrows). The high signal of the fluid on T1W scan, due to the thyroglobulin secreted by a papillary carcinoma, provides the clue to these cystic metastatic nodes from papillary carcinoma.

- Areas of necrosis in 78% and dense amorphous calcification in 58% [48] (Figure 10.17).
- Nodal or distant metastases in 80% of patients [49]. Necrotic nodes in 50% [32].
- Often seen against a background of nodular goitre (47%).
- Extracapsular spread and vascular invasion in a third of patients [49] (Figures 10.18 and 10.19).
- Multiple small vessels on colour flow, however, necrotic tumours may be hypovascular.

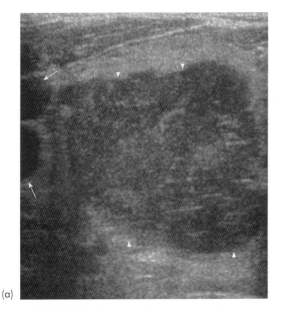

(a)

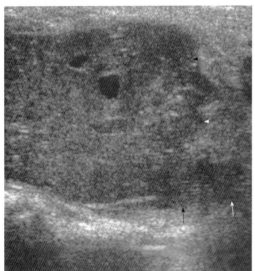

(b)

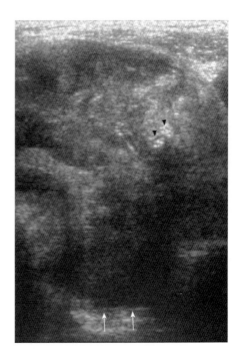

Fig. 10.17 Transverse sonogram shows diffuse, hypoechoic, heterogeneous thyroid with areas of focal calcification (arrowheads). Appearances are of an anaplastic carcinoma against a background of multinodularity. Note the extrathyroid extension of the tumour posteriorly (arrows).

Fig. 10.16 (a) Transverse sonogram showing a solid, hypoechoic, ill-defined mass in the thyroid (arrowheads). Arrows identify adjacent vessels (CCA and IJV). (b) Longitudinal sonogram showing ill-defined edges (arrowheads) and extrathyroid extension (arrows) of anaplastic carcinoma.

CT in anaplastic carcinoma

- Metastatic cervical nodes.
- Mediastinal involvement.
- Define tumour extent (involvement of larynx, trachea and adjacent vessels).

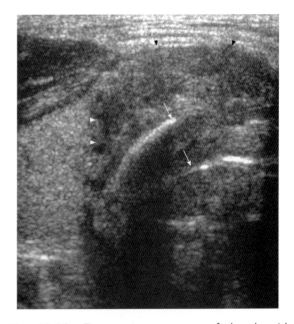

Fig. 10.18 Transverse sonogram of the thyroid showing an ill-defined, anaplastic carcinoma (arrowheads) with extensive tracheal invasion (arrows).

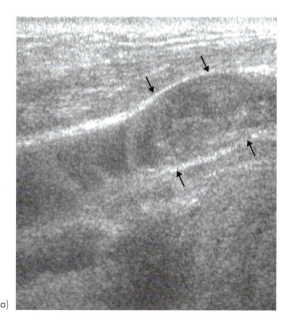

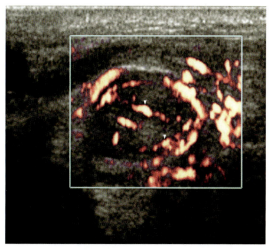

(a)

(b)

Fig. 10.19 Longitudinal grey scale sonogram (a) showing a thrombus in the IJV (arrows) expanding the lumen of the vessel. Note the vessels within the thrombus (arrowheads) on the transverse power Doppler sonogram, (b) confirming it is a tumour thrombus.

MRI in anaplastic carcinoma

Often the general condition of these patients is poor and MRI is difficult to perform; however, if it is possible, its role is to evaluate:

- metastatic cervical nodes,
- define tumour extent (involvement of larynx, trachea and adjacent vessels) (Figure 10.20).

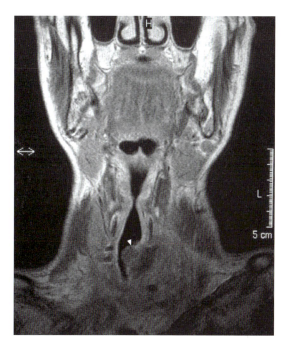

Fig. 10.20 T1W coronal MRI showing tracheal invasion from a thyroid anaplastic carcinoma (arrowhead).

Key points

Anaplastic carcinoma

- Ill defined, hypoechoic, often cystic
- Amorphous calcification
- Background nodularity
- Chaotic vascular pattern on colour flow imaging
- Frequent adjacent vascular invasion
- Frequent associated lymphadenopathy

Medullary carcinoma

Medullary carcinoma arises from the parafollicular C-cells that secrete thyrocalcitonin and represent 5% of all thyroid cancers [41]. The tumour is commonly seen at the site of maximum C-cell concentration, which is the lateral upper two-thirds of the gland [42]. In 10–20% of all cases, there is a family history of phaeochromocytoma or hypercalcaemia. In 50% of cases, nodal metastases are seen at presentation and 15–25% have distant metastases to the liver, lungs and bone [42]. Medullary carcinoma can be associated with MEN syndrome, these patients have a biologically aggressive tumour and may develop metastases earlier with a 55% survival rate at 5 years [50, 51].

Recurrence in the neck and mediastinum is common in medullary carcinoma and an increased serum calcitonin is highly specific for tumour recurrence.

Ultrasound features

- Solid hypoechoic nodule (Figures 10.21 and 10.22).
- Echogenic (Figure 10.23) foci in 80–90% of tumours which represent deposits of amyloid and associated calcification [32,41]. Similar deposits are also seen in 50–60% of associated nodal metastases.
- Chaotic vessels within the tumour, type III vascularity (Figure 10.22).
- Location: focal hypoechoic mass in the upper third of the gland in the sporadic form and diffuse involvement of both lobes in the familial form [41].

CT in medullary carcinoma

- Metastatic cervical nodes.
- Mediastinal involvement.
- Define tumour extent (involvement of larynx, trachea and adjacent vessels).

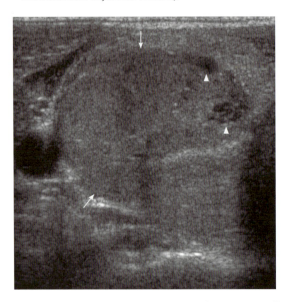

Fig. 10.21 Transverse sonogram showing an ill-defined, hypoechoic, thyroid nodule (arrows) with small cystic areas (arrowheads). Power Doppler demonstrated large intranodular vessels and FNAC confirmed a medullary carcinoma.

MRI in medullary carcinoma

- Metastatic cervical nodes.
- Define tumour extent (Figure 10.24) (involvement of larynx, trachea and adjacent vessels).

Key points

Medullary carcinoma

- Solid, hypoechoic
- Focal or diffuse
- Echogenic foci within
- Chaotic vascular pattern on colour flow imaging
- Associated characteristic lymphadenopathy

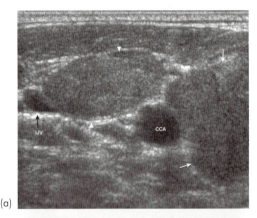

(a)

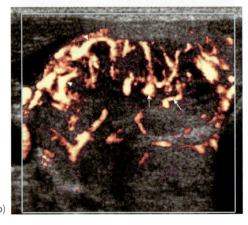

(b)

Fig. 10.22 Transverse sonogram (a) showing an ill-defined, hypoechoic thyroid nodule (arrow) with adjacent abnormal nodes (arrowheads). The power Doppler (b) showing abnormal vascularity within the thyroid tumour (arrows) and the lymph node (arrowheads).

Follicular lesions

It is not always possible to distinguish a benign from a malignant follicular lesion with FNAC or a core biopsy as vascular and capsular invasion (which form the basis for the diagnosis of malignancy in these lesions) can only be evaluated at surgical histology.

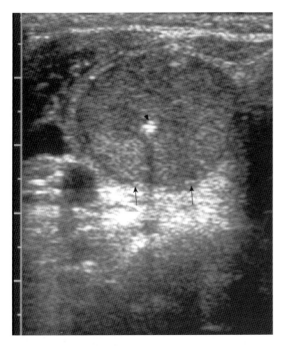

Fig. 10.23 Transverse sonogram of the thyroid showing a fairly well-defined, hypoechoic, medullary carcinoma (arrows) with a dense shadowing focal echogenicity (arrowheads). This represents calcification and amyloid deposition in medullary carcinoma.

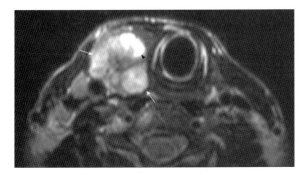

Fig. 10.24 A T2W MRI shows the mass (arrows) as hyperintense compared to adjacent muscle with cystic focal areas within (arrowheads) (same patient as in Figure 10.21).

Some clinicians, therefore, prefer to use the collective term "follicular lesion" for both a benign follicular adenoma and a malignant follicular carcinoma.

While the cytological differentiation between a benign and a malignant follicular lesion is contentious, some cytologists will classify follicular lesions as either microfollicular or macrofollicular. A macrofollicular lesion has a low risk for malignancy whereas a microfollicular lesion may carry a 20–25% risk of being a follicular carcinoma [52].

Follicular carcinoma accounts for 2–5% of all thyroid cancers [37] and is more prevalent (25–30%) in iodine deficient areas [53]. In most cases, it develops from a pre-existing adenoma and has a propensity for haematogenous spread to the lungs, liver, bone and brain. Although patients frequently present with distant metastases, nodal metastases in the neck are rare.

Ultrasound features

- Well defined, haloed in 80%.
- Predominantly solid and homogeneous in 70%.
- Commonly hyperechoic/isoechoic (Figure 10.25); hypoechoic lesions are rare and have a higher risk of being malignant [54] (Figure 10.26).
- Calcification is rare.
- Benign lesions have a type II vascularity whereas malignant lesions have a type III vascularity [37] (Figure 10.27).

Sonography is unable to accurately distinguish a benign from malignant follicular lesion. In some centres a "wait and see" policy may be adopted, if a small follicular lesion is diagnosed on US ± FNAC. This is a further role for US. The suspicion of malignancy is raised, if the nodule is ill defined, hypoechoic, has a thick irregular capsule and has chaotic intranodular vascularity (Figures 10.26 and 10.27). The only certain sign of malignancy is when there is frank vascular invasion (IJV and CCA) and extracapsular spread.

CT and MRI in follicular lesions

- Define tumour extent (involvement of larynx, trachea and adjacent vessels).

Scitnigraphy in follicular lesions

- Identification of bone metastases.

> **Key points**
>
> *Follicular lesion*
>
> • Hyperechoic, homogeneous
> • Haloed
> • Calcification is rare
> • Chaotic vascular pattern on colour flow imaging in follicular carcinoma

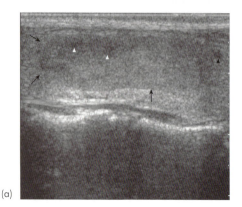

(a)

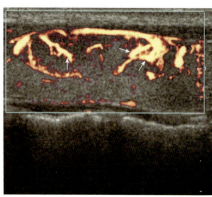

(b)

Fig. 10.25 Longitudinal sonogram (a) showing an ill-defined, isoechoic thyroid mass (arrows) with focal areas of hypoechogenicity (arrowheads). The large intranodular vessels on power Doppler (b) (arrows) suggest the sinister nature of the nodule – follicular carcinoma was identified at surgery.

Hurthle cell tumours

Hurthle cell tumours were previously considered benign, however, these tumours have a potential for malignancy and may metastasise to the lungs and lymph nodes (30%). They are uncommon lesions (3.8%).

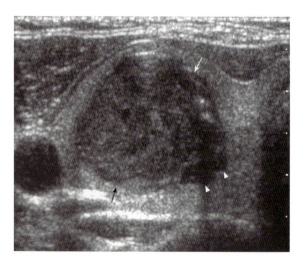

Fig. 10.26 This patient presented with a rib lesion. Biopsy of the lesion suggested metastases from follicular carcinoma. Transverse scan of the thyroid shows a hypoechoic, heterogeneous mass (arrows) with infiltrative edges (arrowheads), follicular carcinoma.

Most Hurthle cell lesions are follicular in pattern and the criteria for differentiating between a benign and a malignant lesion are similar to those for follicular tumours (capsular and vascular invasion).

Ultrasound features

• Non-calcified, mostly solid.
• Ill defined, partially haloed (Figure 10.28).
• Mixed internal echogenicity (Figure 10.28).
• Adjacent malignant nodes may be the only clue to malignancy.

CT and MRI in Hurthle cell tumours

• Define tumour extent (involvement of larynx, trachea and adjacent vessels).
• Identify any adjacent malignant nodes.

> **Key points**
>
> *Hurthle cell tumour*
>
> • Commonly resembles a follicular lesion on US
> • Mixed internal echogenicity (hyperechoic and hypoechoic)
> • Incomplete halo
> • Non-specific vascular pattern on colour flow imaging

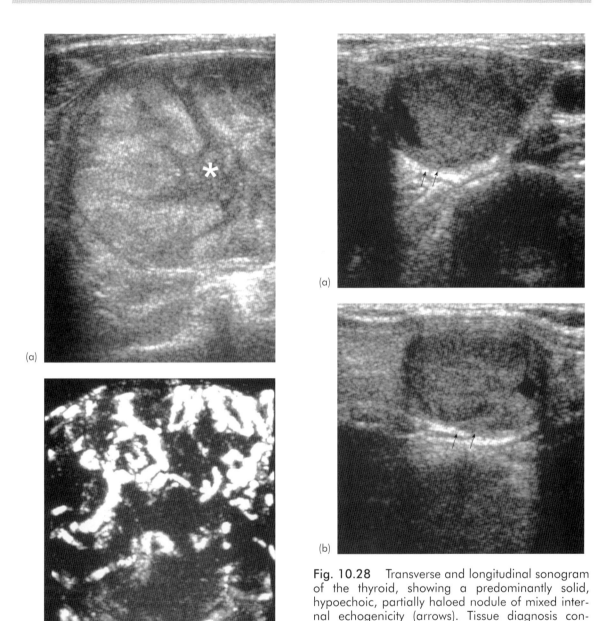

Fig. 10.28 Transverse and longitudinal sonogram of the thyroid, showing a predominantly solid, hypoechoic, partially haloed nodule of mixed internal echogenicity (arrows). Tissue diagnosis confirmed a Hurthle cell tumour.

Fig. 10.27 Large, heterogeneous thyroid mass (a) with a cystic component (haemorrhage and necrosis [*]). Power Doppler (b) shows extensive vascularity within the solid portion suggesting a malignant lesion. Biopsy confirmed a follicular carcinoma.

Thyroid metastases

Thyroid metastases are infrequent and the incidence in patients with a known primary is 2–17%. Metastases to the thyroid are due to haematogenous spread commonly from the following primary sites: melanoma, breast, renal cell carcinoma, lungs and colon.

Ultrasound features [55]

- Non-calcified, homogeneous, hypoechoic mass (Figure 10.29).
- Well defined and predominantly in the lower pole (Figure 10.29).

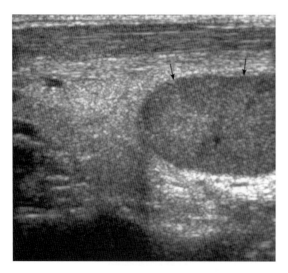

Fig. 10.29 Longitudinal sonogram of the thyroid shows a well-defined, sharply demarcated, hypoechoic, homogeneous thyroid metastases in the lower pole (arrows). This patient had a known primary with disseminated disease.

- Heterogeneous echopattern in diffuse involvement (Figure 10.30).
- Multiple, hypoechoic solid, thyroid nodules (Figure 10.31).
- Invariably associated with disseminated disease.

Key points

Thyroid metastases

- Large and solid focal mass
- Homogeneously hypoechoic mass
- Typically well defined
- Diffuse heterogeneous echopattern
- Non-specific vascular pattern on colour flow imaging
- Invariably associated with disseminated disease

Lymphoma

Lymphoma accounts for 1–3% of all thyroid malignancies and an antecedent history of Hashimoto's thyroiditis is commonly present [32,41]. Non-Hodgkin's lymphoma is more common than Hodgkin's disease. A common presentation is of an elderly female who presents with a rapidly enlarging

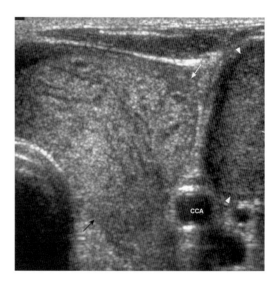

Fig. 10.30 Transverse scan of the thyroid (in a patient with a known primary) showing a diffusely enlarged, hypoechoic gland with heterogneous echopattern consistent with diffuse metastatic involvement (arrows). Note the adjacent associated malignant lymphadenopathy (arrowheads).

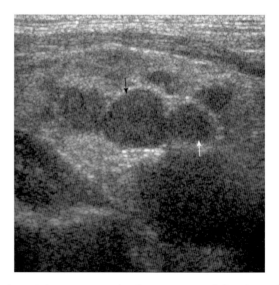

Fig. 10.31 Longitudinal sonogram of the thyroid (in a patient with known disseminated malignancy) showing multiple, solid, hypoechoic thyroid nodules (arrows). These were confirmed to be metastatic following a FNAC.

neck mass. Thyroid involvement may be focal or diffuse and extrathyroid spread and vascular invasion are seen in 50–60% and 25%, respectively [56,57].

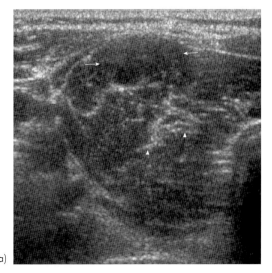

(a)

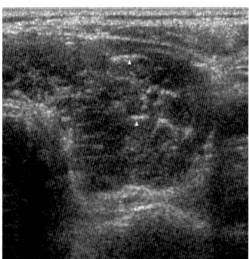

(b)

Fig. 10.32 Transverse sonograms of the thyroid showing rounded outlines, hypoechoic gland with bright fibrotic streaks (arrowheads) suggesting previous Hashimotos thyroiditis. Note the hypoechoic nodule anteriorly (arrow) in (a). Features suggest lymphoma of the thyroid.

Ultrasound features

- Focal thyroid nodules may have a pseudocystic appearance or heterogeneous appearance with or without posterior enhancement (Figure 10.32).
- Diffuse involvement may result in a heterogeneous echopattern (Figure 10.33) or simple enlargement of the gland with no abnormality in echopattern.
- Associated, round, hypoechoic lymphomatous nodes (Figure 10.34).

- Non-specific features on colour flow imaging (Figure 10.35).
- Background of previous Hashimoto's thyroiditis in the form of fibrotic, echogenic streaks within the thyroid (Figure 10.32).

CT in thyroid lymphoma (Figure 10.33c)

- Define tumour extent (involvement of larynx, trachea and adjacent vessels).
- Identify any adjacent malignant nodes.
- To stage the disease.

MRI in thyroid lymphoma

- Define tumour extent (involvement of larynx, trachea and adjacent vessels).
- Identify any adjacent malignant nodes.

Key points

Lymphoma

- Hypoechoic
- Focal or diffuse thyroid involvement
- Pseudocystic appearance
- Heterogeneous echopattern
- Changes of Hashimoto's thyroiditis
- Non-specific vascularity on colour flow imaging
- Associated characteristic lymphadenopathy

Recurrent disease

Evaluation of recurrent disease is often a diagnostic dilemma. Thyroglobulin levels, total body scans and serum calcitonin (for medullary carcinoma) assays form an integral part of detection of tumour recurrence.

In patients with well-differentiated cancers, total body scans using ^{131}I are performed to detect both regional and distant recurrences. Serum thyroglobulin levels as well as total body scans may be difficult to interpret when the patient has undergone a partial resection of the gland and has not undergone post-operative thyroid ablation.

The imaging armamentarium includes US, CT, MRI and PET scanning.

In the post-operative state US may be difficult to perform. However, in experienced hands it can clearly

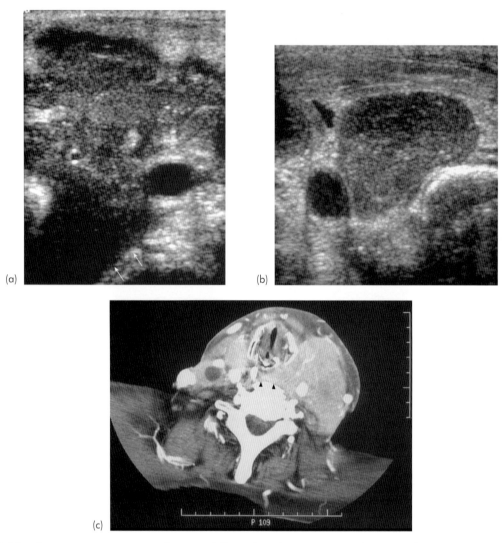

(a)

(b)

(c)

Fig. 10.33 Transverse sonograms showing diffuse, lymphomatous involvement of the thyroid (a and b). Note the extrathyroid extension posteriorly (arrows) in (a). A contrast-enhanced CT (c) shows a markedly enlarged gland with heterogeneous enhancement and posterior extrathyroid infiltration (arrowheads).

evaluate the post-operative thyroid bed and the neck for the presence or absence of any disease (Figures 10.36 and 10.37).

CT and MRI are easier to perform and interpret in the post-operative state (Figure 10.38), and CT has the advantage that it can also evaluate the mediastinum and lungs.

PET scanning is playing an increasing role in the evaluation of recurrent thyroid cancers. In patients where it identifies probable disease it may have to be supplemented by focused US (±FNAC), CT or MRI.

Key points

Evaluation of recurrent disease

- Increasing level of thyroglobulin
- ^{131}I total body scan
- US of the neck, if expertise available
- CT/MRI of neck, if US expertise not available
- PET
- PET directed CT/MRI (neck, thorax and abdomen)

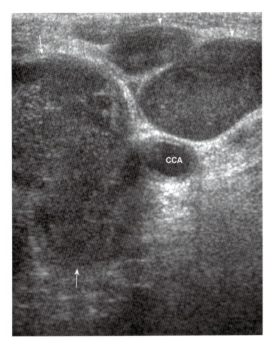

Fig. 10.34 Transverse sonogram showing diffuse lymphomatous involvement of the thyroid (arrow) with extrathyroid spread. Note the adjacent lymphomatous nodes (arrowheads).

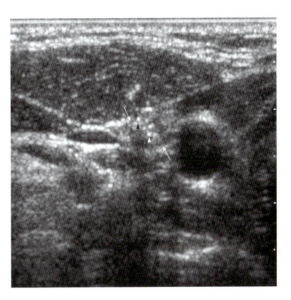

Fig. 10.36 Transverse sonogram (in a patient with previous surgery for papillary carcinoma of thyroid) showing a small nodule (arrows) with echogenic foci (arrowheads) seen in the thyroid bed. Appearances are suggestive of tumour recurrence and FNAC confirmed the recurrent disease.

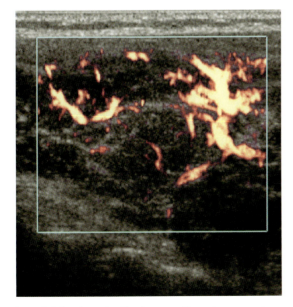

Fig. 10.35 Longitudinal power Doppler scan showing abnormal intrathyroid vascularity in a patient with thyroid lymphoma.

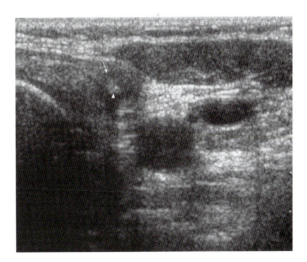

Fig. 10.37 Transverse sonogram (in a patient with previous surgery for papillary carcinoma of thyroid) showing a small nodule (arrow) with dense shadowing echogenic focus (arrowhead). The appearances are suggestive of suture granuloma and FNAC confirmed its nature.

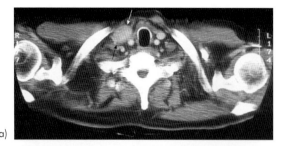

(a)

(b)

Fig. 10.38 (a) Axial contrast-enhanced CT scan (in a patient with previous surgery for medullary carcinoma, with increased calcitonin levels) showing a mildly enhancing mass in the right lower neck (arrows). The mass was clearly identified by US (b) (arrows) and a FNAC-confirmed recurrent medullary carcinoma.

Management of thyroid cancer

The general management of thyroid cancer is surgical resection of the thyroid gland with any involved regional lymph nodes, radioactive ablation of residual thyroid tissue and thyroxine suppression therapy. The specific treatment given is dependent on the local practice of a specialist multidisciplinary team and so differences may exist regarding the indications, extent of thyroidectomy, type of neck

dissection, thyrotropin suppression and the post-operative use of radioactive iodine scanning and therapy. Radiotherapy may play a role whereas the place for chemotherapy is still evolving.

The solitary nodule

All single and multiple thyroid nodules should be evaluated with at least a US or an FNA. Confirmed benign nodules can be followed with serial assessments.

Patients with a suspicious nodule, a follicular neoplasm or a malignant mass should undergo surgery. The minimum excision for both a suspicious nodule and a follicular neoplasm is a lobectomy and isthmusectomy, which may be converted into a total thyroidectomy if the nodule is found to be malignant [58]. In all cases, surgery should minimise avoidable injury to the recurrent and superior laryngeal nerves and preserve functioning parathyroid tissue when appropriate.

Differentiated thyroid carcinoma (papillary and follicular carcinoma)

A solitary papillary carcinoma that is <1 cm in diameter is treated with either a lobectomy and isthmusectomy or a total thyroidectomy, depending on local protocol [59]. A total, sub-total or near-total thyroidectomy is performed for all other differentiated thyroid carcinomas, including bilateral or multifocal carcinomas and in patients with local invasion, regional nodal disease or distant metastases [58,59].

A central compartment lymph node dissection (levels VI and VII) is performed in cases where there are clinically enlarged central nodes, and a modified radical neck dissection is done when there are clinically enlarged or malignant lateral cervical nodes.

Medullary thyroid carcinoma

A total thyroidectomy and central compartment dissection are done to remove all local disease, and a modified radical neck dissection is done to remove clinical regional disease. Serum calcitonin levels are monitored post-operatively [59].

Undifferentiated (anaplastic) thyroid carcinoma

Anaplastic thyroid carcinoma is aggressive and while respectable tumour should be removed, surgery is usually done to relieve airway obstruction. Pre-operative radiotherapy may improve resectability [59].

Recurrent thyroid carcinoma

Locally recurrent disease should be resected, if at all possible. When resection is not feasible, external radiotherapy may be useful [58].

Conclusion

Benign thyroid nodules are common and malignant thyroid nodules rare. The management of a thyroid nodule remains contentious. Conventional FNAC without US guidance is the most cost-effective initial investigation. However, a US scan is widely available and should be performed on patients with a palpable or occult thyroid nodule. Radiologist performing ultrasonography should use the many signs available to evaluate the thyroid, thyroid nodules and regional lymph nodes, and when indicated proceed to biopsy (FNAC) any lesion that appears suspicious for malignancy.

The management of thyroid nodules must be done in conjunction with a clinician, cytologist and surgeon. Local expertise will influence the shape of the diagnostic pathway. A suggested algorithm is

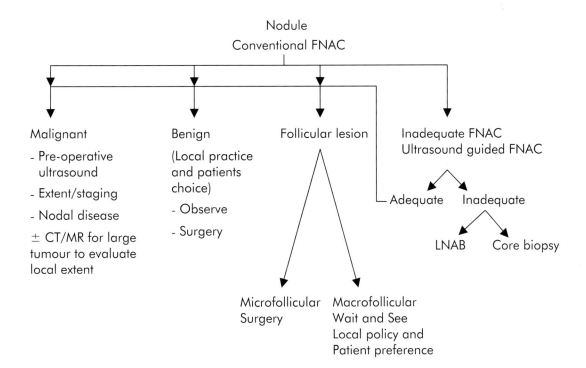

References

1. Tunbridge WMG, Evered DC, Hall R *et al.* The spectrum of thyroid disease in a community: the Whickham survey. *Clin. Endocrinol.* 1977; **7**: 481–493.
2. Vander JB, Gaston EA and Dawber TR. The significance of nontoxic thyroid nodules: final report of a 15-year study of the incidence of thyroid malignancy. *Ann. Int. Med.* 1968; **69**: 537–540.
3. Rojeski MT and Gharib H. Nodular thyroid disease: evaluation and management. *N. Eng. J. Med.* 1985; **313**: 428–436.
4. Rallison MK, Dobyns BM, Meikle AW *et al.* Natural history of thyroid abnormalities: prevalence incidence, and regression of thyroid diseases in adolescent and young adults. *Am. J. Med.* 1991; **91**: 363–370.
5. Brander A, Viikinkoski P, Nickels J and Kivisaari L. Thyroid gland: US screening in a random adult population. *Radiology* 1991; **181**: 683–687.

6. Ezzat S, Sarti Da, Cain DR and Braunstein GD. Thyroid incidentalomas. Prevalence by palpation and ultrasonography. *Arch. Int. Med.* 1994; **154**: 1838–1840.

7. Hopkins CR and Reading CC. Thyroid and parathyroid imaging. *Semin. Ultrasound CT MRI* 1995; **16**: 279–295.

8. Clark KJ, Cronan JJ and Scola FH. Color Doppler sonography: anatomic and physiologic assessment of the thyroid. *J. Clin. Ultrasound* 1995; **23**: 215–223.

9. Mazzaferri EL. Management of solitary thyroid nodule. *N. Engl. J. Med.* 1993; **328**: 553–559.

10. Lahey FH and Hare HF. Malignancy in adenomas of the thyroid. *J. Am. Med. Assoc.* 1951; **145**: 689–695.

11. Leichty RD, Graham M and Freemeyer P. Benign solitary thyroid nodule. *Surg. Gynecol. Obstet.* 1965; **121**: 571–573.

12. Watkinson JC and Maisey MN. Imaging head and neck cancer using radioisotopes: a review. *J. Roy. Soc. Med.* 1988; **81**: 653–657.

13. Gharib H. Fine-needle aspiration biopsy of thyroid nodules: advantages, limitations, and effect. *Mayo Clin. Proc.* 1994; **69**: 44–49.

14. Campbell JP and Pillsbury HC. Management of the thyroid nodule. *Head Neck* 1989; **11**: 414–425.

15. Siperstein A and Clark O. Carcinoma of follicular epithelium: surgical therapy. In: *The Thyroid*, 6th edition. JB Lippincott Co., Philadelphia 1129–1137.

16. Keston Jones M. Management of nodular thyroid disease. *Br. Med. J.* 2001; **323**: 293–294.

17. Kumar H, Daykin J, Holder R *et al.* Gender, clinical findings and serum thyrotrophin (TSH) measurements in the prediction of thyroid neoplasia in 1005 patients presenting with thyroid enlargement and investigated by fine needle aspiration cytology (FNAC). *Thyroid* 1999; **9**(11): 1105–1109.

18. Watkinson JC. The evaluation of solitary thyroid nodule. *Clin. Orolaryngol.* 1990; **15**: 1–5.

19. Walsh RM, Watkinson JC and Franklyn J. The management of the solitary thyroid nodule: a review. *Clin. Otolaryngol.* 1999; **24**: 388–397.

20. Ashcroft MW and Van Herle AJ. Management of thyroid nodules. II Scanning techniques, thyroid suppressive therapy, and fine needle aspiration. *Head Neck Surg.* 1981; **3**: 297–322.

21. Pepper GM, Zwickler D and Rosen Y. Fine needle aspiration cytology of the thyroid nodule: results of a start-up project in a general teaching hospital setting. *Arch. Int. Med.* 1989; **149**: 594–596.

22. The Papanicolaou Society of Cytopathology Task Force on Standards of Practice: Guidelines of the Papanicolaou Society of Cytopathology for examination of fine-needle aspiration specimens from thyroid nodules. *Diag. Cytopathol.* 1996; **15**: 84–89.

23. Giuffrida D and Gharib H. Controversies in the management of cold, hot, and occult thyroid nodules. *Am. J. Med.* 1995; **99**: 642–650.

24. Sabel MS, Haque D, Velasco JM and Staren ED. Use of ultrasound-guided fine needle aspiration biopsy in the management of thyroid disease. *Am. Surg.* 1998; **64**: 738–742.

25. Hatada T, Okada K, Ishii H, Ichii S and Utsunomiya J. Evaluation of ultrasound-guided fine-needle aspiration Biopsy for thyroid nodules. *Am. J. Surg.* 1998; **175**: 133–136.

26. Newkirk KA, Ruigel MD, Jelinek J *et al.* Ultrasound-guided fine needle aspiration and thyroid disease. *Otolaryngol. Head Neck* 2000; **123**: 700–705.

27. McGregor GI, Luomo A and Jackson SM. Lymph node metastases from well-differentiated thyroid cancer: a clinical review. *Am. J. Surg.* 1985; **149**: 610.

28. Solbiati L, Giangrande A, De Pra L *et al.* Percutaneous injection of parathyroid tumours and ultrasound guidance: treatment for secondary hyperparathyroidism. *Radiology* 1985; **155**: 607–610.

29. Takashima S, Fukuda H, Nomura N *et al.* Thyroid nodules: re-evaluation with ultrasound. *J. Clin. Ultrasound* 1995; **23**: 179–184.

30. McIvor NP, Freeman JL and Salem S. Ultrasonography of the thyroid and parathyroid glands. *ORL* 1993; **55**: 303–308.

31. Rago T, Vitti P, Chiorator L, Mazzeo S *et al.* Role conventional ultrasonography and colour flow Doppler sonography in predicting malignancy in "cold" thyroid nodules. *Eur. J. Endocrinol.* 1998; **138**: 41–46.

32. Yousem DM and Scheff AM. Thyroid and parathyroid. In: PM Som and HD Curtin (Eds) *Head and Neck Imaging*, 3rd edition. Mosby, St Louis. 1996, 953–975.

33. Ahuja A, Chick W, King W and Metreweli C. Clinical significance of the comet tail artifact in thyroid ultrasound. *J. Clin. Ultrasound* 1996; **24**: 129–133.

34. Woolner LB, Beahs OH, Black Bm *et al.* Classification and prognosis of thyroid cancer. *Am. J. Surg.* 1961; **102**: 354–387.

35. McCall A, Jarosz H, Lawrence Am and Paloyan E. The incidence of thyroid carcinoma in solitary cold nodules and in multinodular goiters. *Surgery* 1986; **100**: 1128–1131.

36. Lagalla R, Cariso G, Midiri M and Cardinale AE. Echo-Doppler couleru et pathologie thyroidienne. *J. Echograph. Med. Ultrasons.* 1992; **13**: 44–47.

37. Solbiati L, Livraghi T, Ballarati E, Ierace T and Crespi L. Thyroid gland. In: L. Solbiati and G Rizzatto (Eds) *Ultrasound of Superficial Structures*. Churchill Livingstone, London. 1995, 49–85.

38. Carpi A, Nicolini A and Sagripanti A. Protocols for the preoperative selection of palpable thyroid nodules. Review and progress. *Am. J. Clin. Oncol.* 1999; **22**(5): 499–504.

39. Freitas JE and Freitas AE. Thyroid and parathyroid imaging. *Semin. Nucl. Med.* 1994; **24**: 234–245.

40. King AD, Ahuja AT, To EWH, Tse GMK and Metreweli C. Staging of papillary carcinoma of the thyroid: magnetic resonance imaging vs ultrasound of the neck. *Clin. Radiol.* 2000; **55**(3): 222–226.

41. Bruneton JN and Normand F. Thyroid gland. In: JN Bruneton (Ed.) *Ultrasonography of the Neck*. Springer-Verlag, Berlin. 1987, 22–50.

42. LiVolsi VA. Pathology of thyroid disease. In: SA Flak (Ed.) *Thyroid Disease: Endocrinology, Surgery, Nuclear Medicine and Radiotherapy*. Lippincott-Raven, Philadelphia, PA. 1997, 65–104.

43. Simeone JF, Daniels GH, Mueller PR *et al.* High resolution real time sonography of the thyroid. *Radiology* 1982; **145**: 431–435.

44. Solbiati L, Volterrani L, Rizzatto G *et al.* The thyroid gland with low uptake lesions: evaluation with ultrasound. *Radiology* 1985; **155**: 187–191.

45. Propper RA, Skolnick ML, Weinstein BJ and Dekker A. The non-specificity of the thyroid halo sign. *J. Clin. Ultrasound* 1989; **8**: 129–132.

46. Noyek AM, Finkelstein DM and Kirsch JC. Diagnostic imaging of the thyroid gland. In: SA Falk, (Ed.) *Thyroid Disease: Endocrinology, Surgery, Nuclear Medicine, and Radiotherapy*. Raven Press, New York. 1990; 952–975.

47. Ahuja AT, Chow L, Chick W *et al.* Metastatic cervical nodes in papillary carcinoma of the thyroid: ultrasound and histological correlation. *Clin. Radiol.* 1995; **50**: 229–231.

48. Takashima S, Morimoto S, Ikezoe J *et al.* CT evaluation of anaplastic thyroid carcinoma. *Am. J. Roentgenol.* 1990; **154**: 61–63.

49. Compagno J. Diseases of the thyroid. In: Barnes L (Ed.) *Surgical Pathology of the Head and Neck*. Marcel Dekker, New York. 1985; 1435–1486.

50. Kaufman FR, Roe TF, Isaacs H and Weitzman JJ. Metastatic medullary carcinoma in young children with mucosal neuroma syndrome. *Pediatrics* 1982; **70**: 263–267.

51. Norton JA, Froome BA, Farrell RE and Wells SA. Multiple endocrine neoplasia type IIb: the most aggressive form of medullary carcinoma. *Surg. Clin. N. Am.* 1979; **59**: 109–118.

52. Tombouret R, Szefelbein WM and Pitman MB. Ultrasound-guided fine-needle aspiration biopsy of the thyroid. *Cancer* 1999; **87**: 299–305.

53. Williams ED, Doinach I, Bjanarson O and Michie W. Thyroid cancer in a iodide rich area. *Cancer* 1977; **39**: 215–222.

54. Lin JD, Hsueh C, Chao TC, Weng JF and Huang BY. Thyroid follicular neoplasms diagnosed by high-resolution ultrasonography with fine needle aspiration cytology.

55. Ahuja A, King W and Metreweli C. Role of ultrasonography in thyroid metastases. *Clin. Radiol.* 1994: **49**: 627–629.

56. Anscombe AM and Wright DH. Primary malignant lymphoma of the thyroid – a tumour of mucosa associated lymphoid tissue: review of seventy-six cases. *Histopathology* 1985; **9**: 81–87.

57. Burke JS, Butler JJ and Fuller LM. Malignant lymphomas of the thyroid. *Cancer* 1977; **39**: 1587–1602.

58. Singer PA, Cooper DS, Daniels GH *et al*. Treatment guidelines for patients with thyroid nodules and well-differentiated thyroid cancer. *Arch. Int. Med.* 1996; **156**: 2165–2172.

59. Cobin RH, Gharib H, Bergman DA *et al*. Thyroid carcinoma guidelines. *Endocr. Pract.* 2001; **7**(3): 202–220.

Maxilla and Sinuses

HY Yuen, J Kew and CA van Hasselt

Primary malignancies arising in the sinonasal cavities are uncommon. They comprise about 3% of all head and neck tumours [1] and less than 1% of all malignancies [2].

Approximately 50–60% of malignant sinonasal tumours arise within the maxillary sinuses, 10–25% in the ethmoid and 15–30% in the nasal cavity [3–5]. The frontal and sphenoid sinuses are very rarely involved by primary malignancies.

Most sinonasal malignancies are epithelial tumours (Box 11.1). These can be further subdivided into tumours of epithelial origin and tumours of salivary gland origin. Tumours of epithelial origin include papillomas, squamous cell carcinomas (SCCs), adenocarcinomas and anaplastic carcinomas. Tumours of salivary gland origin can be divided into pleomorphic adenoma, adenoid cystic carcinomas, acinic cell carcinomas and mucoepidermoid carcinomas [6].

The most common primary malignant tumour in the paranasal sinuses is SCC of the maxillary sinus. We will concentrate our discussion on this entity

---

Box 11.1   Sinonasal malignancies

A. Malignant epithelial tumours
  1. SCC
  2. Non-SCC
     - Salivary: adenoid cystic,* mucoepidermoid
     - Non-salivary: adenocarcinomas*
       – Adenoid cystic carcinoma
       – Mucoepidermoid carcinoma
       – Adenocarcinoma
       – Neuroendocrine carcinoma
       – Hyalinising clear cell carcinoma
  3. Melanoma

  4. Olfactory neuroblastoma
  5. Sinonasal undifferentiated carcinoma

B. Malignant non-epithelial tumours
  1. Lymphoproliferative tumours
  2. Metastases
  3. Sarcomas

C. Intermediate-type tumours
  1. Schneiderian papillomas
  2. Angiofibroma
  3. Ameloblastoma

*Majority of the non-epidermoid mucous gland malignancies.

and then describe other tumours in the paranasal sinuses.

Maxillary squamous cell carcinoma

Epidemiology

Males are affected twice as commonly as females. This tumour usually develops in patients of age range 50–70 years (Box 11.2).

Occupational exposure to industrial carcinogenic substances is associated with the development of SCC of the sinonasal cavities. These include nickel, softwood dust, leather tan, chromium, isopropyl oils and radium. Thorotrast in the past has been the most frequently identified culprit but is now obsolete.

Tobacco by itself does not appear to be a significant aetiological factor for tumours of the sinonasal cavities, although there may be a synergistic effect between softwood dust and tobacco smoking.

Clinical presentations

The paranasal sinuses are anatomically obscure in location and thus are not openly accessible for inspection. Moreover, the early symptoms of sinus malignancy are non-specific and may be mistakenly regarded as being due to sinusitis, which is often coexisting due to obstructive effect of the tumour. Thus patients with sinus malignancies usually present late with more sinister symptoms when the tumour has infiltrated extensively. There is an average delay of 5–8 months before establishing the diagnosis of maxillary sinus SCC, and 60–97% of patients present with advanced T3 and T4 tumours [8–11]. Late stage disease coupled with the extensive surgical resection required results in the high morbidity associated with sinus malignancies.

The early symptoms of maxillary sinus malignancies include pain and rhinorrhoea. The painful sensation in maxillary lesions is perceived in the cheek. Initially such pain may be mild and intermittent, but with disease progression it tends to become more severe and constant. This is a result of the destructive effect

---

> **Box 11.2   Epidemiology of maxillary SCC**
>
> - $M:F = 2:1$
> - Late middle age 50–70 years
> - Industrial carcinogenic substances: nickel, softwood dust, leather tan, chromium, isopropyl oils, radium and thorotrast
> - Tobacco may have synergistic effect with softwood dust

---

of the tumour, which will lead to another seemingly contradicting symptom, hypoaesthesia or paraesthesia, i.e. numbness. This occurs as a result of tumour erosion involving the neural canals and foramina. If the tumour erodes the orbital floor including the infraorbital canal, the infraorbital nerve (a division of the branch of the trigeminal nerve supplying cutaneous sensation to the cheek) will also be jeopardised resulting in decreased sensation. Therefore, *an increase in severity and consistency of the pain*, as well as the development of *paraesthesia* should raise suspicion of more sinister pathology rather than simply due to sinusitis.

Discharge in the form of rhinorrhoea is another common early symptom. It may be the result of sinusitis caused by the obstructive effect of the tumour or as an underlying associated condition. Such nasal discharge is non-specific but when associated with *persistent blood staining* should again suggest the presence of an underlying aggressive lesion.

Symptoms of more advanced disease can be related to the loco-regional invasion, which depends on the direction of growth, or from cervical nodal or distant metastases.

Advanced loco-regional disease commonly affects the orbit, the alveolar bone and the face. Erosion of the roof of the maxillary antrum/orbital floor permits the tumour to extend into the orbit. At this stage paraesthesia of the cheek is often present due to infiltration of the infraorbital nerve as discussed above. Involvement of the extra-ocular muscles, usually the inferior rectus and the inferior oblique, will result in *diplopia*. Mass effect may cause *exophthalmos* and *visual loss* will occur when the optic nerve is invaded. Facial symptoms are due to anterior antral wall destruction and the tumour mass causing *facial swelling and asymmetry*. Inferior extension of the maxillary sinus tumour will erode the alveolar ridge, which may result in *loosening of the upper premolar and molar teeth*, *ulceration of adjacent palate and gingivobuccal sulcus*, or even *fistulation into the oral cavity*.

About 10% (range 4–21%) of patients with maxillary sinus SCC present with positive regional nodes, most commonly in the upper jugular, submandibular and retropharyngeal regions. Distant metastases, however, are not common at the time of diagnosis and identified in only up to 4% of patients [8,9,12,13].

Diagnosis

Apart from the suspicious symptoms such as persistent severe pain, paraesthesia and epistaxis as discussed above, the presence of symptoms atypical of sinusitis should also alert the clinician to the possibility of an underlying aggressive lesion. These may manifest in the form of recurrent or persistent symptoms resistant to medical treatment or the development of predominant unilateral symptoms.

The advent of fibre-optic endoscopy now allows more direct and complete examination of the nasal cavities and paranasal sinuses. After detailed history taking, whenever there is clinical suspicion, an endoscopic examination must be performed. Any abnormal lesion identified should be biopsied, if it does not appear unusually vascular. Histological confirmation of malignancy is an indispensable function of endoscopy and optimally should be obtained before imaging studies are performed for further evaluation. However, the tumour may not be visually accessible if it is not overtly involving the medial aspect of the maxillary sinus and the absence of a lesion on endoscopic inspection cannot exclude the presence of tumour inside the antrum. In this respect, imaging studies may serve as the diagnostic tool in establishing the diagnosis.

There is no serological marker for SCCs of the maxillary or other sinuses.

The Ohngren's line (also known as the malignant plane) is defined as the line joining the medial

canthus to the mandibular angle (Figure 11.1). Tumours arising below this imaginary line (infrastructure) in the antero-inferior segment tend to have a better prognosis than those arising above (suprastructure) this line in the postero-superior segment [7] (Box 11.3).

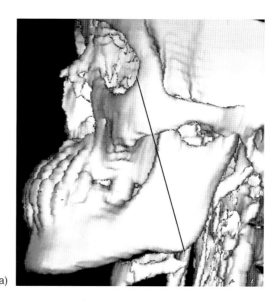
(a)

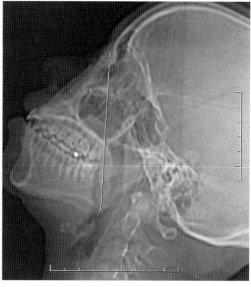
(b)

Fig. 11.1 (a) CT 3D reconstruction image. The Ohngren's line (malignant plane) is defined as the line joining the medial canthus to the mandibular angle, as depicted on a CT 3D reconstructed image. (b) Lateral CT scanogram. The Ohngren's line as depicted on a lateral CT scanogram.

Box 11.3   Diagnosis and staging

Diagnosis

- Endoscopy and biopsy should be performed first to establish the diagnosis of maxillary sinus malignancy whenever possible, then followed by cross-sectional imaging by CT and/or MRI for staging of the disease.
- If no tumour is visually identifiable on endoscopy and the clinical suspicion is high, imaging studies may then serve as the primary diagnostic tool and direct the site for more invasive biopsy to confirm the diagnosis.

Staging

The American Joint Cancer Commission (AJCC) Staging System is the most widely adopted system for staging maxillary sinus malignancy.

Primary tumour (T)

TX	Primary tumour cannot be assessed
T0	No evidence of primary tumour
Tis	Carcinoma *in situ*
T1	Tumour limited to the antral mucosa with no erosion or destruction of bone
T2	Tumour causing bone erosion or destruction, except for the posterior antral wall, including extension into the hard palate and/or the middle nasal meatus
T3	Tumour invades any of the following: bone of the posterior wall of maxillary sinus, subcutaneous tissues, skin of cheek, floor or medial wall of orbit, infratemporal fossa, pterygoid plates and ethmoid sinuses
T4	Tumour invades orbital contents beyond the floor or medial wall including any of the following: the orbital apex, cribiform plate, base of skull, nasopharynx, sphenoid and frontal sinuses

Lymph node (N)

NX	Regional lymph nodes cannot be assessed
N0	No regional lymph node metastasis
N1	Metastasis in a single ipsilateral lymph node (3 cm or less in greatest dimension)
N2	Metastasis in a single ipsilateral lymph node, more than 3 cm but not more than 6 cm in greatest dimension, or in multiple ipsilateral lymph nodes, none more than 6 cm in greatest dimension, or in bilateral or contralateral lymph nodes, none more than 6 cm in greatest dimension
N2a	Metastasis in a single ipsilateral lymph node, more than 3 cm but not more than 6 cm in greatest dimension
N2b	Metastasis in multiple ipsilateral lymph nodes, none more than 6 cm in greatest dimension
N2c	Metastasis in bilateral or contralateral lymph nodes, none more than 6 cm in greatest dimension
N3	Metastasis in a lymph node more than 6 cm in greatest dimension

Distant metastasis (M)

MX	Presence of distant metastasis cannot be assessed
M0	No distant metastasis
M1	Distant metastasis

From *American Joint Committee on Cancer (AJCC) Cancer Staging Manual*, 5th edition. Lippincott Williams & Wilkins, 1997; with permission from the AJCC, Chicago, IL.

Box 11.4   Merits and weakness of CT versus MRI and suggested imaging protocol with reference to maxilla and neck

Merits and weakness of CT versus MRI

CT

- Less expensive; more accessible
- Involves low dose of ionising radiation
- Iodinated contrast incurs risk of anaphylaxis
- Short scanning time thus more tolerable by patient
- Does not incite claustrophobia
- Provides excellent details of osseous anatomy and extent of bone erosion by tumour
- Cannot reliably distinguish tumour component from mucosal inflammation and retained secretions
- Modern multidetector CT provides superb quality reconstruction images in orthogonal planes

MRI

- More expensive; less accessible
- No ionising radiation
- Very low risk of anaphylaxis from gadolinium contrast
- Longer scanning time, so less tolerable by patient
- May cause claustrophobia
- Not very good in delineation of bony details
- Excellent soft tissue contrast – more exact delineation of extent of tumour and differentiation from mucosal inflammation and retained secretions
- Multiplanar imaging

Suggested imaging protocol with reference to maxilla and neck

CT

- Contrast-enhanced axial 3 mm/1 : 1 sections covering the anterior cranial fossa, orbits and maxilla in soft tissue and bone algorithm, then axial 5 mm/1 : 1 sections of the neck down to the suprasternal notch in soft tissue algorithm
- Coronal 3 mm/1 : 1 sections including the pterygoid bones in bone algorithm*
- Contrast: 90 ml Omnipaque (Nycomed, Oslo, Norway) 240, injection rate: 2.5 ml/s, delay time: 30 s

MRI

The coverage is the same as in CT and aims to cover the entire maxilla and the adjacent possible invaded structures including the anterior cranial fossa.

Sequence selected include:

- Maxilla – T_1-weighted (T1W) axial, T_2-weighted (T2W) SPIR axial, T2W coronal, post-gadolinium T1W axial, post-gadolinium T1W coronal with and without fat suppression.
- Neck – T2W SPIR axial, post-gadolinium T1W axial
- Contrast: Omniscan (Nycomed, Oslo, Norway) 1.5 ml/kg

*Single slice CT scan protocol. For multislice CT scans, images only need to be acquired in the axial plane and coronal reconstructions then performed, i.e. not necessary to acquire second coronal set of data.

Imaging

Imaging studies are mandatory in staging and planning the treatment for maxillary sinus malignancy. They provide information which determine resectability of the tumour, the surgical approach, the portal and extent for radiotherapy, as well as baseline with which disease progress is assessed and further surveillance for possible recurrence is compared.

Plain radiographs including tomography nowadays play a very limited role in the evaluation of sinus malignancy. Its major weakness lies in its relatively low sensitivity in detecting bone erosion and inadequacy in delineating the extent of soft tissue lesions and as such has been largely replaced by other cross-sectional imaging techniques.

Computerised tomography (CT) and magnetic resonance imaging (MRI) are the mainstay of imaging studies for the investigation of maxillary sinus malignancy. They are complementary to each other. CT provides excellent details of the bony structures, while MRI can map out accurately the extent and margins of the tumour (Box 11.4).

Although patients with maxillary sinus malignancies usually present late with very advanced stage disease, the occurrence of regional nodal (~10%) and distant metastases (<4%) on first presentation are low. Ultrasound (US) is increasingly being used to assess the cervical nodal status and is promising in providing early diagnosis of cervical nodal metastases. However, the low incidence of regional nodal disease does not justify its routine use in the initial work-up of these patients.

Likewise the search for distant metastases, e.g. chest radiograph or CT thorax for lung metastases, US or CT abdomen for hepatic metastases and bone scintigram for skeletal metastases, should be reserved for patients with tumours that tend more to metastasise haematogenously, including sarcomas, melanoma and adenoid cystic carcinoma, before extensive surgical resection is considered.

Computerised tomography

The cardinal sign of maxillary sinus malignancy on CT is *bone destruction*. Figures 11.2–11.6 are CT images of normal maxillary sinuses with labelling of

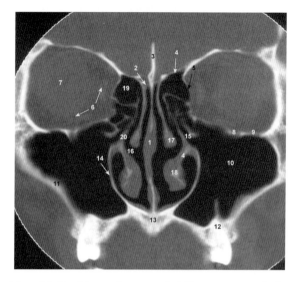

Fig. 11.2 Normal coronal CT anatomy of the maxillary sinus and nasal cavity: 1. nasal septum, 2. cribiform plate, 3. crista galli, 4. fovea ethmoidalis, 5. lamina papyracea, 6. medial and inferior rectus muscles, 7. eyeglobe, 8. infra-orbital canal, 9. orbital floor, 10. maxillary antrum, 11. posterolateral antral wall, 12. alveolar bone, 13. hard palate, 14. medial antral wall, 15. ethmoid infundibulum, 16. middle meatus, 17. middle nasal turbinate, 18. inferior nasal turbinate, 19. anterior ethmoid sinus and 20. uncinate process.

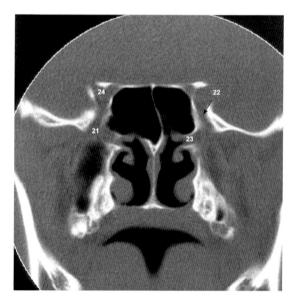

Fig. 11.3 Normal coronal CT anatomy of the sphenoid sinus and pterygopalatine fossa: 21. pterygopalatine fossa, 22. inferior orbital fissure, 23. sphenopalatine foramen and 24. optic canal.

the bony structures of strategic importance, namely the orbital floor, the ethmoid cells, the lamina papyracea, the fovea ethmoidalis, the cribiform plate, all maxillary antral walls, the alveolar bone, the hard palate, and the pterygoid bone attached posteriorly to the maxillary antrum.

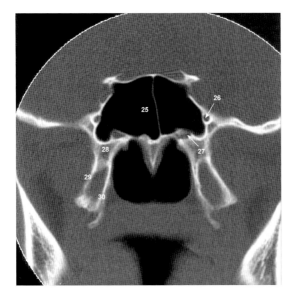

Fig. 11.4   Normal coronal CT anatomy of the sphenoid sinus: 25. sphenoid sinus, 26. foramen rotundum, 27. vidian canal, 28. pterygoid bone, 29. lateral pterygoid plate and 30. medial pterygoid plate.

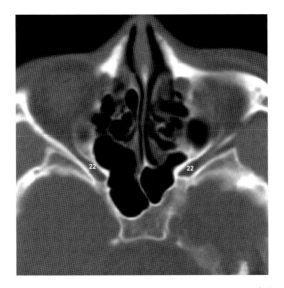

Fig. 11.5   Normal axial CT anatomy image of the posterior ethmoid and sphenoid sinuses: 22. inferior orbital fissure.

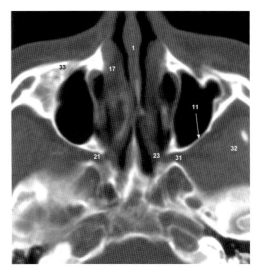

Fig. 11.6   Normal axial CT anatomy of the maxillary sinus and pterygopalatine fossa: 1. nasal septum, 11. posterolateral antral wall, 17. middle nasal turbinate, 21. pterygopalatine fossa, 23. sphenopalatine foramen, 31. pterygomaxillary fissure, 32. infratemporal fossa and 33. anterior antral wall.

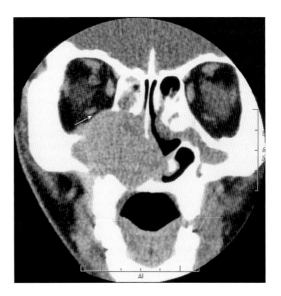

Fig. 11.7   Coronal CT of a right maxillary sinus carcinoma eroding the orbital floor. A clear plane of cleavage can still be identified between the tumour and the inferior rectus muscle. The tumour destroys the medial antral wall and extends into the right nasal cavity and erodes the nasal septum to further extend into the left nasal cavity abutting the left inferior nasal turbinate. The hard palate and the lower anterior wall are also eroded by the tumour.

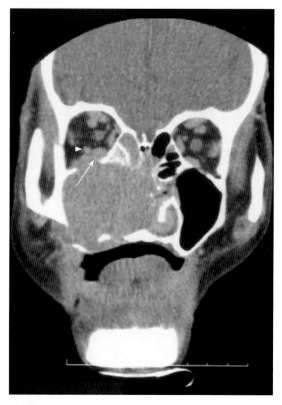

Fig. 11.8 Coronal CT of a right maxillary sinus carcinoma that has eroded the orbital floor. In this case, the tumour has invaded and is inseparable from the inferior rectus muscle (arrow). The right inferior oblique is intact. The right inferior orbital nerve and artery (arrow head) are displaced into the right orbital cavity just lateral to the right inferior rectus muscle. This tumour has also destroyed the medial antral wall, nasal septum, hard palate and posterolateral antral wall, and infiltrated both sides of the nasal cavity.

These bony structures must be meticulously examined and their disruption indicates that the tumour has extended beyond the confines of the maxillary sinuses.

Once the orbital floor is disrupted, the orbital fat and extra-ocular muscles must be examined for signs of tumour invasion. Intraconal extension of tumour may invade the optic nerve and jeopardise vision. Close proximity of the tumour to these structures short of overt invasion may still signify adhesion and unless a clear plane of cleavage can be identified, these structures cannot be regarded as intact (Figures 11.7 and 11.8).

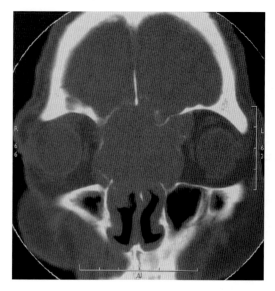

Fig. 11.9 Coronal CT of an anterior ethmoid carcinoma. This case is used to illustrate intracranial tumour extension through erosion of the anterior cranial fossa at the cribiform plate and fovea ethmoidalis. Note that the tumour has also eroded through the lamina papyracea into the orbital cavities bilaterally. Maxillary antral tumour extending into the ethmoid cells may also infiltrate in this pattern.

Breaching of the anterior cranial fossa most commonly at the cribiform plate and the fovea ethmoidalis indicates possible intracranial extension and meningeal or brain parenchymal infiltration must be considered (Figures 11.9 and 11.10). Meningeal extension manifests as enhancing irregular thickening and brain parenchymal infiltration as direct extension in continuity with the main tumour bulk.

Erosions of the medial and the inferolateral walls of the maxillary sinus allow the tumour to invade the nasal cavity and the buccal space, respectively (Figure 11.10). Inferiorly, destruction of the alveolar part of the maxilla may result in loosening of the teeth, most commonly the upper premolar and molar, and the hard palate may also be eroded, if there is further medial extension. If there is full thickness destruction, a fistular tract will develop connecting the antrum to the oral cavity (Figure 11.11).

Posteriorly, the integrity of the pterygopalatine fossa is of utmost importance. This is because this fossa is an anatomical cross-road from where the tumour can spread in multiple directions (Figures 11.12 and

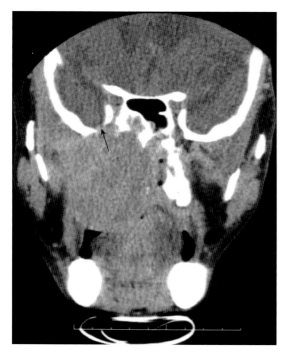

Fig. 11.10 Coronal CT of a right maxillary sinus carcinoma. Same case as Figure 11.8. Posteriorly, the tumour has destroyed the entire posterior and postero-lateral walls of the antrum, and the entire right ptery-goid bone. The tumour extensively infiltrates the right buccal, masticator and parapharyngeal spaces. The right infratemporal fossa is also invaded by tumour. There is erosion of the right middle cranial fossa just lateral to the right inferior orbital fissure (arrow).

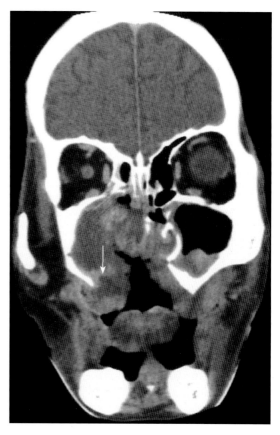

Fig. 11.11 Coronal CT of a right maxillary sinus carcinoma eroding the superior alveolar ridge and destroying the medial maxillary antral wall and the right side and mid-portion of the hard palate resulting in a fistular tract into the oral cavity.

11.13). Anterosuperiorly, the fossa is communicating with the inferior orbital fissure and tumour spread can result in optic nerve compression at the orbital apex. Posteriorly, there are the foramen rotundum and the pterygoid (vidian) canal which transmit the maxillary division of the trigeminal nerve from Meckel's cave and the artery of the pterygoid canal (vidian artery) branching from the maxillary artery, respectively. These two foramina are a potential portal of entry for the tumour to spread into the middle cranial fossa, especially as perineural spread along the foramen rotundum. Laterally, the tumour can extend from the fossa via the pterygomaxillary fissure into the infratemporal fossa. Medially, the tumour can spread through the sphenopalatine foramen into the posterosuperior nasal cavity. Inferiorly, the fossa communicates with the oral cavity via the pterygopalatine canal, which transmits the palatine

vessels and nerves and this is again a potential channel of tumour spread (Figure 11.14).

Magnetic resonance imaging

MRI provides superb soft tissue contrast resolution allowing differentiation of tumour from retained secretions and inflammatory mucosal and soft tissue thickening, while these all show similar densities on CT. The other advantages of MRI include multiplanar imaging capability and lack of radiation (Boxes 11.5 and 11.6).

MRI makes use of the phenomenon of free water in distinguishing the various types of soft tissues. Retained secretions and mucosal oedema will be expected to show low signal on T1W images and high

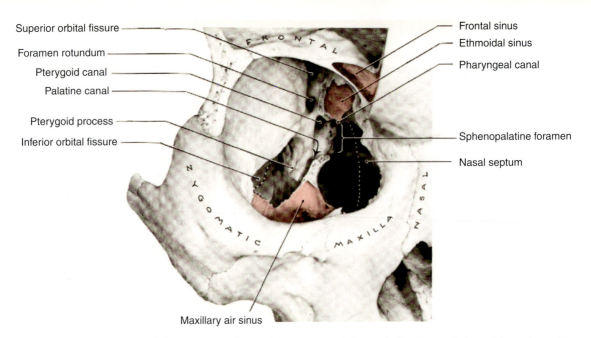

Superior orbital fissure
Foramen rotundum
Pterygoid canal
Palatine canal
Pterygoid process
Inferior orbital fissure

Frontal sinus
Ethmoidal sinus
Pharyngeal canal
Sphenopalatine foramen
Nasal septum

Maxillary air sinus

Fig. 11.12 Frontal view of the pterygopalatine fossa exposed through the floor of the orbit and maxillary sinus. Reproduced with permission from James E. Anderson. *Grant's Atlas of Anatomy*, 8th edition. Williams & Wilkins. 1983, Figure 7.47.

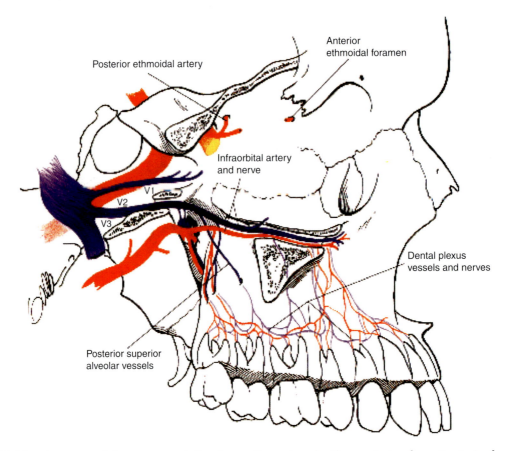

Posterior ethmoidal artery
Anterior ethmoidal foramen
Infraorbital artery and nerve
V1
V2
V3
Dental plexus vessels and nerves
Posterior superior alveolar vessels

Fig. 11.13 Anatomy of the pterygopalatine fossa. Reproduced with permission from Parviz Janfaza *et al.*, *Surgical Anatomy of the Head and Neck*. Lippincott Williams & Wilkins. 2000, Figure 8.6 (p. 339).

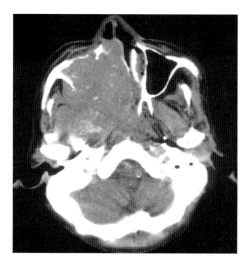

Fig. 11.14 Axial CT of a right maxillary sinus carcinoma. Same case as Figures 11.8 and 11.10. Posteriorly, the tumour destroys the entire posterior and posterolateral walls of the antrum, and the entire right pterygoid bone. The tumour extensively infiltrated the right buccal, masticator and parapharyngeal spaces, the right pterygopalatine fossa, pterygomaxillary fissure and infratemporal fossa.

Box 11.5   Invaluable MRI

MRI is invaluable for

- Assessing intracranial spread into the orbit and anterior cranial fossa: intracranial spread – malignant tumour spread tends to be flat and broad based compared to benign tumours which tend to be polypoid
- Identifying perineural spread
- Differentiating tumour from inspissated mucus/secretions

Box 11.6   Imaging checklist

- Orbital floor and orbital contents
- Ethmoid cells, lamina papyracea, fovea ethmoidalis and cribiform plate
- Anterior cranial fossa
- All maxillary antral walls
- Alveolar bone, hard palate, pterygoid bone, nasal cavity and buccal space
- Pterygopalatine fossa and its communications

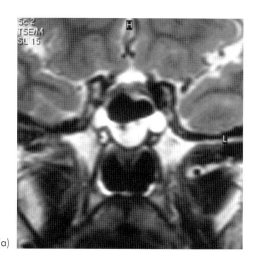

(a)

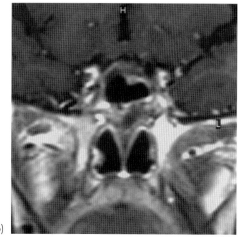

(b)

Fig. 11.15 (a) Coronal MRI of sphenoid sinus mucosal inflammatory thickening. (a) Inflammatory mucosal thickening in the sphenoid sinus shows very high signal on T2W images. (b) Inflammatory mucosal thickening in the sphenoid sinus shows only surface thin rim enhancement on post-gadolinium T1W images.

signal on T2W images because of the high content of free water in secretions and interstitial fluid. Maxillary sinus tumour on the other hand shows low to intermediate signal on both T1W and T2W images. However, long-standing obstruction is commonly present in maxillary sinus tumour, which results in fluid absorption and inspissation. This causes varying degrees of T1 and T2 shortening and the end result is usually a mixture of different signals on both T1W and T2W images. Tumours usually enhance vividly after gadolinium administration because

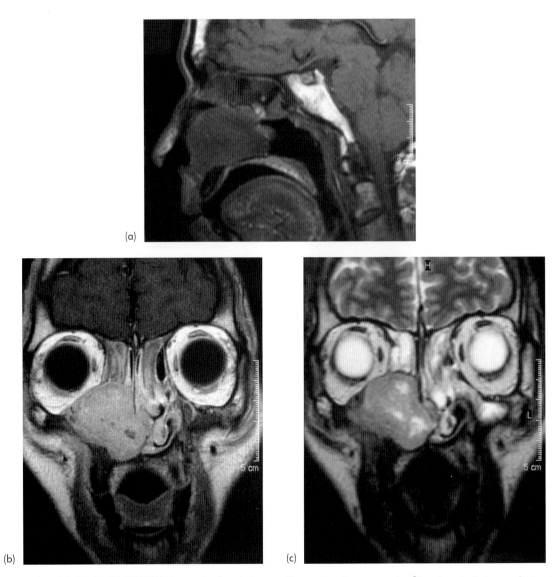

Fig. 11.16 (a) Sagittal MRI (T1W image) of a right maxillary antral tumour showing low to intermediate signal on T1W image. (b) Coronal MRI (post-gadolinium T1W image) of the right maxillary antral tumour showing avid enhancement after gadolinium on T1W image. Note the excellent soft tissue contrast which gives more exact delineation of extent of tumour and differentiation from mucosal inflammation and retained secretions. (c) Coronal MRI (T2W image) of the right maxillary antral tumour showing low to intermediate signal on T2W image.

of their prominent vascularity differentiating this against the background inflammatory change. Retained secretions, inspissated or not, will not enhance. Inflammatory mucosa shows mainly surface rim enhancement and is predominantly non-enhancing [14] (Figures 11.15 and 11.16). Similarly, when the tumour has extended beyond the confines of the antral walls into the surrounding soft tissues, such as into the subcutaneous tissues of the cheek,

the margins of the infiltration is much better delineated on MRI than on CT (Figures 11.17).

In addition, MRI can detect perineural spread with much higher sensitivity (Figure 11.18). Intracranial tumour extension also demonstrates characteristic broad-based, flat surface in contrast to the polypoid surface seen in benign process such as polyps and papillomas [15].

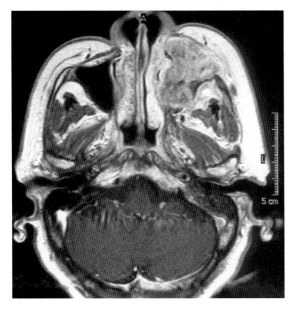

Fig. 11.17 Axial MRI (post-gadolinium T1W image) of a left maxillary antral adenoid cystic carcinoma showing anterior erosion through the anterior antral wall to invade the subcutaneous tissues of the left cheek including the left nasolabial fold.

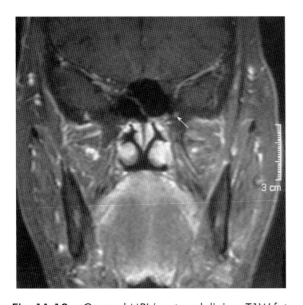

Fig. 11.18 Coronal MRI (post-gadolinium T1W fat-saturation image) showing tumour infiltration from the left pterygopalatine fossa into the left foramen rotundum. Same case as Figure 11.17. There is abnormal enhancement on the post-gadolinium images in the left pterygopalatine fossa which extends into the left foramen rotundum and indicates tumour infiltration.

Management

Treatment plan for maxillary antral tumour depends largely on the stage of the disease and tumour histopathology. Early stage tumours (stage T1, T2 or tumours confined to the infrastructure) can achieve equally good local control rates by surgery or radiotherapy alone. More advanced tumours (stage T3, T4 or tumours involving the suprastructure) will require combination therapy of surgery and radiotherapy. Chemotherapy, in general, is used as an adjunct therapy or when there are systemic metastases.

Surgery

Surgical resection is the mainstay of curative treatment for tumours of the maxillary antrum. Even for tumours too large to be completely resected, debulking surgery can provide symptomatic control of pain relief and rapid decompression. For early stage tumours confined to the infrastructure, complete resection with clear margins can often be obtained with satisfactory local control. Reported 5-year survival rates range from 19% to 86% for malignant sinonasal tract tumours treated solely by surgical resection alone [16–18]. When tumours involve the suprastructure, especially the orbits and the pterygopalatine fossae, or when there is perineural spread, complete resection is more difficult to achieve and combination therapy with radiotherapy will be required.

There is still controversy about the indication for orbital exenteration. Previously quoted indications for orbital exenteration include bone erosion, posterior ethmoid, orbital apex or infraorbital nerve invasion, and various degrees of periorbital invasion [19]. A number of studies [20–23] have concluded that bone erosion is not an absolute indication for orbital exenteration and pre-operative radiotherapy enhances the chance of preservation of the globe. However adjuvant radiotherapy, either before or after surgery, does not improve the survival. Meta-analysis of these studies also shows no statistically significant difference between the orbital sparing group and the orbital exenteration group [19].

The low incidence of cervical nodal metastatic deposits from maxillary antral tumours does not justify the routine performance of elective neck dissection or irradiation. The presence of cervical nodal disease on initial presentation does not affect survival [24, 25] and should not preclude radical treatment of the primary tumour.

Radiation therapy

Radiotherapy is commonly given together with surgery or with chemotherapy as combined modality treatment.

Pre-operative radiotherapy is associated with more post-operative complications than post-operative radiotherapy (29% versus 14%) but higher survival (64% at 5 years) has been demonstrated in the pre-operative patient group than post-operative patient group (26% at 5 years) [26]. On the other hand, satisfactory survival rate (overall 42–48% 5-year actuarial survival) has also been demonstrated in patients receiving radiotherapy after surgery [27], with emphasis on clinical stage being an important prognostic factor [28].

Many surgeons prefer post-operative radiotherapy because the non-irradiated tumour margins are better delineated intra-operatively, the post-operative wound healing is more predictable and the post-operative targeted tumour volume is smaller [29].

Unresectable T4 malignant tumours have been treated with aggressive chemoradiotherapy with a 3-year local control rate of 78% [30].

Chemotherapy

Multimodality treatment protocols including induction chemotherapy, followed by surgical resection and then concomitant radiotherapy and chemotherapy have been reported to produce favourable results compared to historic controls treated by surgery and radiotherapy only [31].

Chemotherapy delivered intra-arterially via selective catheterisation of the dominant supplying artery to the tumour has also been reported with favourable response [32–34]. The aim of intra-arterial chemotherapy is to attain the highest possible concentration of the chemotherapeutic agent in the tumour while minimising the systemic toxicity. With the development of newer cisplatin-based regimens the full potential of intra-arterial chemotherapy, either alone or in combination with other modalities, require further studies for evaluation.

Other tumours of the maxilla
Other malignant epithelial tumours

Non-squamous cell carcinoma
Adenoid cystic carcinoma
Adenoid cystic carcinoma tends to be slow growing. It appears as an invasive tumour mass similar to SCC on CT but shows increased T2W signal on MRI because of the glandular component (Figure 11.19). *Perineural spread* is the hallmark of this tumour and may occur either retrograde (e.g. intracranially) or antegrade (e.g. to infratemporal or pterygopalatine fossa) (Figure. 11.18). For this tumour haematogenous spread to the lungs and bones is also more common than lymphatic spread. Recurrence can occur up to 10–20 years after initial treatment and long-term follow-up is required.

Adenocarcinoma
Adenocarcinoma has a much higher incidence among woodworkers (1000-fold increased risk) and is thus more common in males with a peak incidence at age 55–60 years. On endoscopy, they may show

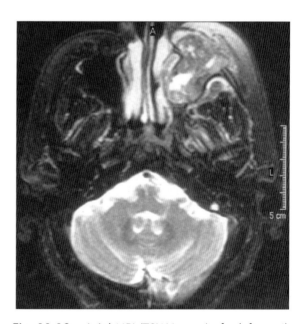

Fig. 11.19   Axial MRI (T2W image) of a left maxillary antral adenoid cystic carcinoma. Same case as Figures 11.17 and 11.18. Note the high T2W signal component of the tumour because of the glandular component (compare Figure 11.16c).

three different growth forms: papillary, sessile or alveolar-mucoid.

Melanoma

Melanoma accounts for 3.5% of sinonasal neoplasms. It tends to occur during the fifth to eighth decades and appears as a heavily pigmented or pink polypoid or fleshy mass. It arises more commonly from the nasal cavity, particularly the anterior nasal septum, and also the middle and inferior nasal turbinates than from the sinuses where the maxillary sinus is more often affected than the ethmoid. It appears on CT as a soft tissue mass with mucosal infiltration. On MRI, melanotic tumour shows hyperintensity on T1W images and hypointensity on T2W images while amelanotic tumour shows hypointensity on T1W images and hyperintensity on T2W images. 10–20% of patients develop lymphatic spread and 50–75% will develop local recurrence or metastases within 1 year. Wide local resection is the treatment of choice and may be supplemented by radiotherapy. Neck dissection is indicated when there is neck nodal disease.

Olfactory neuroblastoma

Olfactory neuroblastoma (esthesioblastoma) shows a bimodal age distribution with one peak at 11–20 years and the other at 51–60 years. Common presentations include epistaxis and nasal obstruction. It appears as an enhancing soft tissue mass in the nasal vault, which may erode through the cribiform plate and extend into the anterior cranial fossa and as such coronal scans are mandatory in the investigation (Figure 11.20). It appears hypointense to brain on T1W images and hyperintense on T2W images. Spread is via lymphatics and deposits may occur in the parotids, skin, lung, liver, eye, spinal cord and canal. Local recurrence rate is as high as 50%. Treatment requires adequate surgical resection, which often entails combined craniofacial resection. Postoperative radiotherapy is also indicated.

Clinical staging system proposed by Kadish [35]:

- Group A: Tumour confined to nasal cavity.
- Group B: Tumour extending into paranasal sinuses.
- Group C: Tumour spread beyond nasal cavity and paranasal cavity.

New staging system using CT/MRI scan proposed by Dulguerov and Calcaterra [36]:

- T1: Tumour involving the paranasal cavity and/or paranasal sinuses (excluding sphenoid), sparing the most superior ethmoid cells.
- T2: Tumour involving the nasal cavity and/or paranasal sinuses (including the sphenoid) with extension to or erosion of the cribiform plate.
- T3: Tumour extending into the orbit or protruding into the anterior cranial fossa.
- T4: Tumour involving the brain.

Sinonasal undifferentiated carcinoma

Sinonasal undifferentiated carcinoma is often associated with paucity of symptoms at the time of diagnosis. However, at times it may be hormonally active and produce paraneoplastic symptoms. Endoscopy often reveals an ill-defined large tumour most often in the ethmoid sinus and superior nasal cavity. It

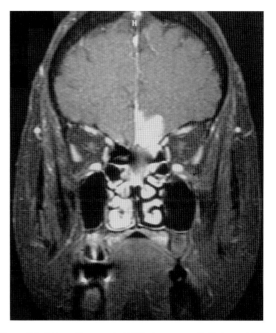

Fig. 11.20 Coronal MRI (post-gadolinium T1W fat saturation image) of an olfactory neuroblastoma arising from the left superior nasal vault eroding through the cribiform plate and extending into the anterior cranial fossa with invasion of the left frontal lobe parenchyma.

appears as an ill-defined soft tissue mass on CT which frequently invades adjacent structures including the anterior cranial fossa, orbits, pterygopalatine fossa, parapharyngeal space, cavernous sinus, and adjacent paranasal sinuses. It is iso-intense to muscles on T1W images and iso- to hyperintense on T2W images of MRI.

Malignant non-epithelial tumours

Lymphoma

Non-Hodgkin's lymphoma is more common than Hodgkin's lymphoma in the maxillary sinus. It may present with nasal obstruction, rhinorrhoea, epistaxis, sinusitis or more sinister symptoms such as visual loss and paraesthesia, as well as systemic symptoms of lymphoma including generalised lymphadenopathy. Paranasal sinus lymphoma is associated with disseminated lymphoma and AIDS.

It appears on imaging as soft tissue opacification with expansion, erosion or infiltration, which may mimic sinusitis, polyposis, granulomatous processes and other benign or malignant neoplasms (Figure 11.21).

Management is by chemotherapy and radiotherapy.

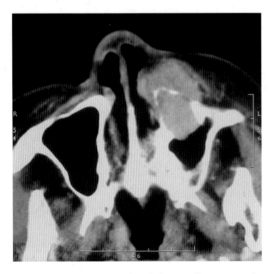

Fig. 11.21 Axial CT of a left maxillary sinus lymphoma. Soft tissue tumour arising from the anterior portion of the left maxillary antrum infiltrating anteriorly into the left nasolabial fold and left medial cheek. Biopsy revealed lymphoma.

Metastases

Metastases to the paranasal sinuses may originate from the kidney, lung, breast, gastrointestinal tract, and less commonly the cervix and liver. The maxillary sinus is the most commonly involved among the paranasal sinuses.

They usually present as mass lesions resulting in nasal obstruction with other signs of secondary disease. Bone scintigram often reveals other sites of osseous deposits. Treatment is aimed at palliation for relief of pain, bleeding and orbital complications.

Sarcomas
Osteosarcoma

Osteosarcoma is seen in patients in the second and third decades and is associated with Paget's disease, previous irradiation, giant cell tumour, fibrous dysplasia and ossifying fibroma. It tends to stimulate periodontal disease resulting in a mass effect, swelling, pain, loose teeth and bleeding gums. Paraesthesia may also develop if there is nerve invasion. It may appear as a lytic or blastic lesion with typical sunburst periosteal reaction with or without an associated soft tissue mass. It shows low and inhomogeneous signal on both T1W and T2W images.

Chondrosarcoma

Chondrosarcoma is most commonly seen in patients in the fourth decade but 10% may be seen in children. Males are affected twice as commonly as females. Hyperglycaemia is a known associated paraneoplastic syndrome.

On CT, it appears as an expansile osteolytic lesion with the sphenoid bone more commonly involved. Punctate or snowflake-like calcifications may be seen within. A soft tissue mass is often seen, which shows low signal on T1W images and appears hypo- or isointense to brain on T2W images. Treatment is by early wide excision.

Intermediate-type tumours

Schneiderian papilloma

Patients with Schneiderian papilloma usually present at age 40–60 years and males are three to five times more likely affected than females. Common presenting symptoms include *unilateral* nasal obstruction, epistaxis, postnasal drip, recurrent sinusitis and sinus headache, especially with the distinct absence of an allergic history. This tumour appears as a firm, bulky red or vascular mass with polypoid growth and convoluted cerebriform mucosa. It is almost always unilateral (less than 5% are bilateral) (Figure 11.22) and is occasionally multicentric. It commonly arises from the lateral nasal wall in the vicinity of the middle turbinate and the maxillary antrum is the most frequently involved among the paranasal sinuses. On CT it appears as an enhancing soft tissue density mass. Bone destruction usually involves the medial antral wall. The origin of the tumour may not be apparent as the tumour may be pedunculated. Foci of calcification may be seen within. On MRI, it is iso- to slightly hyperintense to muscle on unenhanced T1W images, hyperintense to muscle on T2W images, with curvilinear hyperintense striations throughout tumour mass on T2W images and contrast-enhanced T1W images. Central T1W hypointensity and T2W hyperintensity suggests necrosis associated with coexistent SCC (5–27%). Direct contiguous spread usually extends into the ethmoid and maxillary sinuses and less commonly into the frontal and sphenoid sinuses. It may involve the orbit, nasopharynx, but rarely violates the meninges and intracranial structures.

Treatment is by complete *en bloc* surgical excision with frozen section. Endoscopic excision may also be performed. In suspected recurrence, CT can show the bony defects and soft tissue masses but cannot differentiate between recurrence and inflammation; MRI, which is the best for soft tissue depiction, also cannot differentiate between recurrent tumour and inflammation but can give an indication for directing the biopsy.

Juvenile angiofibroma

Juvenile angiofibroma is most commonly seen in young boys with an average age of 15 years who present with recurrent and severe epistaxis, nasal obstruction, nasal speech and sometimes facial deformity. It appears as a soft red mass in the nasopharynx or posterior nares and biopsy is absolutely contraindicated. CT will confirm its location in the nasopharynx or posterior nares and typical appearances include

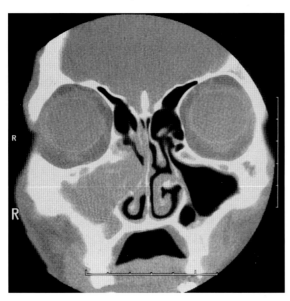

Fig. 11.22 Coronal CT of an inverted papilloma. Complete opacification of the right maxillary antrum and OMU. The other paranasal sinuses are all clear. The unilateral, solitary involvement raises the suspicion of the underlying lesion. Biopsy revealed inverted papilloma.

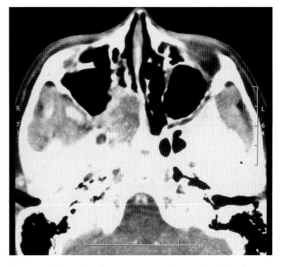

Fig. 11.23 Axial contrast-enhanced CT showing a juvenile angiofibroma. Large mass lesion extends from the right nasopharynx via the right posterior choana into the right nasal cavity. The mass shows moderate heterogeneous enhancement after contrast. The mass is bowing and deviating the nasal septum to the left. The mass is also eroding the posterior part of the medial wall of the right maxillary antrum, and mildly bulging into the antrum. There is also extension laterally into the right pterygopalatine fossa.

Box 11.7　Staging/classification of juvenile angiofibroma

Sessions *et al.*, 1981 [37]
IA　Limited to nose and/or nasopharyngeal vault
IB　Extension into one or more sinus
IIA　Minimal extension into pterygomaxillary fossa
IIB　Full occupation of pterygomaxillary fossa with or without erosion of orbital bones
IIC　Infratemporal fossa with or without cheek
III　Intracranial extension

Fisch, 1983 [38]
I　　Tumours limited to nasal cavity nasopharynx with no bony destruction
II　　Tumours invading pterygomaxillary fossa, paranasal sinuses with bone destruction
III　Tumours invading infratemporal fossa, orbit and parasellar region remaining lateral to cavernous
　　　sinus
IV　Tumours with invasion to cavernous sinus, optic chiasmal region and pituitary fossa

Chandler *et al.*, 1984 [39]
I　　Tumour confined to nasopharyngeal vault
II　　Tumour extending into nasal cavity or sphenoid sinus
III　Tumour extending into antrum, ethmoid sinus, pterygomaxillary fossa, infratemporal fossa, orbit
　　　and/or cheek
IV　Intracranial tumour

---

a highly vascular mass with associated anterior bowing of the posterior antral wall, widening of the pterygopalatine fossa, superior and/or inferior orbital fissures (Figure 11.23). Regions to look for spread include the sphenoid sinuses, posterolateral wall of nasal cavity, pterygopalatine fossa, retroantral region, orbit, middle cranial fossa and infratemporal fossa (Box 11.7).

On MRI, juvenile angiofibroma shows intermediate signal on T1W images with discrete hypointense punctate foci due to flow voids (Figure 11.24). Conventional angiogram will show the supply by the internal maxillary artery. Pre-operative embolisation will help to decrease the intra-operative blood loss (Figure 11.25).

Ameloblastoma (adamantinoma)

Ameloblastoma is seen equally between male and female patients usually in the fourth or fifth decade. It presents as a slow growing mass causing deformity of the face/nose. Endoscopy usually reveals a mass in the nose. Twenty-five percent are located in the maxilla in the region of bicuspids and molars. CT shows a uni- or multi-loculated lytic lesion with

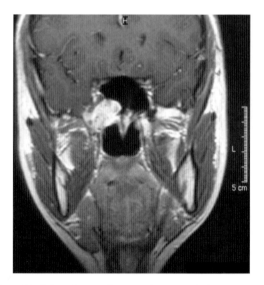

Fig. 11.24 Coronal MRI (post-gadolinium T1W image) of a juvenile angiofibroma. Same case as Figure 11.23. The juvenile angiofibroma shows intense and homogeneous enhancement on MRI.

scalloped margins and cortical expansion. There may be an associated impacted tooth or resorption of the root of a tooth. Treatment is by complete

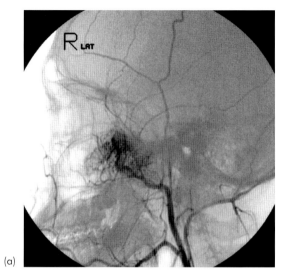 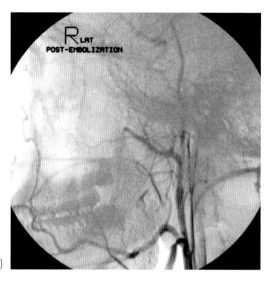

(a) (b)

Fig. 11.25 Pre-embolisation right external carotid arteriogram (lateral). Same case as Figures 11.23 and 11.24. (a) Right external carotid arteriogram showing a hypervascular mass supplied by the right internal maxillary artery consistent with angiofibroma. (b) Following embolisation with Ivalon particles showing almost complete devascularisation of the tumour.

Box 11.8

Ultimately, diagnosis is made on histology and the role of the radiologist is to image the extent of the tumour in areas undetectable by the clinicians for accurate staging.

en bloc excision. Local recurrence frequently becomes more aggressive after excision and CT is best suited for assessment of any bony changes.

Acknowledgements

The authors would like to thank Dr. Brian KH Yu, FRCR, FHKAM (Clinical Oncology) for reviewing the manuscript and contributing to the section on radiotherapy.

References

1. Vijay MR and Khaled IE. Sinonasal imaging. *Rad. Clin. N. Am.* 1998; **36**(5): 921–939.
2. Lalitha Shankar, Kathryn Evans, Michael Hawke and Heinz Stammberger. *An Atlas of Imaging of the Paranasal Sinuses.* Martin Dunitz. 1994, 109.
3. Som P and Brandwein M. Tumours and tumour-like conditions of sinonasal cavity. In: P Som and HD Curtin (Eds) *Head and Neck Imaging,* 3rd edition. Mosby Year Book, St Louis. 1996, 185–187.
4. Gullane PJ and Conley J. Carcinoma of the maxillary sinus. *J. Otolaryngol.* 1983; **12**: 141–145.
5. Gadeberg CC, Hjelm-Hansen M, Soggard H *et al.* Malignant tumors of the paranasal sinuses and nasal cavity. A series of 180 patients. *Acta Radiol.* 1984; **23**: 181–187.
6. Hill JH, Scboroff BJ and Applebaum EL. Nonsquamous tumors of the nose and paranasal sinuses. *Otolaryngol.Clin. N. Am.* 1986; **19**: 723–729.
7. Baredes S, Cho HT and Som ML. Total maxillectomy. In: A Blitzer, W Lawson and WH Friedman (Eds) *Surgery of the Paranasal Sinuses.* WB Saunders Co., Philadelphia, PA. 1985, 204–216.
8. St-Pierre S and Baker SR. Squamous cell carcinoma of the maxillary sinus: analysis of 66 cases. *Head Neck Surg.* 1983; **5**: 508–513.
9. Lavertu P, Roberts JK, Kraus DH, Levine HL, Wood BG, Medendorp SV and Tucker HM. Squamous cell carcinoma of the paranasal sinuses: the Cleveland Clinic experience 1977–1986. *Laryngoscope* 1989; **99**: 1130–1136.
10. Sisson Sr GA, Toriumi DM and Atiyah RA. Paranasal sinus malignancy: a comprehensive update. *Laryngoscope* 1898; **99**: 143–150.
11. Spiro JD, Soo KC and Spiro RH. Squamous carcinoma of the nasal cavity and paranasal sinuses. *Am. J. Surg.* 1989; **158**: 328–332.
12. Miyaguchi M, Sakai S-I, Takashima H and Hosokawa H. Lymph node and distant metastases in patients with sinonasal carcinoma. *J. Laryngol. Otol.* 1995; **109**: 304–307.
13. Robin PE and Powell DJ. Regional node involvement and distant metastases in carcinoma of the nasal cavity and paranasal sinuses. *J. Laryngol. Otol.* 1980; **94**: 301–309.
14. Tessell PV and Lee YY. Gd-DTPA enhanced MR for detecting intracranial extension of sinonasal malignancies. *J. Comput. Assist. Tomogr.* 1991; **15**: 387–392.
15. Som P. Tumors and tumor-like conditions of sino-nasal cavity. In P Som and RT Bergeron (Eds) *Head and Neck Imaging,* 2nd edition. Mosby Year Book, St. Louis. 1990, 169–227.

16. Frazell E and Lewis JS. Cancer of the nasal cavity and accessory sinuses: a report on the management of 416 patients. *Cancer* 1963; **16**: 1293.

17. Sisson GA, Toriumi DM and Atiyah RA. Paranasal sinus malignancy: a comprehensive update. *Laryngoscope* 1989; **99**: 143.

18. Jackson RT, Fitzhugh GS and Constable WC. Malignant neoplasms of the nasal cavities and paranasal sinuses (a retrospective study). *Laryngoscope* 1977; **87**: 357.

19. Ricardo L Carrau and Eugene N Meyers. Neoplasms of the nose and paranasal sinuses. In *Head and Neck Surgery – Otolaryngology*, 2nd edition. Lippincott-Raven Publishers, Philadelphia, PA, 1998, 1461.

20. Gullane PJ and Conley J. Carcinoma of the maxillary sinus: a correlation of the clinical course with orbital involvement, pterygoid erosion, or pterygopalatine invasion and cervical metastases. *J. Otolaryngol.* 1983; **12**: 141.

21. Som ML. Surgical management of carcinoma of the maxilla. *Arch. Otolaryngol.* 1974; **99**: 270–273.

22. Perry C, Levine PA, Williamson BR and Cantrell RW. Preservation of the eye in paranasal sinus cancer surgery. *Arch. Otolaryngol. Head Neck Surg.* 1988; **114**: 632–634.

23. Xuexi W, Pingzhang T and Yongfa Q. Management of the orbital contents in radical surgery for squamous cell carcinoma of the maxillary sinus. *Chin. Med. J. (Engl.)* 1995; **108**: 123–125.

24. Kondo M, Ogawa K, Inuyama Y et al. Prognostic factors influencing the relapse of squamous cell carcinoma of the maxillary sinus. *Cancer* 1985; **55**: 190–196.

25. St. Pierre S and Baker SR. Squamous cell carcinoma of the maxillary sinus: analysis of 66 cases. *Head Neck Surg.* 1983; **5**: 508–513.

26. Yu-Hua H, Gui-Yi T, Yu-Quin Q et al. Comparison of pre- and post-operative radiation in the combined treatment of carcinoma of the maxillary antrum. *Int. J. Radiat. Oncol. Biol. Phys.* 1982; **8**: 1045.

27. Ogawa K, Toita T, Kakinohana Y, Adachi G, Kojya S, Itokazu T, Shinhama A, Matsumura J and Murayama S. Postoperative radiotherapy for squamous cell carcinoma of the maxillary sinus: analysis of local control and late complications. *Oncol. Rep.* 2001; **8**(2): 315–319.

28. Zaharia M, Salem L, Travezan R et al. Post-operative radiation therapy in the management of cancer of the maxillary sinus. *Int. J. Radiat. Oncol. Biol. Phys.* 1989; **17**: 967.

29. Ricardo L Carrau and Eugene N Myers. Neoplasms of the nose and paranasal sinuses. In: Byron J Bailey (Ed.) *Head and Neck Surgery – Otolaryngology*, 3rd edition. William & Wilkins. 2001, 1258. Philadelphia, PA.

30. Harrison LB, Raben A, Pfister DG, Zelefsky M, Strong E, Shah JP, Spiro RH, Shaha A, Kraus DH, Schantz SP, Carper E, Bodansky B, White C and Bosl G. A prospective phase II trial of concomitant chemotherapy and radiotherapy with delayed accelerated fractionation in unresectable tumors of the head and neck. *Head Neck* 1998; **20**(6): 497–503.

31. Lee MM, Vokes EE, Rosen A et al. Multimodality therapy in advanced paranasal sinus carcinoma: superior long term results. *Cancer J. Sci. Am.* 1999; **5**: 219.

32. Robbins KT, Storniolo AM, Kerber C et al. Phase I study of highly selective supradose cisplatin infusions for advanced head and neck cancer. *J. Clin. Oncol.* 1994; **12**: 2113.

33. Robbins KT, Kumar P, Regine WF et al. Efficacy of targeted supradose cisplatin and concomitant radiation therapy for advanced head and neck cancer: the Memphis experience. *Int. J. Radiat. Oncol. Biol. Phys.* 1997; **38**: 263.

34. Samant S, Kumar P, Wan J et al. Concomitant radiation therapy and targeted cisplatin chemotherapy for the treatment of advanced pyriform sinus carcinoma: disease control and preservation of organ function. *Head Neck* 1999; **21**: 595.

35. Kadish S, Goodman M and Wang CC. Olfactory neuroblastoma, a clinical analysis of 17 cases. *Cancer* 1976; **37**: 1571.

36. Dulguerov P and Calcaterra T. Esthesioneuroblastoma: The UCLA experience 1970–1990. *Laryngoscope* 1992; **102**: 843.

37. Sessions RB, Bryan RN, Naclerio RM and Alford BR. Radiographic staging of juvenile angiofibroma. *Head Neck Surg.* 1981; **3**: 279–283.

38. Fisch U. The infratemporal fossa approach for nasopharyngeal tumors. *Laryngoscope* 1983; **93**: 36–44.

39. Chandler JR, Goulding R, Moskowitz L and Quencer RM. Nasopharyngeal angiofibromas: staging and management. *Ann. Otol. Rhinol. Laryngol.* 1984; **93**: 322–329.

Cancer of the Skull Base

AD King and AC Vlantis

Role of imaging

In the past, cancer of the skull base was extremely difficult to treat. At that time, the role of radiology was simply to make a diagnosis based on site and appearance, and where possible, to identify a site for biopsy. With recent major advances in surgical techniques and when combining the skills of otolaryngologists, neurosurgeons and plastic surgeons, there are almost no areas of the skull base that are not amenable to surgery. Even those deep-seated tumours involving the cavernous sinus, clivus, superior orbital fissure and infratemporal fossa are now surgically accessible. Recent advances in radiotherapy allow conformal and stereotactic techniques to deliver high-dose radiation to small precise areas. As a result of these advances in surgery and radiotherapy, the principle role of radiology has expanded to include not only the diagnosis but also the mapping of the extent of a tumour in relationship to vital neurological and vascular structures. Diagnostic features of skull base tumours and important radiological anatomy are discussed below. For further detailed anatomy of the skull base, please refer to Chapter 5.

Which imaging modality should be employed to image skull base tumours?

Cross-sectional imaging using magnetic resonance imaging (MRI) is the technique of choice for evaluating tumours of the skull base. This is because it offers excellent tissue contrast in multiple scanning planes. Specific advantages of MR over computed tomography (CT) are listed in Table 12.1.

There are a few specific advantages of CT over MRI listed in Table 12.2. In these cases, CT is required in addition to MRI.

Other imaging techniques used to evaluate head and neck cancer include position emission tomography (PET) scanning (please refer to Chapter 4) and conventional angiography. Conventional angiography is performed pre-operatively to demonstrate the

Table 12.1 Advantages of MRI for skull base tumours.

Sinonasal region
Distinction of inflammatory mucosal changes from tumour. Most tumours of the head and neck are of intermediate or mildly increased signal on T2, whereas inflammatory mucosa and retained secretions give a very high signal. On T1 after contrast most tumours in the sinonasal region enhance but not as intensely as mucosa

Nervous system
Demonstration of the relationship of a tumour to neurological structures such as dura, brain, cranial nerves (including perineural tumour extension) and optic chiasm

Vascular system
Demonstration of the relationship of a tumour to major vascular structures including the carotid arteries and cavernous sinus. Demonstration of tumour vascularity

Bone
Demonstration of the extent of bone marrow invasion

Table 12.2 Advantages of CT for skull base tumours.

Bone
Demonstration of cortical invasion, particularly, in the paranasal sinuses and petrous temporal bone
Calcification
Demonstration of the pattern of tumour calcification which aids in the characterisation of tumours such as a chondrosarcoma

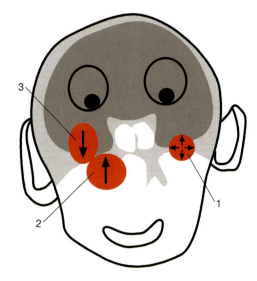

Fig 12.1 Diagnostic imaging of skull base tumours: 1. tumours arising within the skull base, 2. tumours arising below the skull base (extracranial) and 3. tumours arising above the skull base (intracranial).

vascular supply of a tumour and to embolise feeding vessels of a tumour to reduce the intra-operative blood loss. In cases where there is tumour involvement and/or encasement of the internal carotid artery, temporary occlusion of the artery using an angiographically inserted balloon, and the subsequent measurement of objective and subjective parameters, can determine whether the artery can be safely resected or not [1].

Imaging of skull base tumours

For treatment purposes, tumours are divided into three groups according to whether they involve the anterior, middle (medial or lateral) or posterior skull base. For diagnostic imaging purposes, skull base tumours may be divided into three groups according to the origin of the tumour as shown in Figure 12.1. Discussion of individual skull base tumours in this chapter is based on this radiological system of classification.

Tumours arising within the skull base

Tumours arising within the skull base, depicted in Figure 12.2, include:

- Tumours arising from bone: chondrosarcoma, chordoma, radiation-induced sarcoma, metastases and carcinoma of the petrous temporal bone.
- Tumours arising from nerves: schwannoma and neurofibroma.
- Tumours arising from chemoreceptor tissue: glomus jugulare, glomus tympanicum and glomus vagale.

Chondrosarcoma

Diagnostic imaging features

Chondrosarcomas (Figure 12.3) [2] arise within the skull base at the site of a synchondrosis and so are

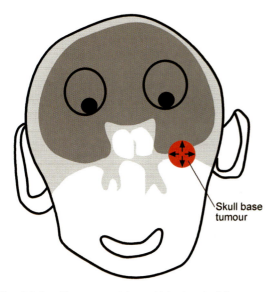

Fig. 12.2   Tumours arising within the skull base.

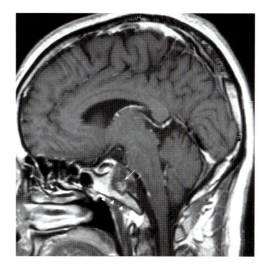

Fig. 12.4   Sagittal T1-weighted MRI with contrast showing a chordoma (arrow) in the posterior aspect of the clivus (arrowheads).

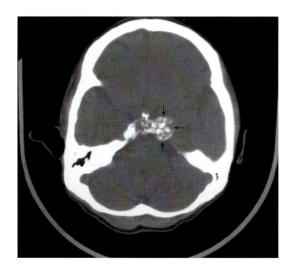

Fig. 12.3   Axial CT of a chondrosarcoma (arrows) arising at the synchondrosis between the clivus and petrous temporal bone.

usually off the midline and found most frequently between the clivus and petrous temporal bone. They show bony destruction without a sclerotic rim, and the soft tissue component may demonstrate small rings of calcification on CT.

Treatment

Chondrosarcomas are best managed by complete surgical excision followed by radiotherapy; currently,

fractionated proton therapy is favoured. If complete excision is not possible, then near-total or partial tumour excision is done to relieve symptoms.

Important imaging points for treatment

To accurately plan surgery, CT and MRI are used to evaluate the tumour because it involves soft tissue and bony structures at the skull base. CT delineates bone destruction and MRI defines the tumour margin from the brain, soft tissues such as the pharynx and visualises blood vessels which it may displace [3]. The relationship of the tumour to vital neurological structures, vasculature and bone must be determined.

Key points for diagnosis

- Off midline, between the clivus and petrous temporal bone
- Small rings of calcification on CT

Chordoma

Diagnostic imaging features

Chordomas (Figure 12.4) arise from the embryonic remnants of the notochord, usually in the midline along the clivus. By virtue of the sites of the tumours, they present with headaches and cranial nerve palsies. The tumour erodes the clivus without a sclerotic rim, and destroys portions of bone. Calcification may be identified within the tumour. Chordomas show variable enhancement patterns, and on MRI they may have cystic regions of high signal on T1-weighted images.

Treatment

Chordomas are relatively radioresistant. Surgical resection is the treatment of choice followed by proton beam irradiation. Despite complete resection, recurrence is frequent. Metastases occur in 10% of cases.

Important imaging points for treatment

Define the extent of the tumour in relationship to the cavernous sinus, carotid artery and posterior fossa.

> ### Key points for diagnosis
>
> - Midline (along the clivus)
> - Destroyed portions of bone. Calcification may be identified. Variable enhancement pattern
> - Cystic regions of high signal on T1-weighted MR images

Radiation-induced sarcoma

Diagnostic imaging features

Radiation-induced sarcomas (Figure 12.5) [4] are being encountered more frequently as a result of the improved long-term survival of patients treated with radiotherapy. They are usually high-grade sarcomas with a wide range of histological elements. At diagnosis, they are large tumours arising within or at the margin of the radiation field which cause extensive bony destruction and have a large soft tissue component.

Treatment

Complete surgical resection offers the only possibility of cure. Surgery is followed by adjuvant chemotherapy and radiotherapy.

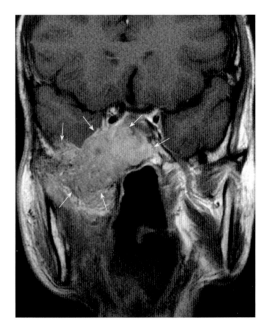

Fig. 12.5 Coronal T1-weighted MRI with contrast of a radiation-induced sarcoma (arrows) in the right slide of the skull base.

Important imaging points for treatment

Dependent upon the site and size of the tumour.

> ### Key points for diagnosis
>
> - Within the radiation field
> - Extensive bony destruction with a large soft tissue component

Metastases

Diagnostic imaging features

Metastases (Figure 12.6) to the skull base are infrequent. They usually arise from carcinoma of the prostate, lung, breast or kidney. The radiological appearance (osteolytic or sclerotic) depends upon the primary tumour.

Treatment

Radiotherapy is usually employed but treatment options are influenced by the histology, site and overall condition of the patient.

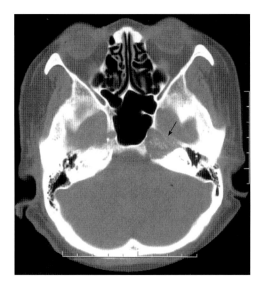

Fig. 12.6 Axial CT bone window showing a lytic metastasis (arrow) in the left petrous apex.

In general, patients with systemic metastases are thought not to be curable, and the role for surgery would be palliative in nature. Surgery of an isolated symptomatic metastasis at the skull base may be attempted to relieve symptoms.

Carcinoma of the petrous temporal bone

Diagnostic imaging features
Carcinoma of the petrous temporal bone is most frequently a squamous cell carcinoma that arises from the spread of carcinoma of the external auditory canal. Carcinoma of the middle and inner ear is rare and includes papillary carcinoma that arises from the endolymphatic sac. Carcinomas have non-specific soft tissue components and show bony destruction.

Treatment
Carcinoma of the petrous temporal bone is best treated with surgery and post-operative radiotherapy. This may be a subtotal petrosectomy, with meningeal resection if needed. Involvement of the facial nerve should be determined on imaging and carries a poor outcome [5].

Important imaging points for treatment
Radiology has an important role in demonstrating the extent of the tumour and of spread beyond the temporal bone. Invasion may occur anteriorly into the carotid canal and temporomandibular joint, inferiorly into the jugular fossa and soft tissues of the infra-temporal fossa, posteriorly into the mastoid, medial into the otic capsule and superiorly into the cranium.

> **Key points for diagnosis**
> * Non-specific soft tissue component and bone destruction

Nerve sheath tumours (schwannomas and neurofibromas)

Diagnostic imaging features
Nerve sheath tumours are related to the cranial nerves as they pass through the skull base. The most frequently involved nerves are the vestibular branch of the VIII nerve, the so-called acoustic neuroma which is usually a vestibular schwannoma (Figure 12.7a), the vagus nerve (vagal schwannoma) and the facial nerve (facial neuroma) (Figure 12.7b and c). Nerve sheath tumours expand the neural foramina before causing destruction. Most are well-defined solid homogeneous tumours with moderate or marked contrast enhancement. However, large schwannomas may have a cystic component and neurofibromas may have a cystic or fatty component.

Treatment
Acoustic neuromas are divided into those confined to the internal auditory canal and small, medium or large tumours that extend beyond it into the cerebellopontine angle. The lateral extent of the tumour in the internal auditory canal will influence the surgical approach used. The best outcome of acoustic neuroma surgery is retention of serviceable hearing, usually only possible for small tumours confined to the internal auditory canal approached by the middle fossa or retrosigmoid route. The next goal is preservation of the facial nerve. Once hearing preservation is not possible, the translabyrinthine approach has the lowest morbidity.

Facial nerve neuromas are usually resected via a middle fossa or translabyrinthine approach and grafted at the time of resection.

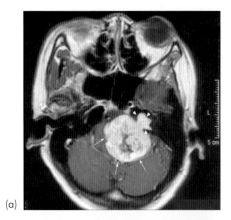

(a)

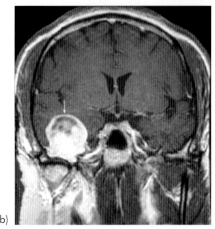

(b)

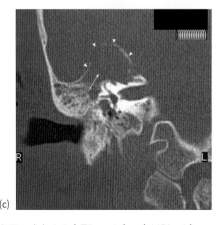

(c)

Fig. 12.7 (a) Axial T1-weighted MRI with contrast showing a large acoustic neuroma in the left cerebellopontine angle (arrows) extending into the internal auditory canal (arrowheads). (b) Coronal T1-weighted MRI with contrast of a schwannoma (arrow) arising from the facial nerve. (c) Coronal CT bone window of the seventh nerve schwannoma causing expansion and destruction of the petrous temporal bone (arrow). A thin rim of bone is lifted superiorly (arrowheads).

Important imaging points for treatment of acoustic neuroma

- Dimensions of the tumour.
- Lateral limit of the tumour in the internal auditory canal.
- Medial extension into cerebellopontine angle.

Key points for diagnosis of nerve sheath tumours

- Expand the neural foramina before causing destruction
- Well-defined solid homogeneous tumours
- Moderate/marked contrast enhancement
- May have cystic or fatty component

Glomus tumours (chemodectomas or paragangliomas)

Diagnostic imaging features

Glomus tumours [6] that involve the skull base arise in the jugular bulb (glomus jugulare) (Figure 12.8), the middle ear cavity (glomus tympanicum) and around the vagus nerve (glomus vagale). They are indolent locally destructive tumours. Glomus jugulare tumours erode the jugular fossa and then extend into the middle ear, mastoid, labyrinth, external auditory canal, occipital bone, posterior fossa and middle cranial fossa via the carotid canal and foramen lacerum. Glomus jugulare tumours causing destruction of the ear may be difficult to distinguish from large glomus tympanicum tumours that arise over the promontory of the middle ear. Glomus vagale tumours arise at or just below the skull base and present as a parapharyngeal mass. The extent of bone destruction is shown best by fine section CT, while MR is better for demonstrating the soft tissue component, especially when there is inferior extension below the skull base and intracranial extension above the skull base. MRI and MR angiography demonstrate the relationship of the tumour to the jugular vein and carotid artery. Glomus tumours are highly vascular, showing multiple small signal voids on MRI and marked early contrast enhancement on dynamic CT and MRI. The early enhancement pattern allows glomus tumours to be distinguished from inflammatory tissue.

Ten per cent are multiple and can be detected using radionuclide scintigraphy (octreotide or MIBG). A small percentage secrete vaso-active substances.

Treatment

In general, complete surgical resection is performed but radiotherapy may be used for the control of inoperable cases.

Important imaging points for treatment

CT or MRI is required to distinguish glomus tumours from other causes of a pulsatile mass, such as a high jugular bulb and aberrant carotid artery.

Small, localised tumours (i.e. glomus tympanicum) can be resected with limited surgery. Large tumours (i.e. glomus jugulare) may require extensive resection and pre-operative embolisation. In these cases, the relationship to major vessels, the inferior extent (below the skull base) and the superior extent (intracranial) need to be carefully mapped by MRI.

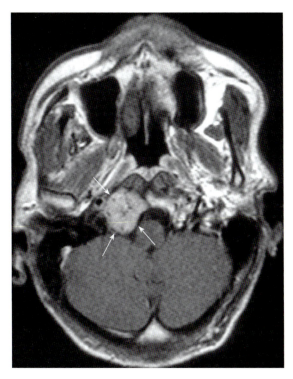

Fig. 12.8 Axial T1-weighted MRI with contrast of a glomus jugulare tumour (arrows).

Key points for diagnosis

- Locally destructive tumour
- Arise around the jugular bulb, middle ear and vagus nerve
- Highly vascular showing multiple small signal voids on MRI and marked early contrast enhancement

Tumours arising below the skull base

Tumours arising below the skull base, depicted in Figure 12.9, include:

- Tumours arising below the anterior skull base: sinonasal carcinoma and esthesioneuroblastoma.
- Tumours arising below the middle skull base: juvenile angiofibroma, nasopharyngeal tumours and parotid tumours.
- Tumours arising at any site: metastases, nerve sheath tumours, lymphoma and rhabdomyosarcoma.

Sinonasal carcinoma

Diagnostic imaging features

The histology of sinonasal carcinoma (Figure 12.10) is varied but most show a non-specific intermediate

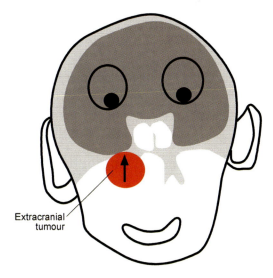

Extracranial tumour

Fig. 12.9 Tumours arising below the skull base.

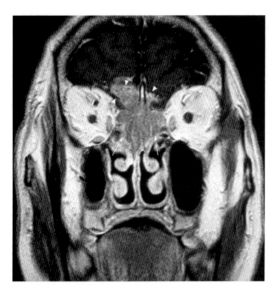

Fig. 12.10 Coronal T1-weighted MRI with contrast of a sinonasal carcinoma (arrows) extending through the cribriform plate into cranium (arrowheads).

attenuation on CT and intermediate or mildly increased signal on T1- and T2-weighted MRI images with mild contrast enhancement. MRI has a particular advantage in distinguishing the tumour from mucosal inflammatory changes and retained secretions. Carcinomas in this region cause bone destruction and may invade the skull base. Tumours in the maxillary sinus invade posteriorly into the pterygopalatine fossa and pterygomaxillary fissure, while those in the ethmoid sinuses and superior nasal cavity have a propensity to invade through the cribriform plate and fovea ethmoidalis into the cranium. The intracranial tumour may be flat and broad based or may be more of a dumbbell shape. Early extension into the dura of the cranium is demonstrated best by MRI.

Treatment
Surgical resection and radiotherapy.

Important imaging points for treatment
Accurately map the tumour extent and distinguish it from mucosal inflammatory change with MRI.

Local failure is the commonest type of recurrence and so all possible sites of local extension should be examined including the orbit, the skull base especially the cribriform plate, the cranium (dura and brain), the pterygopalatine fossa and pterygomaxillary fissure, other sinuses (frontal and sphenoid) and the floor of the nose.

> ### Key points for diagnosis
> - Non-specific soft tissue mass with bone destruction

Esthesioneuroblastoma (olfactory neuroblastoma)

Diagnostic imaging features
Esthesioneuroblastoma (Figure 12.11a) [7] arises from the olfactory epithelium of the superior nasal cavity. In later stages, it may become bilateral, invade the paranasal sinuses and extend through the cribriform plate into the cranium. The tumour remodels or destroys bone. The soft tissue component is non-specific, being homogeneous or slightly heterogeneous, with occasional calcification. All tumours enhance with contrast on CT and MRI. MRI has the advantage of superior depiction of early tumour spread through the cribriform plate. When the intracranial component of the tumour enlarges, it may have a characteristic peripheral cystic component (Figure 12.11b).

Treatment
This is a persistent tumour with a tendency to recur. Craniofacial resection is indicated even when imaging shows no invasion through the cribriform plate because microscopic disease at this site is common. Adjuvant radiotherapy with or without chemotherapy is given.

Important imaging points for treatment
Invasion of cribriform plate and cranium.

> ### Key points for diagnosis
> - Superior nasal cavity mass
> - Remodels or destroys bone
> - Relationship to the cribriform plate and cranium
> - Intracranial component may have a characteristic peripheral cystic component

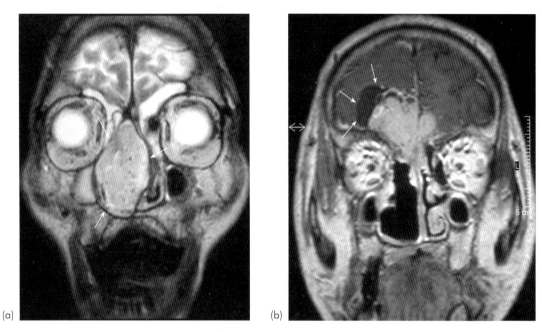

(a)   (b)

Fig. 12.11   (a) Coronal T2-weighted MRI of an esthesioneuroblastoma of the right side of the nasal cavity (arrows). (b) Coronal T1-weighted MRI with contrast of a recurrent esthesioneuroblastoma. The crainal portion has a peripheral cystic component (arrows).

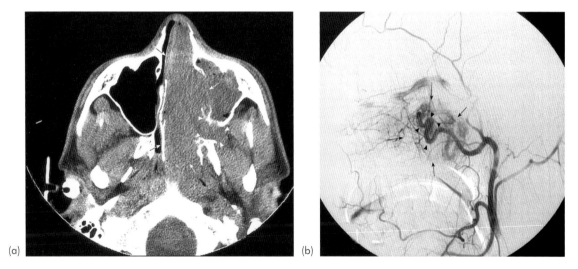

(a)   (b)

Fig. 12.12   (a)   Axial CT scan without contrast of a juvenile angiofibroma (arrows) in the nasal cavity and nasopharynx with invasion into the maxillary sinus and into the skull base causing widening of the pterygopalatine fossa and pterygomaxilliary fissure (arrowheads). (b) Angiogram showing a tumour blush (arrows) of the juvenile angiofibroma which is supplied by the maxillary artery (arrowheads).

Juvenile angiofibroma

Diagnostic imaging features

A juvenile angiofibroma (Figure 12.12) is a benign but highly vascular and aggressive tumour occurring in young males. Angiofibromas are thought to arise in the region of the pterygoid canal in the pterygopalatine fossa. In the nasal cavity, they are usually based in the region of the sphenopalatine foramen. Imaging reveals a tumour with intense contrast enhancement, and signal voids are identified on MRI. The tumour has a propensity to involve the skull base, eroding the pterygoid bone, expanding the ptery-gopalatine fossa and extending along the pterygo-maxillary fissure and bowing the posterior wall of the maxillary sinus anteriorly. Further invasion of the skull vault involves the maxillary, ethmoid and sphe-noid sinuses, infratemporal fossa, orbit and the mid-dle cranial fossa. The radiological appearance is characteristic and biopsy, which may lead to torren-tial bleeding, should not be performed.

Treatment

Treatment is surgical with or without pre-operative embolisation of the feeding vessels to decrease the intra-operative blood loss that occurs from branches of the external carotid, distal maxillary artery and ascending pharyngeal artery (Figure 12.12b), and later from branches of the internal carotid artery.

Important imaging points for treatment

The main determinant of tumour recurrence after surgery is involvement of the pterygoid canal and invasion of the greater wing of the sphenoid.

The tumour can spread laterally to the infratemporal fossa and superiorly via the infra-orbital fissure to the orbit and then to the middle cranial fossa. Rule out cavernous sinus, internal carotid artery and intracranial involvement.

Prior to surgery, which is the treatment of choice, knowledge of the blood supply of the tumour is essential.

Key points for diagnosis

- Young males
- Arises from the junction of the nasophar-ynx and posterior nasal cavity
- Highly vascular with signal voids (MRI) and intense contrast enhancement
- Propensity to involve the skull base along pterygomaxillary fissure, eroding the ptery-goid bone, expanding the pterygopalatine fossa

Nasopharyngeal tumours

Nasopharyngeal carcinoma, minor salivary gland tumours, rhabdomyosarcoma and lymphoma. Please refer to Chapter 5.

Parotid tumours

Diagnostic imaging features

Parotid gland tumours (Figure 12.13) may extend into the temporal bone at the skull base either directly from the superficial lobe or via the parapharyngeal space from the deep lobe. Care is needed when imag-ing parotid tumours because of their tendency to spread along nerves, especially the facial nerve, to the skull base. This is most notable with adenoid cystic carcinoma which has a propensity for perineural spread leading to infiltration of the nerves running through the skull base.

Treatment

Surgery is the primary treatment for malignant parotid tumours. Radiotherapy is given post-operatively when indicated to improve local control and survival, for inoperable tumours and to those patients unfit for surgery. Please refer to Chapter 9.

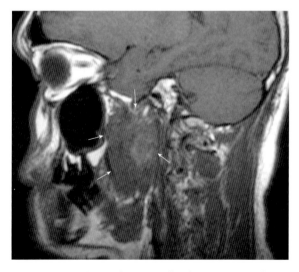

Fig. 12.13 Sagittal T1-weighted MR image show-ing a deep lobe parotid tumour (arrows) extending up to the skull base.

Important imaging points for treatment

Perineural tumour spread. MRI with fat saturation is required to show the perineural tumour spread.

> ### Key points for diagnosis
> - Tumour involving deep lobe of parotid and/or parapharyngeal space
> - Perineural tumour spread

Tumours arising above the skull base

Tumours arising above the skull base, depicted in Figure 12.14, include:

- Meningioma, invasive pituitary adenoma and craniopharyngioma.

Meningioma

Diagnostic imaging features

Meningiomas (Figure 12.15) related to the sphenoid bone of the skull base exhibit a more aggressive clinical behaviour than those related to the skull vault. Bony hyperostosis and direct bony invasion are more common, as is malignant transformation. Apart from direct bony invasion meningiomas also spread along the arachnoid cells that accompany the nerves as they traverse the neural foramina in the skull base. Imaging reveals an extra-axial intracranial tumour that is homogeneous and isointense to brain on MRI and displays marked contrast enhancement, often with a "dural tail" of enhancement. Hyperostosis of adjacent bone is found on both CT and MRI, but it is more easily detected by CT. Meningiomas arising along the planum sphenoidal may show "blistering" of the underlying bone.

Treatment

This slow growing tumour invades bone and dura and is best treated with complete excision and post-operative radiotherapy. Subtotal resection preserving cranial nerves and important vessels, followed by RT to the residual tumour, preserves function and offers acceptable long-term control of meningiomas.

Those meningiomas arising in the medial aspect of the sphenoid around the cavernous sinus represent a difficult surgical challenge because of the close proximity of vital neurovascular structures. Those

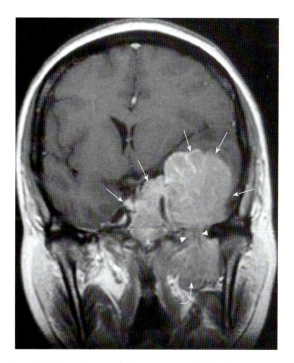

Fig. 12.15 Coronal T1-weighted MRI with contrast showing a large intracranial meningioma (arrows) extending into the cavernous sinus and through the skull base (arrowheads) into the parapharyngeal region (curved arrow).

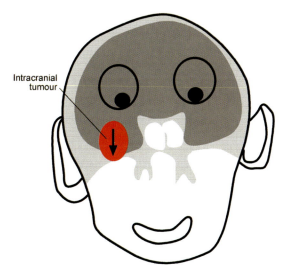

Intracranial tumour

Fig. 12.14 Tumours arising above the skull base.

in the lateral aspect arise in a more "silent" area and often present late.

Important imaging points for treatment

Relationship of the meningioma to the internal carotid artery, which may be encased and narrowed, cavernous sinus, optic chiasm and cranial nerves.

Key points for diagnosis

- Extra-axial intracranial tumour that is homogeneous (isointense to the brain on MRI)
- Marked contrast enhancement and dural tail
- Bony hyperostosis and direct bony invasion

Invasive pituitary adenoma and craniopharyngioma

Not discussed further.

Summary of important imaging points for management

Resection of skull base tumours must be balanced with the anticipated minimum residual acceptable function. Surgery is undertaken only when it is feasible. The ICA cannot usually be resected or occluded if there is poor collateral circulation. The contents of one orbit, but not both, can be sacrificed, as can one temporal bone. The morbidity from cranial nerve palsies can be significant. Gross CNS involvement is a relative contraindication to surgery. Bearing this in mind the radiologist must clearly delineate the bone and soft tissue involvement by the tumour. The relationship of the tumour to major blood vessels, cranial nerves and structures above and below the skull base is essential for the appropriate management of the patient.

References

1. Adams GL, Madison M, Remley K and Gapany M. Preoperative permanent ballon occlusion of the internal carotid artery in patients with advanced head and neck squamous cell carcinoma. *Laryngoscope* 1999; **109**: 460–466.
2. Korten AGGC, ter Berg HJW, Spincemaille H, van der Laan RT and Van de Wel AM. Intracranial chondrosarcoma: review of the literature and report of 15 cases. *J. Neurol. Neurosurg. Psychiat.* 1998; **65**: 88–92.
3. Weber AL, Liebsch NJ, Sanchez R and Sweriduk ST. Chordomas of the skull base. Radiologic and clinical evaluation. *Neuroimag. Clin. N. Am.* 1994; **4**: 515–527.
4. King AD, Ahuja AT, Teo P, Tse GMK and Kew J. Radiation induced sarcomas of the head and neck following radiotherapy for nasopharyngeal carcinoma. *Clin. Radiol.* 2000; **55**: 684–689.
5. Liu FF, Keane TJ and Davidson J. Primary carcinoma involving the petrous temporal bone. *Head Neck* 1993; **15**: 39–43.
6. Vogel TJ and Balzer JO. Base of skull, nasopharynx and parapharyngeal space. *Neuroimag. Clin. N. Am.* 1996; **6**: 362–364.
7. Li C, Yousem DM, Hayden RE and Doty RL. Olfactory neuroblastoma: MR evaluation. *Am. J. Neuroradiol.* 1993; **14**: 1167–1171.

Cervical Mass – Cancer?

RM Evans and AT Ahuja

Introduction

This chapter will deal with a common clinical problem, i.e. what is the diagnosis of a patient who presents with a palpable cervical mass? Which is the best imaging modality to use to try and solve the question will depend on local expertise, availability of equipment, referral pathways, etc. This chapter will deal with the different pathologies that present as a mass in the neck, highlighting the signs that allow a radiologist to make a diagnosis, with reference to all the major imaging modalities, i.e. computed tomography (CT), magnetic resonance imaging (MRI) and ultrasound (US).

Our preference is for US as the initial investigation for a cervical mass. US is widely available, is cost effective, and the near field resolution that can be obtained is superior to both CT and MRI and allows for excellent resolution of superficial cervical pathology. The depiction of colour flow within a mass at the flick of a switch is a major advantage of US over CT and MRI. US lends itself to image-guided biopsy, allowing a rapid (one-stop) cytological or histological diagnosis to be obtained via either fine needle aspiration cytology (FNAC) or core biopsy. The disadvantages of US include its limitation in depicting the full extent of deep or complex masses and its limitation in the depiction of anatomical information in a format that is intelligible to surgeons and clinicians.

> **Key points**
>
> - US: ideal initial investigation for a cervical mass
> - US lends itself to biopsy techniques: one-stop approach
> - MRI or CT allows deep extent of tumours to be assessed
> - MRI or CT – more easily interpreted by surgeons/clinicians

While we feel that US is the optimal choice in dealing with a cervical mass, we realise that with the sub-specialisation that has now evolved in most radiology departments, barriers may have developed. Not all head and neck radiologists have either access to, or an interest in US. However, if US expertise and availability is present – this chapter will show the benefit of using US as the initial investigation, allowing a cost-effective triage of patients and more efficient utilisation of other imaging modalities, namely MRI and CT.

Whatever imaging modality is adopted, be it US, MRI or CT, the diagnostic approach should be similar. The radiologist should seek to answer the following four key questions regarding clinical dilemma about cervical mass:

1. Is the mass nodal in origin?
2. If nodal – is it benign or malignant?
3. If non-nodal – can a specific diagnosis be made on imaging alone?
4. If a specific diagnosis cannot be made – is there a need to proceed to a biopsy?

Is the mass nodal in origin?

When presented with a patient who has a neck lump the first question that imaging must answer is "Is the mass a lymph node?" This question is answered using

1. knowledge of major lymphatic pathways in the neck,
2. known appearances of lymph nodes on imaging, both benign and malignant.

These two topics have been dealt with previously in Chapter 1.

If nodal – is it benign or malignant?

For differentiating between benign and malignant lymph nodes, the criteria have been dealt earlier in Chapter 1 and they are annotated in Table 13.1 for ease of reference. There are US signs that can point to a particular diagnosis, e.g. round, diffusely hypoechoic nodes, possibly containing a hilus, with a florid colour flow pattern – are highly suggestive of lymphoma. Identification of these signs will, therefore, influence further investigations and management. A decision can be taken to carry out a core biopsy under US control or excision biopsy (as dictated by local practice) and if a histological diagnosis is confirmed, the patient will need staging by CT.

This differs from the management of a patient with a known squamous cell carcinoma (SCC) primary in

Table 13.1   Diagnostic pathways.

	Signs/site	Probable diagnosis	Further investigation
1	Rounded, hypoechoic nodes, hilus, enhanced "benign" colour flow pattern	Lymphoma	Core biopsy If lymphoma confirmed – CT staging
2	Rounded, necrotic node, peripheral colour flow, ill defined	SCC	FNAC Known primary – stage Unknown primary – CT/MRI + endoscopy
3	Matted nodes, cystic degeneration, apex posterior triangle, displaced hilar vascularity	TB	FNAC →Cytology →Microbiology
4	Rounded, hyperechoic nodes with punctate calcification, paratracheal chain, along IJV	Metastatic papillary carcinoma thyroid	FNAC Evaluate thyroid for primary tumour
5	Small, ovoid node, heterogeneous, no specific colour flow pattern. Post-radiotherapy field. Previous primary	? Recurrent disease	Excision biopsy (FNAC and core biopsy – low diagnostic yield)
6	Large cystic mass, containing echogenic fluid. Posterior to the submandibular space	Second branchial cleft cyst Metastatic SCC Metastatic thyroid papillary carcinoma	FNAC

whom a cervical mass is detected. US may identify a necrotic ill-defined node with peripheral vascularity, areas of vascular displacement and subcapsular vessels – features that point to a diagnosis of a metastatic SCC node. FNAC is excellent for confirmation of SCC, and a core biopsy is usually not required. A US-guided FNAC can be performed, allowing the patient's neck to be accurately staged by imaging with cytological confirmation.

In combination with the node characteristics, the site of the node detected may also point the radiologist to search a particular area if the primary tumour site is unknown. US can identify the typical fine punctate calcification of a papillary carcinoma metastasis, these nodes are typically found in the paratracheal and lower deep cervical lymph node chains. FNAC will usually confirm the diagnosis and careful search of the thyroid for the primary tumour can then be carried out.

While no radiological sign is absolute, the combination of a cluster of signs in conjunction with a typical site may help suggest the diagnosis and will influence the choice of biopsy technique to be carried out, e.g. FNAC or core biopsy.

The choice of technique will be influenced by local practices, e.g. the local policy for the histological diagnosis and typing of lymphoma. If lymphoma is suspected and local pathological expertise is available to diagnose and classify the type of lymphoma on a core biopsy rather than on an open excision biopsy, then a decision can be made to proceed to a core biopsy. This will reduce morbidity, reduce the waiting time from referral to treatment and is more cost effective [1].

The question of the unknown primary needs to be considered if one is looking at patients presenting with a cervical mass, as this is a common clinical problem. Approximately 5.5% of patients with metastatic disease in cervical lymph nodes fail to have a primary tumour site identified, despite extensive evaluation [2]. These patients are considered to have an "unknown primary". The role of imaging is to direct the clinician to specific subsites in the neck to enable site directed biopsies to be taken. While the lymphatic drainage patterns are fairly constant in the neck, be aware that a previous lymph node dissection, or resection, or radiotherapy or a previous biopsy may alter lymph node drainage. Lymph can "skip" through metastatic nodes or can shunt across the neck to a contralateral side.

If the lymph node is in the lower deep cervical chain or supraclavicular chain, then the primary lesion is likely to be located below the clavicles [3]. If the FNAC confirms a SCC or poorly differentiated carcinoma then the prognosis is dismal. If it is adenocarcinoma then the primary is invariably in the chest or abdomen. If the node is situated higher in the neck the node may be draining parotid or thyroid and one must look at these sites for a primary.

For nodes in the upper cervical region, a primary tumour will be found in approximately 40% of patients. Eighty per cent of the patients will be found to have a primary tumour in the oropharynx: common sites being tonsillar fossa, base of tongue and pyriform sinus (hypopharynx) [3]. The diagnostic workup for a patient with an unknown primary is: clinical history and examination including examination of the oral cavity, oropharynx, nasopharynx, hypopharynx and larynx by laryngoscopy and naso-endoscopy. A chest X-ray should be performed in addition to either a CT or MRI study from the skull base to clavicles. Once the cytology of an FNA is known and the imaging has been reviewed, then a panendoscopy is carried out. Multiple biopsies of the nasopharynx, both tonsils, tongue base, both pyriform sinuses and any suspicious or abnormal mucosal areas are done. An ipsilateral tonsillectomy is also performed as the incidence of occult carcinoma in the tonsil ranges from 26% to 35% [4,5].

If positron emission tomography (PET) (discussed earlier in the book in Chapter 4) is available, the PET scan should be performed before panendoscopy to allow for any suspicious areas to be biopsied. The elusive goal for PET is to find the unknown primary tumour in this group of patients, and recent papers have reported success rates ranging from 25% to 30% for FDG-PET in the search for the unknown primary [6–8].

Key points

Unknown primary

- Cervical lymph nodes – US-guided FNAC
- History, examination, indirect laryngoscopy and naso-endoscopy
- Chest X-ray

- CT/MRI
  Skull base to clavicle
  Check – tongue base, tonsil, nasopharynx and pyriform fossae.
- PET: if available
- Pan endoscopy + biopsies
- Ipsilateral tonsillectomy

Having dealt with nodal masses the next question that must be answered is: what is the likely diagnosis if we have determined that the cervical mass is non-nodal?

If non-nodal – can a specific diagnosis be made on imaging alone?

We will look at the common congenital lesions that present as a mass in the neck and also at the other common pathologies that may present in this region. Although benign, the radiologist must be aware that several conditions can mimic malignancy. A second branchial cleft cyst (BCC), a metastatic papillary carcinoma node and a metastatic SCC node may all have a location similar to each other. If one is aware of the characteristic appearances of the common non-nodal masses that occur in the neck, potential misdiagnoses may be avoided.

Key points

Non-nodal masses

- Congenital cystic masses
  - BCC
  - Thyroglossal duct cyst (TDC)
  - Cystic hygroma
  - Dermoid, teratoma
- Others
  - Lipoma
  - Nerve sheath tumour
  - Haemangioma
  - Carotid body tumour (CBT)

Branchial cleft cyst

We will deal only with the second BCC which makes up 95% of BCCs. This typically presents as a cystic mass, without a sinus or fistula, at the angle of the mandible. It is usually situated superficial to the carotid bifurcation and posterior to the submandibular gland, often abutting the posterior aspect of the gland.

On sonography BCCs may often appear solid (Figure 13.1) which is a common feature of all congenital cystic lesions in the neck. The cyst contents are echogenic with occasional hyperechoic flecks [9]. This is due to proteinaceous content such as mucus, debris, lymphocytes, epithelial cells and cholesterol crystals. The BCCs may however appear as true anechoic cysts or have a mixed appearance (Figures 13.2 and 13.3).

BCCs typically present in children or young adults either as a painless fluctuating mass or, as a result of repeated infections, as a recurrent swelling. BCCs contain a lymphoid lining in 97% of cases that will hypertrophy with infection.

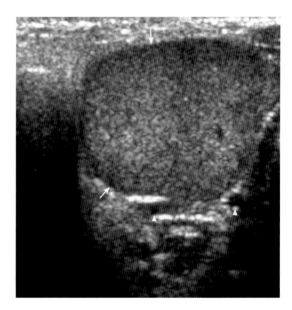

Fig. 13.1 Transverse sonogram of a second BCC (arrows) anterior to the carotid bifurcation (arrowheads), showing homogeneous internal echoes (pseudo-solid appearance). Slight pressure on the mass with the US transducer will reveal swirling motion of the contents suggesting its cystic nature.

CT or MR may be indicated if a sinus or fistula is suspected. If a "beak" is identified on US pointing medially, then it is prudent to obtain further imaging in order to exclude a sinus or fistula. CT reveals a homogenous mass with low attenuation and a thin, well-defined wall. Infected cysts on the other hand can be hyperattenuated with an ill-defined irregular rim, again mimicking a metastatic node [10]. On MR a characteristic high signal is seen within the cyst on a T2-weighted (T2W) series (Figure 13.4); however, there can be a considerable amount of intracystic low signal "debris". The proteinaceous content of the cyst may some times cause it to appear hyperintense (Figure 13.5) or isointense rather than hypointense (Figure 13.4) on T1-weighted (T1W) series.

When a BCC is suspected, even if the history is "typical", an FNA is advised to exclude other cystic malignancies such as a necrotic SCC node or a necrotic metastatic thyroid papillary carcinoma node (Figure 13.6) [11].

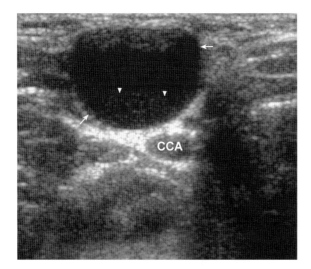

Fig. 13.2 Transverse sonogram of the second BCC (arrows) showing a predominantly anechoic pattern with a few internal echoes from debris (arrowheads). Note the lesion is anterior to CCA.

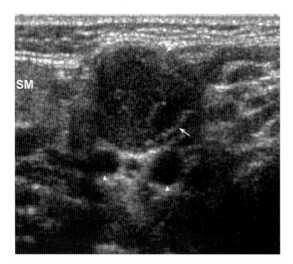

Fig. 13.3 Transverse sonogram showing a second BCC (arrows) with heterogeneous internal echoes. This appearance is seen in patients with previous infection or haemorrhage within the lesion. Note its relationship to the carotid bifurcation (arrowheads) and the submandibular gland (SM).

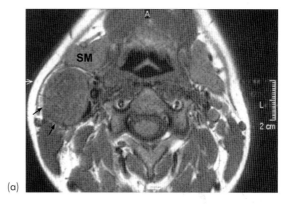

(a)

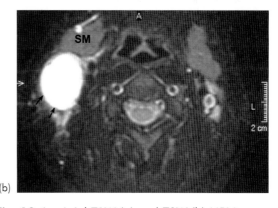

(b)

Fig. 13.4 Axial T1W (a) and T2W (b) MRI images of a second BCC (arrows). Note it is isointense on T1W and hyperintense on T2W sequences. Also note its location posterior to the submandibular gland (SM).

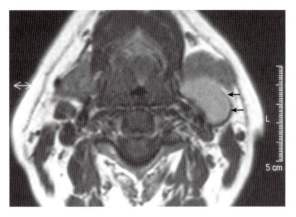

Fig. 13.5 Axial T1W MRI showing a second BCC (arrows). Note it is hyperintense on T1W scans. This is often noted in congenital cystic neck lesions due to the proteinaceous content of the fluid.

Key points

Branchial cleft cysts
- Appearances: pseudo-solid, cystic and mixed
- Posterior to the submandibular space
- Mimics
    Metastatic SCC
    Metastatic papillary carcinoma thyroid
- FNA mandatory

Thyroglossal duct cysts

In the 3rd to 4th week of foetal development the paired thyroid primordia descend into the neck along the thyroglossal duct that runs from the foramen caecum in the base of the tongue to the lower anterior neck, passing the hyoid bone. The duct normally involutes by the eighth week. Persistence of the duct or a portion of the duct can lead to congenital anomalies such as ectopic thyroid tissue or TDCs.

These benign lesions need to be highlighted for two reasons:

1. Appearances can mimic metastatic submental nodes
2. Thyroid carcinoma can develop in a TDC (incidence 1% in adults: 95% papillary adenocarcinoma, 5% SCC) [10].

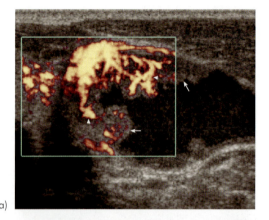

(a)

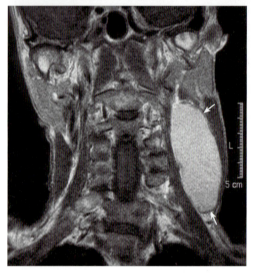

(b)

Fig. 13.6 This patient presented with a large and cystic left neck mass. A previous FNAC suggested haemorrhage into a cyst. A US was performed (a) which showed a large cystic lesion with a solid vascular component (arrows) with large vessels (arrowheads). The sonographic appearances suggested a metastatic lymph node from either a papillary carcinoma or SCC. A careful sonographic examination of the thyroid showed a typical papillary carcinoma on the ipsilateral side. A T1W coronal MRI (b) shows a large cystic lesion (arrows) hyperintense to adjacent muscle due to thyroglobulin secreted by the tumour consistent with a metastasis from papillary carcinoma. FNAC of the solid portion and thyroid nodule under US guidance confirmed a papillary carcinoma.

The majority of TDCs are infrahyoid (25–65%), 15–50% occur at the level of the hyoid and 20–25% are suprahyoid in location. The information the surgeon requires is the location of the cyst in relation

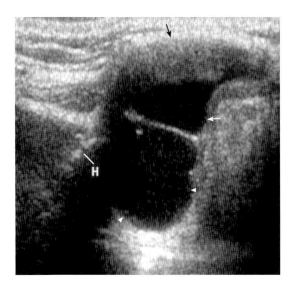

Fig. 13.7 Longitudinal sonogram of a infrahyoid TDC (arrows) which is predominantly anechoic with faint internal echoes. Note its posterior extension into the prelaryngeal space (arrowheads). H identifies the hyoid bone.

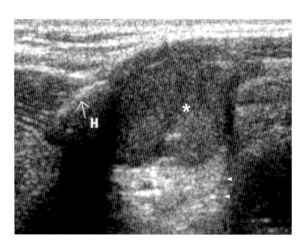

Fig. 13.8 Longitudinal sonogram of a infrahyoid TDC (*) showing homogeneous internal echoes. Swirling motion on transducer pressure and posterior enhancement (arrowheads) suggest the cystic nature of the lesion. This "pseudo-solid" appearance is caused by the proteinaceous content of the lesion. H identifies the hyoid bone.

to the hyoid. If it is intimate with the hyoid, he will need to remove the central portion of the hyoid in order to fully excise the suprahyoid portion of the tract, (Sistrunk procedure). The surgeon also needs the presence of normal thyroid tissue to be confirmed by US.

TDCs may appear frankly cystic, solid/cystic or again have a pseudo-solid appearance due to the proteinaceous content of the cyst secreted by the epithelial lining (Figures 13.7–13.9) [12, 13]. If one sees a solid component within a cyst, and given that the incidence of malignancy is 1%, an FNA needs to be carried out if the cyst is not to be excised. The variable cyst contents account for the varied appearances on CT and MRI (Figures 13.10 and 13.11) [14]. If a mural nodule or mass is identified, malignancy should be suspected.

Differentiating TDCs from lymph nodes can be difficult. One should remember that in the suprahyoid region a TDC pierces the mylohyoid, while nodes are superficial. Infrahyoid, a TDC will be embedded in the strap muscle and be off midline, whereas lymph nodes will be superficial or deep to strap muscles. While a dermoid can be mistaken for a suprahyoid TDC it should move independently of the tongue.

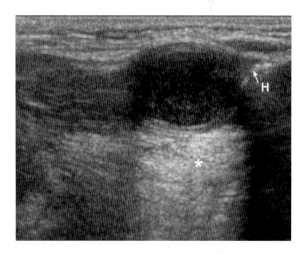

Fig. 13.9 A longitudinal sonogram of a suprahyoid TDC with heterogeneous internal echoes and posterior enhancement (*). H identifies the hyoid bone.

Key points

Thyroglossal duct cyst

- Relationship to hyoid
- Mimics metastatic nodes
- Malignancy occurs in 1%

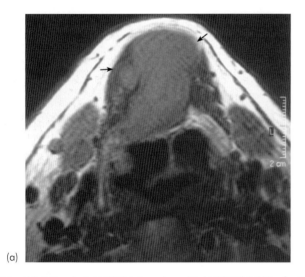

(a)

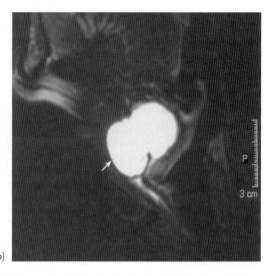

(b)

Fig. 13.10   Axial T1W (a) and sagittal T2W (b) MR of a TDC (arrows). Note the lesion is slightly hyperintense on T1W and hyperintense on T2W scans. Also note its extension posteriorly into the prelaryngeal space.

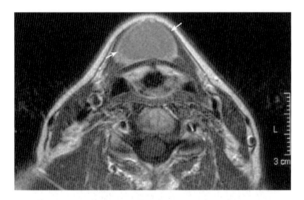

Fig. 13.11   Axial T1W MR showing a TDC (arrows). Note the "cystic lesion" is hyperintense on T1W scan, a feature frequently seen in congenital neck cysts due to their proteinaceous content.

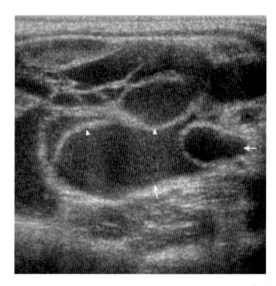

Fig. 13.12   Longitudinal sonogram showing the typical appearance of a cystic hygroma with multiple cystic spaces (arrows) and internal septation (arrowheads).

Cystic hygroma

A cystic hygroma is a lymphatic malformation that typically presents in children. On US it is multiloculated with thin septae and is trans-spatial (Figure 13.12). While it can be diagnosed on US, MR (Figure 13.13) or CT is mandatory to demonstrate its trans-spatial relationship to the many compartments of the neck that it can involve. This is a paediatric condition, 50–60% present at birth and another 30% present by the age of two. The classical appearances

and typical age distribution mean that this condition is unlikely to be mistaken for a malignancy.

Dermoid and teratoma

The dermoid is the most common of the teratomatous cysts. Approximately 7% occur in the head and

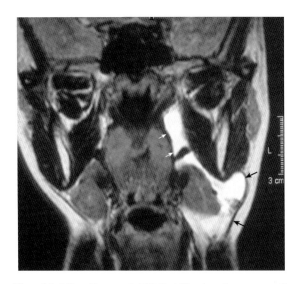

Fig. 13.13 Coronal T2W MR showing a cystic hygroma (arrows). The lesion is clearly seen as a hyperintense lesion. Note its parapharyngeal extension (small arrows). US identifies the nature of the lesion, however, MR delineates its entire anatomical extent better than US.

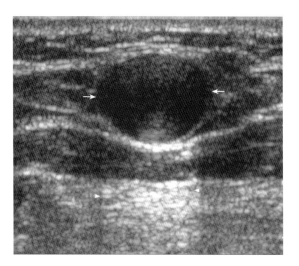

Fig. 13.14 Transverse sonogram showing a well-defined, cystic mass (arrows) with posterior enhancement (arrowheads) in the submental region. The appearances and location are consistent with a dermoid.

neck. They are frequently midline in location, typically in the floor of mouth, deep to the mylohyoid but they can occur anywhere in the midline as well as in the orbit, nasal and oral cavities. They are composed of two germ cell layers and contain skin appendages such as sebaceous glands, which are not present in epidermoid tumours [15]. The sebaceous secretions produced cause a slow enlargement. On US the cyst may appear cystic, pseudo-solid (Figures 13.14 and 13.15) and echogenic solid elements may be seen floating within. On CT, globules of fat floating within the lesion may produce a characteristic "sack of marbles" appearance [16]. Fat and/or fluid levels may be present on CT and MR. Both CT and MR clearly define their anatomical location, extent and internal appearance (Figure 13.16).

Cervical teratomas are rare with only 3% of teratomas being found in the cervical region [17]. They contain all three germ cell layers and may contain fat, teeth, hair, etc. Imaging reflects their composition and CT can optimally demonstrate the bizarre calcification that is often seen in teratomas.

The midline location and their composition does not usually cause confusion in differentiating these tumours from malignancy.

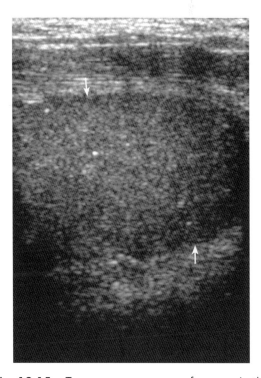

Fig. 13.15 Transverse sonogram of a mass in the sternal notch (arrows) showing uniform internal echoes. Transducer pressure revealed swirling motion within the lesion and suggested the cystic nature of the mass (pseudo-solid appearance). The sternal notch is a common site for a dermoid.

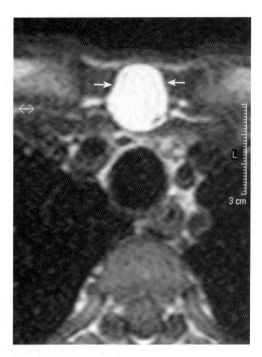

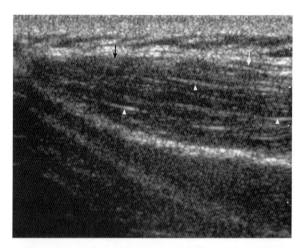

Fig. 13.17   Longitudinal sonogram showing a well-defined lipoma (arrows) with a characteristic "striped/feathery" appearance. Note the bright striations (arrowheads) fairly parallel to the transducer surface.

Fig.13.16   Axial T2W MR showing a cystic mass (arrows) in the sternal notch, the location consistent with a dermoid.

Key points

Dermoid tumours and teratomas

- Midline location, cystic
- Dermoid – sebaceous material
- Teratoma – teeth/calcification

We now need to consider the remaining masses in the neck that may present as a cervical mass and which may mimic cancer, namely:

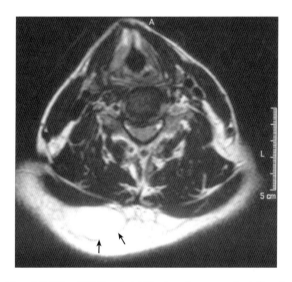

Fig. 13.18   T1W axial MR showing a well-defined lipoma (arrows) with a signal intensity similar to adjacent subcutaneous fat.

Lipoma

The head and neck is a typical site for lipomata (13%). On US there is a classic "feathered" appearance whereby echogenic striae are seen orientated parallel to the transducer (Figure 13.17) [18]. There is no significant distal acoustic enhancement or attenuation and vascularity is sparse. If confirmation is needed, low attenuation of fat is demonstrated on CT and fat suppression techniques on MR (Figure 13.18) will also confirm its composition.

Nerve sheath tumours

These are the great impersonators in the head and neck – both neurofibromas and schwannomas can appear as diffusely hypoechoic masses with marked vascularity, mimicking lymphomatous lymph nodes. They can also undergo cystic change mimicking

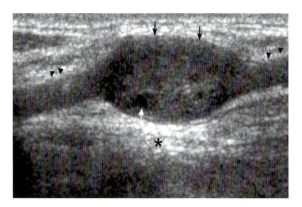

Fig. 13.19 Transverse sonogram of a nerve sheath tumour (arrows) showing associated thickened nerve (arrowheads). Note the enhancement posterior to the mass (*) and small cystic areas within (small arrow).

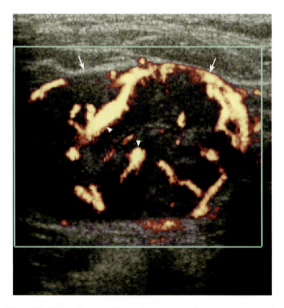

Fig. 13.20 Power Doppler scan of a nerve sheath tumour (arrows) showing multiple large intranodular vessels (arrowheads) within the lesion.

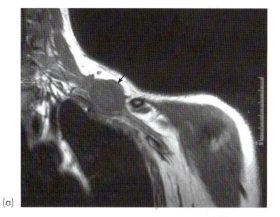

(a)

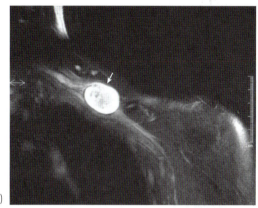

(b)

Fig. 13.21 Coronal T1W (a) and fat-suppressed T2W (b) MR showing a brachial plexus neuroma (arrows), isointense to muscle on T1W and markedly hyperintense on T2W scans.

metastatic lymph nodes. Differentiation between a nerve sheath tumour and lymph node is a common dilemma, major nerve trunks often run in close proximity to lymph node chains, e.g. spinal accessory nerve and accessory lymph nodes. The key in differentiating the entities on US is to try and find the characteristic "tail" of the nerve sheath tumour (Figure 13.19). This is where the emerging nerve can be identified with its characteristically thickened sheath [19]. Power Doppler will often demonstrate prominent vessels with the lesion (Figure 13.20). Occasionally FNA or biopsy of a nerve sheath tumour will be precipitated by the US appearances – e.g. neurofibroma mimicking lymphoma. Biopsy of nerve sheath tumours tends to be painful but this is not a consistent finding. Biopsy is, however, best avoided if possible.

On CT these tumours will be of muscle density and they are difficult to differentiate from nodes. On MR neurofibroma can often show marked hyperintensity on T2W series (Figure 13.21). The multiplanar capability of MR should help in depicting the relationship to any associated nerve trunk allowing the correct diagnosis to be made.

Key points

Nerve sheath tumours

- Hypoechoic on US – mimic lymphoma
- Cystic change – mimic metastatic SCC
- Ubiquitous – remember nerve pathways

Haemangioma

Approximately 15% of haemangiomas occur in the head and neck, the masseter muscle being the most common site. While primarily a vascular malformation with large cavernous spaces, there may also be lymphatic elements present.

US appearances are fairly characteristic, namely hypoechoic, heterogeneous, multiple sinusoidal spaces, and phleboliths seen in 22% of cases (Figures 13.22 and 13.23) [20]. In our experience however, with newer high-resolution transducers and by a careful search, phleboliths are seen in more than 60% of head and neck haemangiomas in adults. While Power Doppler may depict the slow flowing nature of haemangiomata (Figure 13.22b), we believe

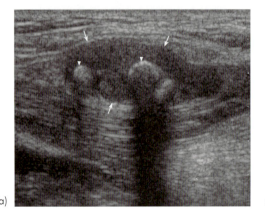
(a)

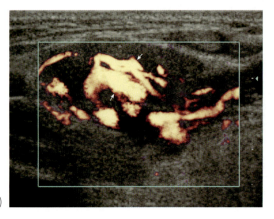
(b)

Fig. 13.22 Transverse sonogram (a) and power Doppler (b) showing a hypoechoic mass (arrows) with multiple phleboliths (arrowheads) and large intranodular vascular spaces (small arrows).

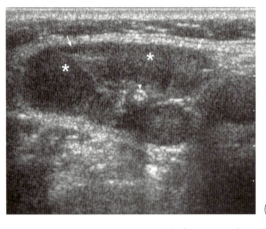
(a)

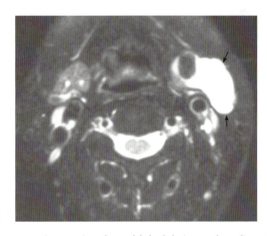
(b)

Fig. 13.23 Transverse sonogram (a) showing a haemangioma (arrows) with a phlebolith (arrowhead) and large vascular spaces with faint internal echoes (*). The faint internal echoes represent slow moving blood seen on real-time grey scale scanning. A T2W MR (b) demonstrates the anatomical location and extent of the haemangioma (arrows).

the flow phenomenon is better demonstrated on real time grey-scale US (Figure 13.23a).

On MR the mass may be indeterminate from muscle on T1W but on T2W fat saturated sequences (Figures 13.23b and 13.24) a characteristic high signal is produced ensuring conspicuity. Although MR may not be as sensitive as US in the identification of phleboliths, it is excellent at depicting the full extent of large haemangiomata which may be trans-spatial. It is superior in this respect to CT and US.

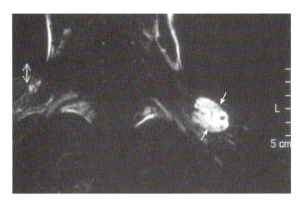

Fig. 13.24 A T2W, fat-suppressed coronal MR of a haemangioma (arrows) showing its typical hyper-intensity on T2W scans.

Key points

Haemangiomata
- Cystic, sinusoidal spaces with slow flow, phleboliths
- Masseter: commonest location
- MR: excellent at depicting trans-spatial extent

Carotid body tumour

Due to their site, CBTs can be mistaken for lymph nodes in the upper portion of the deep cervical chain. One should, however, always remember the relevant anatomy of the lymph node chain and remember the site of origin of the CBT, i.e. the normal carotid body is a 5–6 mm mass on the adventitia of the medial side of the vessels at the carotid bifurcation. Upper and mid-cervical lymph nodes are distributed around the antero-medial and antero-lateral aspects of the internal jugular vein. The subsequent characteristic displacement of either the internal jugular vein or carotid bifurcation should allow for the correct prediction of the origin of the mass.

The characteristic sign of a CBT is a splayed bifurcation (Figures 13.25 and 13.26). A large CBT may

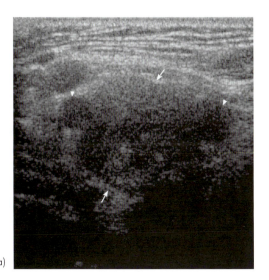

(a)

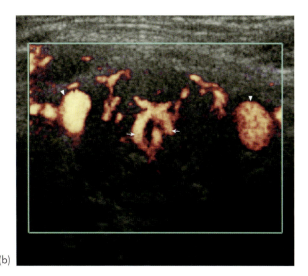

(b)

Fig. 13.25 Transverse sonogram (a) showing a hypoechoic mass (arrows) insinuating the carotid bifurcation (arrowheads). A power Doppler scan (b) clearly shows the large vessels within the lesion (small arrows) and its relationship to the carotid bifurcation.

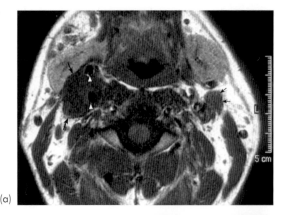

(a)

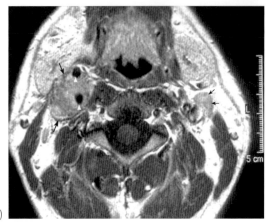

(b)

Fig. 13.26 Axial T1W MR, (a) post-gadolinium T1W image (b) showing a well-defined mass (arrows) insinuating between the carotid bifurcation (arrowheads) on the right. Note it is isointense to muscle on T1W scans and shows uniform enhancement after injection of gadolinium. Also note a similar, smaller, mass on the left (small arrows).

encase the bifurcation. A lymph node mass will displace the internal jugular vein posteriorly and be situated antero-lateral to the carotid bifurcation.

On US the tumour will frequently demonstrate vascularity within (Figure 13.25b). However, in some cases it may not appear particularly vascular on colour flow imaging. This is in apparent contradiction of the marked vascular enhancement seen on contrast-enhanced CT. The bilateral nature of the tumours (between 2% and 10%) [21] means that a diligent search of the contralateral side should always be carried out. While a biopsy of a CBT may have been carried out, sometimes inadvertently, with no apparent complications, a biopsy is not essential to make the diagnosis.

The splaying of the carotid bifurcation by a CBT is well demonstrated by both MR (Figure 13.26) and CT. On CT there is marked enhancement with intravenous contrast reflecting the high vascularity of the tumour. Angiographic techniques on MRI and CT will demonstrate the vascular displacement if necessary. On MRI, CBTs shows a "salt and pepper" appearance on T1W images. The "salt", high signal areas, represents areas of subacute haemorrhage (in small tumours only) whereas the "pepper", low signal areas, represents flow voids of the feeding vessels.

> ## Key points
>
> *Carotid body tumour*
>
> - Location – splaying carotid bifurcation
> - Bilateral in 2–10%
> - Intense vascularity/enhancement on CT
> - "Salt and pepper" appearance on T1W MRI

If a specific diagnosis cannot be made – is there a need to proceed to a biopsy?

The characteristic appearances of non-nodal masses in particular may allow for a specific diagnosis to be made and a management plan to be formulated. There will be many occasions when either a specific diagnosis cannot be made or one suspects a malignancy, which should prompt the next key question – should one proceed to a biopsy? We have dealt with some of the issues earlier in this chapter but any decision has to be made in the light of local practice and expertise. The radiologist must consult with his clinical colleagues and establish a working method or protocol for dealing with this group of patients. A logical progression to image-guided FNA or core biopsy will allow for the rapid initiation of treatment when appropriate.

The decision as to whether an FNA or core biopsy is performed will depend on the level of local cytological support and expertise. If adequate cytological support is available, then the majority of biopsies carried out in the head and neck will be FNA rather than core biopsy. In dealing with patients with head and neck cancer, the majority will have a SCC as the primary tumour. Most cytologists are comfortable in diagnosing metastatic SCC on FNAC if they are given a decent, adequate sample.

Proceeding to a core biopsy rather than an FNA is usually in response to two specific situations:

(a) if lymphoma is suspected,
(b) if the initial attempts at FNA are non-diagnostic.

With the improvements in staining techniques and in immunohistochemistry, pathologists are able to make the diagnosis and accurately type the lymphoma on a core biopsy specimen rather than having to wait for an excision biopsy to be carried out. If this occurs then the decrease in referral-to-treatment time for that particular patient can be significantly reduced. Core biopsy may not be able to give all the answers when dealing with lymphomas, and an excision biopsy may still be required in difficult diagnostic cases.

A lengthy description and discussion of FNA and biopsy techniques is beyond the scope of this section. In our experience there are two items of equipment that are useful if one is to become skilled at both FNA and core biopsy in the head and neck. For FNA, one can use a short piece of flexible tubing between the needle and syringe allowing a second operator to aspirate while the radiologist places the needle under direct guidance into the lesion. If the radiologist attempts to aspirate while controlling the needle and the probe the benefit of US guidance will be lost as the operator will not be able to keep the needle tip under direct vision during the procedure. US guidance means control of the needle tip under direct vision at all times. For core biopsy to be carried out safely in the head and neck, the use of a non-advancing cutting needle is mandatory. A biopsy system that allows the central trochar to either be slowly advanced into the lesion under US control or to be inserted with the cutting "gate" in the fully open position is essential. Once the cutting "gate" is correctly positioned within the mass the biopsy can be taken, safe in the knowledge that the trochar will not advance further. This allows biopsy of masses adjacent to vessels to be carried out safely. The use of advancing cutting needles should be avoided in the head and neck [22].

Approach to management

As detailed above, neck masses may include anything from lipomas to lymphomas, and metastases to malformations. When considering approaches to their management, the strong possibility that the mass may be a metastatic lesion must be borne in mind. The imaging processes described above, with or without an FNA, will almost undoubtedly offer a certain diagnosis. If indeed the diagnosis is that of a metastasis, or if any doubt exists, a diligent search for the primary lesion must be undertaken. It is not advisable to proceed with an excision, incision or a core biopsy of the mass until a full clinical workup has been done.

Search for the primary lesion

This is achieved by a panendoscopy under general anaesthesia. Once the primary tumour is identified it must be carefully evaluated and accurately documented to facilitate staging and management. If, however, no primary can be identified by thorough inspection of the nasal cavity, oral cavity, naso-, oro- and hypo-pharynges, larynx, trachea, bronchi and oesophagus, the tonsil on the side of the mass should be removed and sent for histology together with representative biopsies from the base of the tongue. Particular attention should be paid to the tongue base as accessibility for inspection is difficult and a primary tumour in the tongue base may be deeply situated and not easily visualised.

There are circumstances where tissue, rather than cells, is required to facilitate a definitive diagnosis.

Key points

Biopsy required?

- Formulate plan with clinical colleagues
- FNA
  - Metastatic SCC
  - Papillary carcinoma
  - TB
- Core biopsy
  - "Failed" FNA
  - Lymphoma
- Useful equipment
  - FNA: flexible tubing
  - Core biopsy: non-advancing cutting needle

For tissue typing in lymphomas the mass should preferably be completely excised, such as an enlarged tonsil or lymph node. When the diagnosis remains unclear after a full workup, the mass should be excised and submitted for frozen section analysis, and the surgeon should be prepared to continue with a neck dissection if indicated, the patient having consented to this before surgery.

It is beyond the scope of this text to describe detailed management of the different types of neck masses. Reference should be made to two texts where current concepts and comprehensive descriptions are available for the management of all types of cervical masses [23,24].

Summary

The patient who presents with a cervical mass is a common diagnostic problem. If one can answer the key questions highlighted in this section by the effective use of imaging, if necessary in combination with biopsy techniques, then the radiologist will play a major role in the management of this group of patients. A "team" approach is vital for diagnostic success. Protocols and diagnostic pathways need to be formulated in close consultation with clinical colleagues. The aim of any protocol should be to achieve a rapid and accurate diagnosis of malignancy, which then allows for the appropriate treatment of the patient to occur without delay.

References

1. Cozens NJA and Berman L. Fine needle aspiration or core biopsy. In: *Practical Head and Neck Ultrasound*. Greenwich Medical Media, London. 2000, 131–146.
2. Winegar LK and Griffin W. The occult primary tumour. *Arch. Otolaryngol.* 1973; **98**: 159–163.
3. Mendenhall WM, Mancuso AA, Amdur RJ, Stringer SP, Villaret DB and Cassisi NJ. Squamous cell carcinoma metastatic to the neck from an unknown head and neck primary site. *Am. J. Otolaryngol.* 2001; **22**: 261–267.
4. Lapeyre M, Malissard L, Peiffert D *et al.* Cervical lymph node metastasis from an unknown primary: is a tonsillectomy necessary? *Int. J. Radiat. Oncol. Biol. Phys.* 1977; **39**: 291–296.
5. Mendenhall WM, Mancuso AA, Parsons JT *et al.* Diagnostic evaluation of squamous cell carcinoma metastatic to cervical lymph nodes from an unknown head and neck primary site. *Head Neck* 1998; **20**: 739–744.
6. Kole AC, Niewig OE, Pruim J *et al.* Detection of unknown occult primary tumours using positron emission tomography. *Cancer* 1998; **82**: 1160–1166.
7. Braams JW, Pruim J, Kole PGJ *et al.* Detection of unknown primary head and neck tumours by positron emission tomography. *Int. J. Oral. Max. Surg.* 1997; **26**: 112–115.
8. Jungehulsing M, Scheidhauer K, Damm M *et al.* 2(18F)-fluoro-2-deoxy-D-glucose positron emission tomography is a sensitive tool for the detection of occult primary cancer (carcinoma of unknown primary syndrome) with head and neck manifestation. *Otolaryng Head Neck* 2000; **123**: 294–301.
9. Ahuja AT, King AD and Metreweli C. Second branchial cleft cysts: variability of sonographic appearances in adults. *Am. J. Neuroradiol.* 2000; **21**: 315–319.
10. Lev S and Lev MH. Imaging of cystic lesions. *Radiol. Clin. N. Am.* 2000; **38**: 1013–1027.
11. Ahuja AT, Ng CF, King W and Metreweli C. Solitary cystic nodal metastasis from occult papillary carcinoma of the thyroid mimicking a branchial cyst: a potential pitfall. *Clin. Radiol.* 1998; **53**: 61–63.
12. Ahuja AT, King AD and Metreweli C. Thyroglossal duct cysts: sonographic appearances in adults. *Am. J. Neuroradiol.* 1999; **20**: 579–582.
13. Ahuja AT, King AD and Metreweli C. Sonographic evaluation of thyroglossal duct cysts in children. *Clin. Radiol.* 2000; **55**: 770–774.
14. Glastonbury CM, Davidson HC, Haller JR *et al.* The CT and MR imaging features of carcinoma arising in thyroglossal duct remnants. *Am. J. Neuroradiol.* 2000; **21**: 770.
15. Weissman JL. Non-nodal masses of the neck. In: PM Som and HD Curtin (Eds) *Head and Neck Imaging*, 3rd edition. Mosby Year book, St. Louis. 1996, 794–822.
16. Koeller KK, Alamo L, Adair CF *et al.* Congenital cystic masses of the neck: radiologic-pathologic correlation. *Radiographics* 1999; **19**: 121.
17. Rothschild MA, Catalano P, Urken M *et al.* Evaluation and management of congenital cervical teratoma. *Arch. Otolaryngol.* 1994; **120**: 444.
18. Ahuja AT, King AD, Kew J, King W and Metreweli C. Head and neck lipomas: ultrasound appearances. *Am. J. Neuroradiol.* 1998; **19**: 505–508.
19. King AD, Ahuja AT, King W and Metreweli C. Sonography of peripheral nerve tumours of the neck. *Am. J. Roentgenol.* 1997; **169**. 1695 1698.
20. Yang WT, Ahuja A and Metreweli C. Sonography features of head hemangiomas and vascular malformations: review of 23 patients. *J. Ultrasound Med.* 1997; **16**: 39–44.
21. Enzinger FM and Weiss SW. Paragangliomas. In: *Soft Tissue Tumours*. CV Mosby, St. Louis. 1988, 836–860.
22. Bearcroft PWP, Berman LH and Grant J. The use of ultrasound guided cutting needle biopsy in the neck. *Clin. Radiol.* 1995; **50**: 690–695.
23. van Hasselt CA, Bleach NR and Milford C. *Operative Otorhinolaryngology*. Blackwell Science Ltd, Oxford. 1997.
24. Jones AS, Phillips DE and Hilgers JM. *Diseases of the Head and Neck, Nose and Throat*. Edward Arnold Ltd, London. 1998.

Index